Second
Edition

The
TREATMENT

OF BURNS

CURTIS P. ARTZ, M.D., F.A.C.S.

Professor of Surgery and Chairman of the Department, Medical
College of South Carolina, Charleston, South Carolina; formerly
Commanding Officer and Director, U.S. Army Surgical Research
Unit, Brooke Army Medical Center, Fort Sam Houston, Texas

JOHN A. MONCRIEF, M.D., F.A.C.S.

Colonel, Medical Corps., Commanding Officer and Director, U.S.
Army Surgical Research Unit, Brooke Army Medical Center, Fort
Sam Houston, Texas

W. B. SAUNDERS COMPANY
Philadelphia   London   Toronto

W. B. Saunders Company: West Washington Square
Philadelphia, Pa.   19105

12 Dyott Street
London W.C.1

1835 Yonge Street
Toronto 7, Ontario

Reprinted February, 1969

The Treatment of Burns

TO

Lucy, Susan, John and Joanne

and

Connie, John, Chris and Connie

·with affection

Preface
to Second Edition

It has been ten years since the publication of the first edition of *The Treatment of Burns*. During this decade much new knowledge has been obtained. The original authors have separated and pursued careers in their basic disciplines. Dr. Eric Reiss is currently Chairman of the Department of Medicine at the Michael Reese Hospital in Chicago. Other endeavors in the field of internal medicine have replaced his early research interest in burns.

It seems fitting that a previous commanding officer and the current commanding officer of the United States Army Surgical Research Unit should join in the preparation of this second edition. This effort thereby reflects the experience and thinking in civilian academic medicine as well as that in a military burn center. This volume is entirely a new book. All the chapters have been rewritten; several new ones have been added. These include: Office Treatment of Burns, Burns in Children, and Nursing Care. In addition, three invited authors have contributed new chapters. Dr. Carl Teplitz, a former pathologist at the Surgical Research Unit and currently an associate professor of pathology and pathobiology, Boston University School of Medicine, has supplied a completely new treatise on the pathology of burns. Dr. Burton S. Epstein, now an assistant professor of anesthesiology at George Washington University School of Medicine, Washington, D. C., but previously a member of the Surgical Research Unit, wrote the chapter on anesthesia for burns. Dr. Burke Evans, head of the Division of Orthopedic Surgery at the University of Texas Medical Branch, Galveston, has been interested in the musculoskeletal changes in burns for many years. His chapter on that subject, in this edition, is a monument to his apt studies and abundant clinical experience. Deepest appreciation is expressed to these scientists for their authoritative contributions.

Like the first edition, the chief purpose of this book is to furnish a guide for treatment in accordance with present-day knowledge of burns. An ancillary purpose is to present information about certain practical skills of management which are not discussed in scientific articles. Bibliographies for chapters are largely limited to particularly useful articles, and the text takes into account interpretation of information gained by various investigators throughout the world.

The help of many friends and fellow workers is gratefully acknowledged. Chief among these is that group of physicians who have served on the staff of the Surgical Research Unit. Special thanks go to Miss Mary Nelle Entrekin for her painstaking and exacting editorial work. The photographs are a tribute to the ability of Mr. Claude Dresser and Mr. John Tucker of the Surgical Research Unit and Mr. Robert Brown of the Medical College of South Carolina. The laborious task of typing the manuscript was performed by Mrs. Bia Vallis and Mrs. Barbara Ford of the Medical College of South Carolina and by Miss Goldie Smith, who has had the distinct honor of serving as secretary to all the commanding officers of the Surgical Research Unit since 1953. Finally, it is a pleasure to acknowledge the valuable counsel and cooperation of the staff of the W. B. Saunders Company.

CURTIS P. ARTZ

JOHN A. MONCRIEF

Contents

Chapter One

THE BURN PROBLEM

A burn may vary from a minor first-degree wound to the most severe form of injury to which man is liable. The significant burn evokes a myriad of systemic responses. The magnitude of the injury determines the extent of the physiologic changes. Unlike wounds that can be closed either immediately or in a few days, the deep burn requires time for removal of the dead eschar before closure. The persistence of this dead tissue furthers the injury, and additional systemic derangements occur. This complex disease process has fascinated and stimulated surgeons for decades. Much of our knowledge of the systemic response to surgery has evolved from studies of burns.

The variety of recommendations for treatment makes it clear that there is still no single best treatment for burns. To make the maximum use of modern materials and techniques, the surgeon must be able to choose a method of management which is most suitable under the particular circumstances for each individual patient. The care of all phases of an extensive burn injury taxes the skill and knowledge of the surgeon to the utmost. The difference between success and failure may depend as much upon minute details as it does upon the execution of major operative procedures. The clinician faced with a severely burned patient should have an understanding of the current information concerning the pathophysiology of burn injury to make necessary day-to-day decisions concerning treatment. No two burned patients are alike. Each presents special problems requiring individualization. Several books pertaining to specific aspects of the burn problem are currently available and are listed in the bibliography of this chapter.

HISTORICAL ASPECTS

Historical landmarks in the treatment of burns have followed accomplishments in the field of surgery. Many aspects of the early history of burns have been described by Cockshott of Edinburgh, by Harkins of Seattle, and by Shedd of New Haven.

1

Interest in injuries caused by fire reaches back to the early days of mankind. Hippocrates (*circa* 430 B.C.) suggested the following treatment: "Having melted old swine's seam and mixed it with resin and bitumen, and having spread it on a piece of cloth and warmed it at the fire, apply a bandage." He also proposed the use of warm vinegar-soaked dressings to relieve the burn pain and later treated burns by tanning with solutions of oak bark. Aristotle was interested in the pathogenesis of burns and believed that burns caused by hot ore showed a tendency to heal more rapidly.

Cockshott notes that Paulus of Aegina, a Byzantine of the seventh century A.D. whose writings reflected Greco-Roman thought, utilized various emollient preparations with strange ingredients for treatment. Rhazes and Avicenna, representing ninth- and tenth-century Arabic views, recommended the use of refrigerants locally; this certainly had the virtue of alleviation of pain.

Giovanni de Vigo, a surgeon to Pope Julius II, wrote about the controversy regarding the existence of a toxin in gunpowder burns in 1514. From some of the early writings, it appears that burn wounds occurred more often from the mishandling of gunpowder than from the action of the enemy. This is particularly apparent in the writings of William Clowes, whose book in 1596 was the first devoted primarily to burns. Its title was *A Profitable and Neccessarie Booke of Observations, for All Those That Are Burned With the Flame of Gun Powder.* This work was in the form of a series of case histories and described treatment which consisted chiefly of the use of ointments prescribed by Ambroise Paré. These in turn had been derived from Greco-Roman, Arabic and even Egyptian sources. Clowes was one of the foremost London surgeons of his time and followed a colorful military career. He did not recognize the various degrees of burn, but he did employ five different complex preparations on the different parts of burned individuals.

In 1607, Fabricius Hildanus, of Basel, Switzerland, published a book in Latin entitled *De Combustionibus* in which he recognized three degrees of burn. He also dealt with the problem of management of late burn contractures. In 1797, there appeared a book entitled *An Essay on Burns,* by Edward Kentish, of Newcastle-upon-Tyne (Fig. 1). This was a popular early textbook on burns, and many of the observations that Kentish recorded are relevant today. In 1799, Earle reported the use of crushed ice and ice water for the treatment of burns. His thesis was that ice served as a good analgesic and as a method of preventing local edema. In 1832, Baron Guillaume Dupuytren, a surgeon in Paris, classified burn lesions according to depth into six degrees of injury. In 1833, Syme proposed the use of dry cotton-wool dressing applied with firm pressure. The first burn hospital was operated under the direction of Syme in Edinburgh. The building is still standing.

Sir George Ballingal of Edinburgh published a treatise on military surgery in 1833. His description of the natural history of the burn wound

AN

ESSAY ON BURNS,

IN

TWO PARTS;

PRINCIPALLY

ON THOSE WHICH HAPPEN TO WORKMEN IN MINES, FROM THE EXPLOSIONS OF CARBURETTED HYDROGEN GAS:

CONTAINING ALSO A VIEW OF THE

OPINIONS OF ANCIENT, AND MODERN AUTHORS UPON THE TREATMENT OF ACCIDENTS BY FIRE:

AND INCLUDING

A VARIETY OF CASES CONDUCTED UPON DIFFERENT PRINCIPLES.

THE WHOLE

TENDING TO RESCUE THE HEALING ART FROM EMPIRICISM, AND TO REDUCE IT TO ESTABLISHED LAWS.

The First Part originally published in 1797, the Second Part in 1800.

BY

EDWARD KENTISH, M.D.

Physician to the Bristol Dispensary, and St. Peter's Hospital.

LONDON:

PRINTED FOR LONGMAN, HURST, REES, ORME AND BROWN; AND BARRY AND SON, BRISTOL.

1817.

Figure 1. Title page of an early book on burns by Edward Kentish.

was most accurate, and his account of the fate of the burned patient is quite similar to current-day concepts. Concerning the early death, he stated: "He sinks from causes which we can not explain." The deaths at 10 to 12 days he recognized as being of a febrile nature now recognized as being due to septicemia. He described the later deaths occurring at 3 to 6 weeks after the burn as "sinking in a hectic state, exhausted by a profuse discharge of matter from an extensive suppurating surface." Despite his excellent concept of the fate of the burned patient, he continued the customary treatment of purgation and bloodletting. A layman is credited with the recognition of the fact that purgation, widely practiced at the time, was harmful to the burned patient. This man was David Cleghorn, an Edinburgh brewer who became a recognized expert in the treatment of burns in the early eighteenth century. Many types of local treatment have been used. Oils and waxes have been placed on burns since Roman times. Tannic acid was used with the idea of coagulating the wound as early as 1858. Lizfrank, in 1835, recommended wet dressings containing sodium and calcium chloride. The earliest American reference to exposure of burn wounds was made in a publication by Copeland in 1877. In 1905, Sneve of St. Paul gave an excellent detailed description of the exposure of burns and recorded much that is in accord with present-day concepts of the method.

Curling of London recognized gastroduodenal ulceration as a complication of severe burn injury in 1842. The first case he described was that of a young girl with a burn of 21 per cent of the body surface. In 1863, Baraduc of Paris maintained that the decrease of the circulating blood volume in burns was the most probable cause of death and that the viscosity of the blood was increased in burn cases. In 1881, Tappeiner of Munich recognized from autopsy studies certain fundamental features of the pathophysiology of extensive burns, namely, the concentration of the blood which occurs. This was manifested by reduced water content, increased hemoglobin and decreased bleeding volume. Such observations were very important in the treatment of burns, as they pointed out the need for replacement solutions. By 1901, replacement needs were becoming known. Parascandolo of Naples utilized saline in the treatment of burned patients. He may have learned this from his contemporary, Guido Bacelli, who was at that time a leading figure in Italian medicine and a great promoter of the use of intravenous fluids. Parascandolo also did some work on the development of an antitoxin against alleged toxins from burned skin. This antitoxin is said to have protected the animals used in his experiments. This toxicity theory of burn deaths was widely held.

Complete appreciation of the severity of fluid losses in burns was not apparent until the enlightening studies of Frank P. Underhill (Fig. 2). He was a professor of pharmacology and toxicology who had done excellent work in the study of war gases. During the catastrophic fire at the Rialto Theater in New Haven in 1921, 20 people were seriously burned. Underhill studied the cases, closely following the hemoglobin, hematocrit and serum chlorides. He continued his studies on fluid losses and analyzed

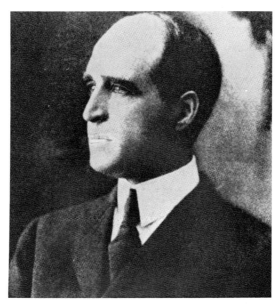

Figure 2.   Frank Pell Underhill, 1877-1932, pioneer in fluid therapy in burns at Yale University.

blister fluid. This led to the recognition of protein losses as being important. His research also showed that the previously held theory that a toxin was released from burned skin was false.

In 1925, Davidson of Detroit renewed interest in the escharotics when he introduced the tannic acid spray (Fig. 3). It was believed that this technique decreased the fluid loss, relieved pain and produced a better eschar. It was finally abandoned in 1944, when McClure pointed out that tannic acid was toxic to the liver. In 1933, Aldridge used gentian violet as an escharotic because he thought it had an additional bacteriostatic effect.

In a book on burns published in 1930, George Pack, later a prominent New York cancer surgeon, recommended the use of blood only in connection with the treatment of shock. His book was a good review of this phase of knowledge of burns at that time. In 1942, Harkins published a scholarly treatise on burns which stood as the standard textbook on the subject for many years (Fig. 4).

The modern era of local burn wound management was initiated by Allen (Fig. 5) and Koch in 1942. They advocated and popularized the use of Vaseline gauze, bulky pressure dressings and strict immobilization. This technique of local care remained the accepted one until Wallace, in 1949, reintroduced the exposure method in Great Britain (Fig. 6). Pulaski, Artz and Blocker evaluated the exposure method in the United States and outlined its indications and contraindications.

One of the greatest recent disasters from fire was the Cocoanut Grove fire in Boston in 1942. This stimulated fundamental research on the sys-

(Text continued on page 11)

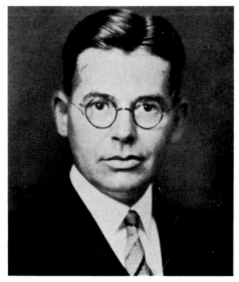

Figure 3.   Edward Clark Davidson, 1894-1933, who at Henry Ford Hospital originated the tannic acid treatment.

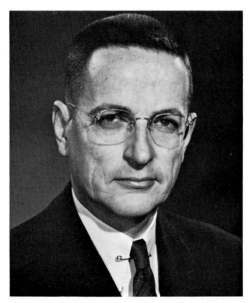

Figure 4.   Henry N. Harkins, author of classic American text on burns.

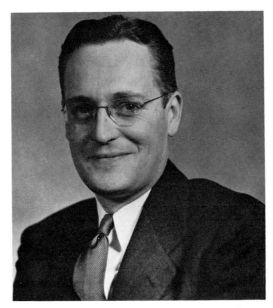

Figure 5. Harvey Stuart Allen, 1906-1955, proponent of Vaseline gauze pressure dressings at Northwestern University.

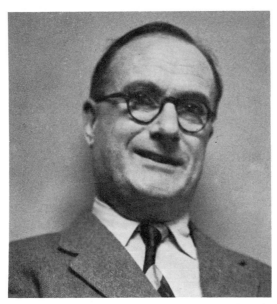

Figure 6. A. B. Wallace, Edinburgh plastic surgeon who reintroduced the exposure method in 1949.

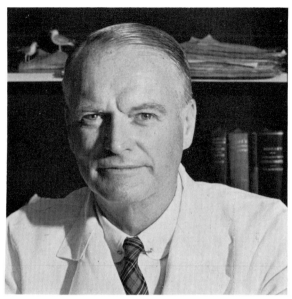

Figure 7.   Oliver Cope, surgeon at Massachusetts General Hospital whose multiple contributions to the study of burns started with studies of victims of the Cocoanut Grove disaster.

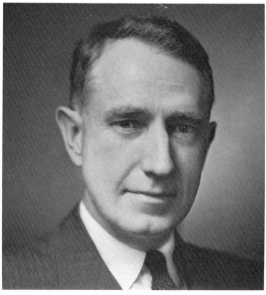

Figure 8.   Francis D. Moore of Harvard University, pioneer over several decades in the response of the body to burn injury.

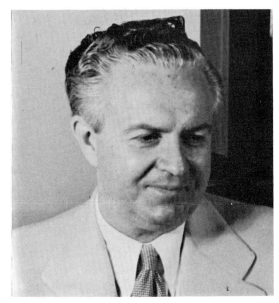

Figure 9.   Everett Idris Evans, 1907-1954, developed early fluid formula for burns.

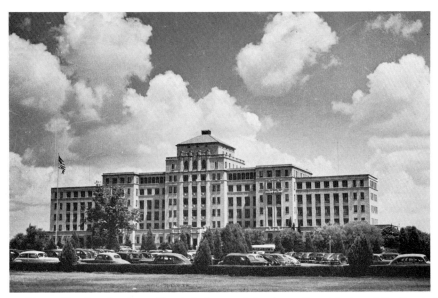

Figure 10.   Brooke Army Hospital—home of the Army Burn Center of the Surgical
Research Unit.

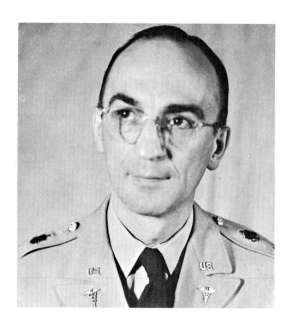

Figures 11 and 12. Col. Edwin J. Pulaski and Col. William H. Amspacher, Commanders of the Surgical Research Unit at the time of the development of the Army Burn Center.

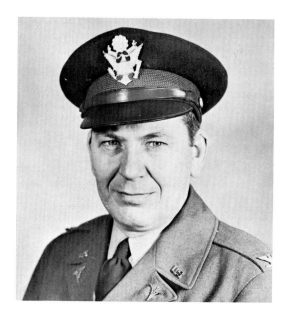

temic response to burning by Cope (Fig. 7) and Moore (Fig. 8). By demonstrating that fluid loss was inside the patient and not exclusively outside, they provided an explanation for the hidden fluid loss in burns. In 1947, Cope emphasized the early, aggressive removal of eschar and closure of the burn wound. The contributions of these two men to the problem of burns over the years are legion. In 1952, Evans of Richmond developed a surface area–weight formula for computing fluid replacement in burns (Fig. 9). The currently popular Brooke fluid formula is a modification of Evans' suggestion.

Studies of the U.S. Army Surgical Research Unit at the Brooke Army Medical Center have produced some advances of historical interest (Fig. 10). The use of the exposure method in the treatment of donor sites was reported in 1952. In 1953, they emphasized for the first time that septicemia was a cardinal problem in burns and the most common cause of death. It was this organization that pointed out the value and necessity of a team concept in burns. Their findings showed that in such a complex injury as burn injury a multidisciplinary approach is necessary. The Surgical Research Unit, under the direction of Col. Edwin J. Pulaski at first and later, Col. William H. Amspacher, developed into an institute for the study and treatment of burns (Figs. 11 and 12). In 1962, the Shriners of North America, stimulated by the work of the Unit, initiated a program of building civilian institutes for burned children. These were to be associated with medical schools. Blocker has developed an outstanding burn team in the Division of Plastic Surgery at the University of Texas Medical Branch,

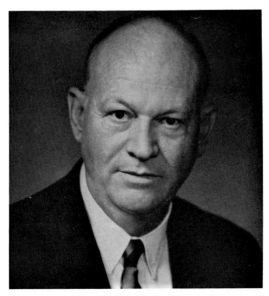

Figure 13. Truman G. Blocker, Jr., a professor at the University of Texas Medical Branch who has been a leader in burn research among the plastic surgeons of America.

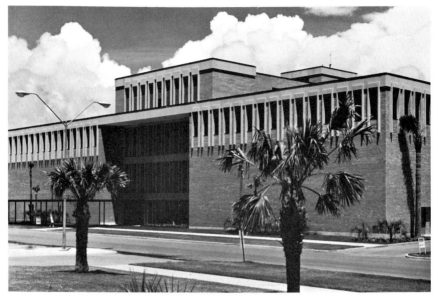

Figure 14.   First Shriners Burn Institute, Galveston, Texas.

Galveston (Fig. 13). His leadership provided the stimulus for the decision by the Shriners to build the first civilian burn institute in America at that school (Fig. 14). Other Shriners institutes have since been developed at the University of Cincinnati and Harvard University.

History of Skin Grafting

Skin grafting is so necessary in treating burns that its history is relevant. The earliest recorded method of skin grafting is the ancient Indian method. The Tilemaker Caste in India is said to have successfully utilized free grafts of skin, including the subcutaneous fat taken from the gluteal region, after it had been beaten with wooden slippers until a considerable amount of swelling had taken place. They used a secret cement for adhesion of the grafts, and they ascribed specific healing power to this substance. Padgett, in his book entitled *Skin Grafting*, tells of a nineteenth-century charlatan named Gamba Curta who cut off a piece of skin, passed it around among onlookers and then reapplied it. This was done to demonstrate the healing powers of an ointment she was recommending. In 1804, G. Boronio conclusively demonstrated free full-thickness autografting by experiments performed on sheep. Bunger, in 1823, moved grafts from thigh to nose, and Mason of Boston did the same in 1843. Both hair root and blister epithelium had been tried as methods of skin grafting.

Skin grafting, as it is known today, had its beginning with the Swiss surgeon Reverdin, who in 1869 used what he termed the "epidermic graft." He reported having transferred two little morsels of epidermis in a patient who had lost the skin of his thumb. Each of these was a thin bit of skin about 2 mm. square placed upon the granulating surface of the injured finger; this method is now referred to as epithelial, or thin razor, grafting. At the time of his fundamental discovery, Reverdin was a house physician on Guyon's service at the Hospital Necker in Paris. In 1872, Ollier reported success with larger and thicker pieces (up to 4 by 8 cm.). Thiersch, in 1874, described the use of deeper pieces of skin. He deliberately took some dermis along with the epidermis.

In 1875, John R. Wolfe, of Glasgow, Scotland, reported the plastic repair of a defect about the lower eyelid with a free, whole-thickness graft from the arm. He is generally credited with the initiation of this method. Fedor Krause, of Germany, however, is given the credit for bringing the whole-thickness graft into practical use. In looking for a simpler technique for grafting which could be used without difficulty by most anyone, John Staige Davis, of Baltimore, Maryland, described what he called the "small deep graft" in 1914. This was based upon Reverdin's idea, but instead of being the thinnest bit of superficial skin that could be cut, it included the full thickness of the skin at its center. This graft proved to be of great practical value and became known as the "pinch graft."

Prior to 1930 almost all grafting in burns was done by the pinch graft technique. The skill necessary to cut freehand a large sheet of skin of appropriate depth was not possessed by many surgeons. Blair and Brown, of St. Louis, popularized the split-thickness skin graft. These grafts were cut by the use of a long, thin knife, which became known as the Blair-Brown knife. In 1939, a drum-type dermatome was developed by Padgett and Hood at the University of Kansas. This instrument facilitated the cutting of large sheets of split-thickness skin to cover the burn wounds. It has remained popular over the years. A real advantage in burn management was the introduction of the electric dermatome by Brown of Indianapolis in 1948. This instrument was modified by Hargest in 1965. He utilized an air-driven motor in place of electricity. This provided a safer instrument with a smoother cut.

INCIDENCE OF BURNS

Burns are an ever present problem. An extensive burn is a catastrophic injury — catastrophic in the overwhelming insult to the patient, catastrophic in its psychological aspects and catastrophic in cost and suffering to the family involved.

Data from the National Health Survey for the years 1957–1961 show that the average number of burn injuries annually is 1,973,000. Of these, 937,000 are activity-restricting injuries, and 268,000 are classed as bed-disabling injuries. In 1962 the U.S. Department of Health, Education, and Welfare, Public Health Service, Division of Vital Statistics, listed 7534 deaths for that year due to accidents caused by fire and the explosion of combustible material and 849 deaths from accidents caused by electric current. During that same year, the number of deaths per 100,000 population caused by fire was 4.1; males outnumbered females 4421 to 3293. The breakdown according to age is shown in Table 1.

Each year in the United States about 7.5 persons per 1000 population are injured by coming into contact with hot objects or open flames. Mr. Edward F. Sands, Assistant Chief, Family Safety Branch, Division of Accident Prevention, United States Public Health Service, states that fire and explosion are the most frequent causes of fatal accidents among children and the elderly. Children under 15 years of age (31 per cent of the population) experience 29 per cent of the deaths from fire and explosion. Persons over 65 (9 per cent of the population) experience 28 per cent of the deaths from fire and explosion. Accidents in the home are responsible for more than three-fourths of all of the deaths from fire and explosion.

According to the U.S. Department of Health, Education, and Welfare's Accidental Deaths and Injury Statistics for the year 1960, there were 7645 deaths due to accidents caused by fire and explosion. The rate during this period was 4.3 deaths per 100,000 population. This is very similar to the 1962 figures. In different sections of the country, burns are more prevalent, especially in the South. The number of deaths and the rates in various areas of the country are shown in Table 2.

Moyer, in writing about the sociologic aspects of trauma, states that in 1 year (1940) accidents destroyed 17.04 years of human life for every 1000 inhabitants of the United States. Cancer was less destructive; it took 15.5 years of life per 1000 persons during the same year. The total working years of life lost to accidents during 1940 was 1,769,000 years, and thermal injuries accounted for 7.7 per cent of this loss, or 135,000 working years. Moyer estimates that the burned and scalded occupy more than 6000 hospital beds during the year. In the 1958 report of the Oklahoma

Table 1. THE BREAKDOWN ACCORDING TO AGE OF THE NUMBER
OF DEATHS CAUSED BY FIRE IN 1962

AGE (IN YEARS)	NUMBER OF DEATHS (PER 100,000 POPULATION)
Under 1	264
1–4	1082
5–14	726
15–24	318
25–34	505
35–44	717
45–54	937
55–64	858
65–74	966
75 and over	1151

Table 2. THE NUMBER OF DEATHS BY FIRE AND THE RATE BY GEOGRAPHICAL AREA FOR THE YEAR 1960

AREA	NUMBER OF DEATHS	RATE (PER 100,000 POPULATION)
New England	394	3.7
Middle Atlantic	1144	3.3
East North Central	1174	3.2
West North Central	543	3.5
South Atlantic	1509	5.8
East South Central	901	7.5
West South Central	1105	6.5
Mountain	225	3.3
Pacific	650	3.1

Crippled Children's Commission, Foerster found that the burn is the leading single diagnosis when ranked by the number of cases, the number of days hospitalized or Commission dollars expended. Thermal burns exceeded the next two ranking diagnoses—acute rheumatic fever and spina bifida—by 90 per cent and 40 per cent respectively. Bull estimates that about 700 to 900 persons die from burns and scalds in England and Wales each year.

From the foregoing statistics, it is obvious that burns are a major injury entity in the United States. Although the number of deaths is small in comparison to the number caused by the great killers—heart disease, cancer and stroke—the number of working years lost is appreciable because of the younger age group in which burns take their toll.

CAUSES OF BURNS

Foerster reviewed the records of 231 burned patients hospitalized at the University Hospital, Oklahoma City, between 1945 and 1959. He found that the burns were caused by stoves in 69 cases, inflammable liquids in 43, open fires in 49, scalding liquids in 33, miscellaneous causes in 29 and causes unknown in 19. Gas heaters and stoves accounted for 40 of the 69 stove burns. Of the 231 patients burned, 153, or 66 per cent, involved ignition of clothing. This figure increased to 78 per cent when scalds were excluded. Of the 231 burns, 141 occurred in children under the age of 12.

Moyer points out that in Dallas, Texas, among 166 serious thermal injuries (covering 15 per cent or more of the body surface), 50 were attributable to the direct contact of clothing with an open flame, and 44 of these were due to contact with a flame of natural gas or butane. Skoog reviewed 789 patients admitted to the burn unit of the University Hospital, Uppsala, Sweden, from 1951 to 1962. The primary cause of injury was scalding in 299 cases, fire in 265, hot objects in 135, electricity in 53 and chemical agents in 31. Although fire and scalding were equally common causes of burns in this study, there was a significant difference in age groups; in children, 54 per cent of the burns were due to scalding (13 per cent in adults) and 20 per cent were due to fire (49 per cent in adults). Seven per cent of the burns were produced by electricity. This high figure is probably a result of the fact that electricity is the predominant source of power in Sweden.

From England, Bull reports that of the 300 to 400 cases admitted annually to the burn unit of the Birmingham Accident Hospital two-thirds are due to domestic accidents and one-third to industrial accidents. The outstanding feature of the domestic burns is that those accidents in which clothing catches fire produce the most extensive and severe injuries. He also reported that between 1945 and 1955, 615 patients with burns due to clothes igniting were admitted to the hospital. For these, the case mortality was 23 per cent, and the mean treatment time was 48 days. In the remaining 810 patients with burns serious enough to demand hospital admission during this time, not associated with burning clothing, the case mortality was only 3.6 per cent and the mean treatment time 27 days.

In general, it may be stated that for children under 3 years of age the most common cause of burns is scalding. From 3 to 14 years, flame burns due to ignited clothing predominate; from 15 to 60 years, industrial accidents account for a large number of burns; for those over 60 years of age, accidents associated with momentary blackouts, smoking in bed or a house catching on fire are the most common. About 80 per cent of burn accidents occur in the home. The common burn in the southern part of the United States is seen in the little girl who, clothed only in a flammable housecoat, backs up to an open fire. The housecoat catches fire and the child runs, fans the flames and becomes the victim of a severe burn. In young children scalds are probably more common in boys because boys are more curious. Clothing burns are more common in girls because their clothing is more flammable. More children's deaths occur in girls because of the large number of clothing burns in this group.

In warfare that does not involve thermonuclear weapons, burns are rare in comparison with other forms of serious trauma. Burns due to flamethrowers are apt to be fatal instantaneously. Phosphorus burns occur, but not commonly. Vesicant gases such as mustard gas are a potential source of burns, but they have not been used in recent wars. Many combat burns occur when buildings catch on fire. A high percentage of burns in military medical practice occur as a result of plane crashes. Deep burns of the exposed portions of the body, namely the face and hands, are common. In addition to these patients, whose injuries are the result of the hazards of military life, there are many patients in the armed forces who are burned because of simple carelessness in everyday activities, such as in the handling of gasoline and the use of field stoves.

PREVENTION OF BURNS

It is obvious from the causes of burns that two major factors should be noted when prevention is considered, namely, the type of heating appliance in the home and the type of clothing. Greater emphasis must be placed upon the adequate guarding of household heating units. Improvement in the design of these units, with the safety of the child as well as the safety of the house in mind, will reduce the number of burn accidents.

The other main line of preventive action, at present, is that safer clothing should be used. The most critical garments are the night clothes of children and the aged and girls' and women's dresses. Certain fabrics are highly combustible, while others are not. It is now practical to treat various flammable fabrics with chemicals that make them sufficiently flame resistant. Legislation should be promoted that requires labeling of various garments as to their flammability. The manufacture of certain garments from flammable fabrics should be prohibited. Moyer states: "There is no surer or less costly approach toward the reduction in burn deaths than the education of women as to the flammability characteristics of fabrics. Should non-flam textiles be generally adopted for clothing it would likely reduce the deaths in the United States by at least 70 per cent because such action would reduce the area and depth of most burns in as much as the most important cause of extensive burns is clothing fire."

TEACHING PROBLEMS IN BURNS

In general, there is no injury that is treated less expertly by the medical profession at large than a burn. This is tragic in view of the extraordinary degree of suffering, financial loss and loss of social usefulness caused by the injudicious treatment of burns. Many patients with third-degree burns who could be healed within 3 or 4 weeks occupy hospital beds for months and even years. Some patients who could be quickly rehabilitated by energetic therapy develop avoidable deformities that prevent them from working; others are unnecessarily disfigured; and some actually die because of neglect.

It is clear that the teaching of burn therapy is not adequate at any level of medical education. Although a senior medical student or an intern may not be expected to be an expert in the art of skin grafting, he should be well grounded in the fundamental principles of therapy and capable of giving adequate emergency care. General practitioners, internists and pediatricians must learn that the limitations of their particular interests demand the skill of the general or the plastic surgeon for the management of a third-degree burn. Nonsurgical specialists may treat second-degree burns, but it is essential for them to recognize the characteristic features of the deeper injury. The sooner the surgeon can treat the patient with third-degree burns, the better for all concerned. Transfer of responsibility to the surgeon several months after injury results in waste of time, money and energy and needless suffering.

It is deplorable, but many well trained surgeons may be incapable of properly managing a deep burn. Too often, surgeons shy away from taking responsibility for the care of burned patients during the period of residency training. This is understandable, for the surgical resident is notoriously busy, and the treatment of only a single severely burned patient is an extremely time-consuming task. Other factors that steer the resident away from burns are the complexities of burn care, most surgeons' preference for clean surgery and lack of encouragement from senior attending surgeons. There must remain a continuing interest in burns on the part of the general surgeon. Among some educators there is a feeling that burns should become the property of plastic surgeons. Unfortunately, in America, there are not enough plastic surgeons to handle all severely burned patients. As a general rule burns are referred to the general surgeon in the community. Postgraduate educational programs in surgery must continue to emphasize the importance of training in burns to general surgical residents. The physiologic derangements that occur in a burned patient are more akin to the problems seen by the general surgeon than they are to those handled by the plastic surgeon. A severe burn involves fluid and electrolyte therapy, infection, nutrition and removal of dead tissue, all areas in which the general surgeon has frequent experience. In some well established training programs, the acute burns are divided between general surgery and plastic surgery, and reconstructive burn problems are assigned to the plastic service.

The urgent need for improving the teaching of the therapy of burns is principally the responsibility of the professors of surgery who exert a dominant influence in medical school as well as residency training. Chiefs of surgical services in hospitals not affiliated with universities must also share in this responsibility.

IMPROVING COMMUNICATIONS CONCERNING BURNS

During the past decade, communications among physicians interested in burns have improved throughout the world. The First International Congress on Research in Burns was held in Washington, D.C., in 1960 and the Second International Congress in Edinburgh in 1965. During the Second Congress, Mr. A. B. Wallace, F.R.C.S.E., the coordinator, proposed the organization of the International Society for Burn Injuries. This group was founded with the hope that it might promote and coordinate research and provide better communications among physicians interested in burns throughout the world. Mr. Wallace was elected general secretary and now has offices in the building of the Royal

College of Surgeons on Nicholson Street in Edinburgh. The Executive Committee of the Society is composed of the following:

A. A. Vishnevsky (U.S.S.R.), Vishnevsky Institute of Surgery of the Academy of Medical Sciences of U.S.S.R., Moscow, U.S.S.R.

A. Monsaingeon (France), 11 Cité Vaneau, Paris, France.

Tord Skoog (Sweden), Plastic Surgery Clinic, University Hospital, Uppsala, Sweden.

F. Zdravic (Algeria), Floriana D/IV, Parc de Pons, El Bier, Algeria.

N. H. Antia (India), Ben Nevis, B. Desia Road, Bombay, India.

Simon Sevitt (England), Department of Pathology, Birmingham Accident Hospital, Birmingham, England.

Mario Dobrkovsky (Czechoslovakia), Burn Unit, Legerova 63, Prague, Czechoslovakia.

Curtis P. Artz (U.S.A.), Department of Surgery, Medical College of South Carolina, Charleston, South Carolina.

F. Benaim (Argentina), Avenida del Liberator, San Martin 6662, Buenos Aires, Argentina.

Joshua S. Horn (Chinese Peoples' Republic), 12, Tung Sung Shu Hutung, He Ping Men L1, Peking 12, China.

S. Ohmori (Japan), Plastic Surgical Service, Tokyo University and Metropolitan Police Hospital, Tokyo, Japan.

A. W. Reda Mabrouk (United Arab Republic), 25 Yacoub Street, Malliah, Cairo, Egypt.

Martin Allgöwer (Switzerland), Ratischen Kantonsspitals, Chur, Switzerland.

Michael Tempest (Nigeria), University College Hospital, Ilbadan, Nigeria.

The national representative for the United States of America is Boyd W. Haynes, of Richmond, Virginia.

Surgeons, nurses and other medical personnel have organized the American Burn Association, which meets yearly. This promotes excellent communication among all workers interested in burns. In addition, the American Association for the Surgery of Trauma has always included as part of its program several papers on burns. For many years the Committee on Trauma of the American College of Surgeons has had a subcommittee on burns that has been active in the improvement of burn care. Almost all surgical organizations are interested in burns, and when particularly good papers on the subject are presented, they are well received. Most plastic surgery organizations place special emphasis on burns.

BURN UNITS AND BURN INSTITUTES

Since a severe burn is such a complicated illness, it requires a specialized team of people for expert care. Obviously, small burns are easily managed in a community hospital. Major burns should be referred to an appropriately staffed and well equipped institution.

There is a great need for the development of specialized centers for burns. It is impractical to assume that all major burns can be handled in institutes. Burn units or burn wards in major medical centers representing a region should be able to provide the ideal in patient care. These units could have a multidisciplinary approach and be properly equipped and adequately staffed. The professional staff of many hospitals and teaching centers have the knowledge for expert burn care, but ancillary help and organization are lacking. Because of the tremendous cost, many hindering compromises in therapy are frequently made. Although building, equipping and staffing of burn units would be quite expensive, such specialized arrangements would afford the most economic and efficient method of managing severe burns. There is a great need for federal and state support for burn units in major hospitals.

An institute for the study and treatment of burns seems extremely reasonable when one considers the many unsolved problems associated with burns and the multidisciplinary approach that seems necessary not only for treatment but also for further research. Advances in burn therapy will come primarily from new knowledge in the fields of biochemistry and physiology. As more is known about the body's response to an overwhelming insult, the treatment of burns can be expected to improve. The concept of basic scientists conducting investigative studies in the same institution in which scientific clinicians are caring for a large number of burns seems wise. It always is a great stimulus to the basic scientist to have first-hand information about clinical problems. At the same time, the thoughtful clinician receives many provocative ideas about patients' reactions to injury from scientists of other disciplines. Certainly the excellent standard of care and the numerous contributions made by the Surgical Research Unit attest to the value of an institute program.

The expansion of philanthropy by the Shriners of North America to the field of burned children in the initiation of three burn institutes is a pioneering effort in civilian medicine toward the improvement of our knowledge of burns. The Board of Trustees of the Shriners organization has wisely associated all the institutes with medical schools. In so doing, the institutes will receive from the university permanent supervision of the technical aspects and provision of the appropriate scientists to achieve the objectives of the institutes. The first three institutes are to be associated with the University of Texas Medical Branch, Galveston, the University of Cincinnati, Cincinnati, and Harvard Medical School, Boston. Each of the three institutes will have 30 beds and an abundant amount of space for research and teaching. The first institute opened in Galveston in 1966. These units may well serve as models for other philanthropic organizations to join forces with medical schools for the solution of difficult problems in the health science field. It would be gratifying if similar institutes could be developed for the treatment and study of burns in adults.

Not every city should have a burn institute. It would be wise to have a few institutes strategically located throughout the country that would conduct broad basic and clinical research programs in addition to caring for patients. Research should be given highest priority. In spite of many advances in the past two decades, the mortality for patients with severe burns is still high. If more burned patients are to be saved, broad investigational programs must be developed.

REFERENCES

Allgöwer, M., and Seigrist, J.: *Verbrennungen.* Berlin, Springer-Verlag, 1957.

Artz, C. P. (ed.): *Research in Burns.* Philadelphia, F. A. Davis Company, 1962.

Artz, C. P.: The Shriners Burn Institute at Galveston. *Bull. Am. Coll. Surgeons* **50**:93, 1965.

Bull, J. P.: Causes, prognosis and prevention of burns. *The Medical Press* **239**:205, 1958.

Cockshott, W. P.: The history of the treatment of burns. *Surg. Gynec. & Obst.* **102**:116, 1956.

Colebrook, L.: *A New Approach to the Treatment of Burns and Scalds.* London, Fine Technical Publications, 1950.

Crews, E. R.: *A Practical Manual for the Treatment of Burns.* Springfield, Illinois, Charles C Thomas, 1964.

Foerster, D. W., and Richardson, W. R.: Causes of burns in Oklahoma. *J. Oklahoma M. A.* **52**:713, 1959.

Goldman, L., and Gardner, R. E. (eds.): *Burns: A Symposium.* Springfield, Illinois, Charles C Thomas, 1965.

Harkins, H. N.: *The Treatment of Burns.* Springfield, Illinois, Charles C Thomas, 1942.

Haynes, B. W., Jr., and others: *Bahama International Conference on Burns.* Philadelphia, Dorrance & Company, 1964.

Holubec, K., and Karfik, V.: *Chirurgicke Lečení Popalenin.* Praha, Statni Zdravotnicke Nakladatelstvi, 1956.

Lorthioir, J. (ed.): *Physiopathologie et Traitement des Brûlures.* Bruselles, Presses Academiques Européennes, 1964.

Monsaingeon, A.: *Les Brules: Etudes Physiopathologiques et Thérapeutiques.* Paris, Masson & Cie, 1963.

Moyer, C. A.: The sociologic aspects of trauma. *Am. J. Surg.* **87**:421, 1954.

Muir, I. F. K., and Barclay, T. L.: *Burns and Their Treatment.* Chicago, Year Book Medical Publishers, Inc., 1962.

Order, S. E., and Moncrief, J. A.: *The Burn Wound.* Springfield, Illinois, Charles C Thomas, 1965.

Pack, G. T., and Davis, A. H.: *Burns.* Philadelphia, J. B. Lippincott Company, 1930.

Padgett, E. C.: *Skin Grafting.* Springfield, Illinois, Charles C Thomas, 1942.

Petrov, B. A.: *Svobodnaya Pyeresadka Kozhi pri Bolshikh Defectakh.* Moskva, Gosudarstvenoye Izdatyelstvo Meditsinskoy Literaturi, 1950.

Rhoads, J. E., and Howard, J. M.: *The Chemistry of Trauma.* Springfield, Illinois, Charles C Thomas, 1963.

Sevitt, S.: *Burns—Pathology and Therapeutic Applications.* London, Butterworth & Company, Ltd., 1957.

Shedd, D. P.: Historical landmarks in the treatment of burns. *Surgery* **43**:1024, 1958.

Skoog, T.: *The Surgical Treatment of Burns.* Stockholm, Almqvist and Wiksells, 1963.

Underhill, F. P.: The significance of anhydremia in extensive surface burns. *J.A.M.A.* **95**:852, 1930.

Chapter Two

PATHOLOGY
OF BURNS

by Carl Teplitz, M.D.

Fatal burns are relatively common in the United States. The annual mortality for burns is comparable to that of malignant lymphomas. The gravity, diversity and complexity of the pathogenetic factors involved in burn illness have captured the imagination of only a few pathologists, while studies by surgeons and physiologists perfuse the literature with ever increasing frequency. Save for the excellent reports and the erudite monograph, *Burns—Pathology and Therapeutic Applications*, by Sevitt and an additional handful of studies by pathologists based on experimental evidence or autopsy observations, the information on burn pathology is based on retrospective analyses of data extracted from general hospital routine autopsy protocols. The serious inadequacies of the routine autopsy with respect to accurate and comprehensive assessment of burn death, even when retrospectively reviewed by a panel of eminent pathologists, has been the subject of a detailed report (Medical Research Council, American Academy of Science). Studies limited to retrospective routine autopsy analyses that deal with the relative frequency, severity or importance of various pathogenetic factors involved in burn death do not therefore always provide meaningful, interpretable results.

Between 1961 and 1963, the author performed 88 autopsies on cases of consecutive fatal burn injury at the U.S. Army Surgical Research Unit. These were performed as part of a prospective study designed to evaluate a host of pathogenetic factors of suspected importance. This series had inherent noteworthy qualities. The subjects generally were young military personnel or their dependents. The accumulated information was therefore derived from cases that only occasionally showed antecedent disease and thus allowed a clear assessment of pathophysiologic factors not obscured or altered by the presence of pathologic factors unrelated to burn injury. The autopsy rate approached 100 per cent at this burn treatment center, and thus there was excellent clinicopathologic correlation, with no factor of autopsy selection in the study of this patient population. Postmortem examinations were performed soon after death. The mean death-autopsy interval was unusually short, and this factor markedly reduced the problem of postmortem tissue autolysis, which occurs at greatly increased rates in burns and sometimes results in difficult and misleading interpretations. Likewise, interpretation of postmortem bacteriologic examinations could be made with confidence because the mean death-autopsy interval in the burn wound sepsis series was 2.9 hours. Each autopsy was treated as a special research project, and exhaustive quantitative bacteriologic and special morphologic examinations of the burn wound and viscera were routinely performed. Giemsa (bacterial) stain was routinely used on the 3-micra sections. Particular attention was also given to the study of the respiratory, gastroduodenal and genitourinary tracts.

Because of the foregoing considerations and because the bulk of these observations have not hitherto been reported, the use of this large autopsy series as the framework for the discussion to follow on the pathology of burns appears justified. This chapter is thus intended as an original contribution to the literature on burns. It is hoped that it will also serve as a comprehensive presentation of burn pathology to both surgeon and pathologist.

Pathologic findings resulting from antecedent disease are hereby acknowledged as considerations in the evaluation of some fatal burn outcomes, particularly in the elderly, but these will not be treated in this discussion.

THE ROUTINE AUTOPSY IN THE EVALUATION OF BURN DEATH

The following routine autopsy deficiencies must be carefully considered and avoided in the endeavor to improve the usefulness of the burn autopsy:

1. *Incisions into the skin of cadavers are an implied autopsy restriction unless otherwise specifically indicated.* As a result, burn wounds are frequently not examined in a manner that produces meaningful information. At the time of this writing, there is a rapidly growing consensus that serious subcutaneous infection subjacent to the burn wound is perhaps the single most important pathogenetic consideration in the evaluation of burn death. Failure to examine the burn wound and its subjacent tissue in cases after the fourth or fifth postburn day virtually invalidates any definitive conclusions that may be drawn concerning the mechanism(s) of death.

2. Controversy presently exists as to the prevalence and pathogenetic importance of respiratory tract alterations in fatal thermal burn injury. Gross autopsy descriptions of the upper respiratory tract and lungs in routine autopsy protocols are frequently insufficient as to the precise extent and severity of the alterations. Microscopic sections are often too few in number, insufficiently representative, not cross sectional in scope and not designated as to the site of selection. The slough of tracheobronchial epithelium, which results from the marked autolysis frequently seen in burn autopsies, renders the evaluation of direct respiratory tract injury in the early burn death difficult. Finally, the differentiation between antecedent chronic lung disease and damage directly incident to burn injury,

although an exceedingly difficult point to evaluate, is perhaps given insufficient consideration.

3. The viscera of burn fatalities often contain few if any significant pathologic alterations to which death can be convincingly ascribed. In such circumstances, findings such as bronchopneumonia (which is terminal and microscopic) or mucus or mucopurulent secretions in the tracheobronchial tree (frequently found in any general nonburn autopsy series) may be listed as the first and therefore the implied major finding in the final anatomic diagnosis. Such practice may mislead the protocol reviewer to the conclusion that such alterations were significantly contributory causes of death.

4. An important problem relates to the assessment of sepsis. The frequently long death-autopsy interval makes interpretation of visceral and heart blood bacteriologic examinations exceedingly difficult. Heart blood cultures are easily contaminated by the wound flora, even when care is exercised, and cultures of liver and spleen, which are very much more meaningful in the evaluation of burn death, are generally not performed. Basal lung cultures, performed as routine procedures in some laboratories, often yield a mixed bacterial flora, even in the absence of infection, and undoubtedly reflect the postmortem descent of the wound flora that has gained tracheobronchial entrance via contaminated suction tubes or through the frequently present tracheostomy stoma. When sepsis is suspected on clinicobacteriologic grounds, such inconsequential lesions as focal traumatic, catheter-induced hemorrhage of the urinary bladder trigone (usually called hemorrhagic cystitis), terminal microscopic bronchopneumonia or perhaps microscopic focal acute prostatitis, are not infrequently implicated as the portal of entry when it is all too probable that significant burn wound infection has been overlooked.

Thus it is inevitable that a given set of prosectors who are performing an autopsy or a given set of observers who are reviewing a routine autopsy protocol might arrive at significantly different conclusions on the basis of the observed findings.

The Role of the Clinician in the Burn Autopsy

The resident prosector may have little awareness of many of the complexities of the burn autopsy that already have been and will be discussed. It is important for the surgeon to consult with the prosector before and during the autopsy procedure. It rests with the surgeon to obtain proper consent for special examination of the burn wound. This should include the written statement, "complete autopsy including multiple long incisions throughout the extent of the burn with exception of face, neck and hands." The pathology of burns most often rests in the burn wound, and thus the importance of this special examination cannot be overemphasized.

A frank discussion with the family indicating the necessity of the special burn wound examination is necessary. Since the undertaker will have to perform an immersion procedure, which is more difficult and time consuming than an injection embalming, the physician should advise the undertaker prior to the performance of the autopsy lest he later notify the family that the body has been mutilated.

GENERAL CLINICOPATHOLOGIC CONSIDERATIONS

A general discussion of burn pathology should include the prefatory statement that the pathophysiologic factors responsible for the grave circulatory and metabolic imbalance present during the first few days after extensive burn injury have no explanatory morphologic counterpart at the light microscopic level. At the present state of knowledge, the elucidation of most pathogenetic factors responsible for the early burn death (days 1 to 4) must rest with the demonstration of physiologic, biochemical and perhaps ultrastructural alterations.

Certain anatomic alterations in the resuscitative phase deserve comment. (1) Severe pulmonary edema with congestion was a constant finding in this series and has been widely reported by others. Its severity is generally greater than that observed in congestive heart failure incident to primary cardiac disease. Pulmonary edema, however, may be an expression of altered physiologic processes and anoxemia, which, might of themselves lead to death even in the absence of the observed intra-alveolar transudation. (2) Asphyxia from carboxyhemoglobinemia or hemorrhagic laryngotracheobronchitis resulting from inhalation of carbon monoxide or other noxious irritant fumes received wide attention following the reports described in the Cocoanut Grove disaster. Such dramatic causes of early death are peculiar to those cases of burn injury occurring under very special environmental conditions.

Extensively burned patients now generally survive the resuscitative period. They often show signs of clinical improvement. Sometime thereafter, the patient's condition may deteriorate and death ensues. Although it is true that a certain base line level of circulatory and metabolic dysfunction is operative long after the resuscitative period, one is justified in assuming that certain additional pathogenetic factors come into play which are responsible for the dramatically altered clinical course. Indeed, it is in this group of patients that the pathologist may elucidate the probable mechanism(s) of death if the postmortem examination is performed in a satisfactory manner.

Inherent in all published statistics on burn mortality are the vital considerations of severity of burn and age distribution of the studied population. However, statistics from various institutions bearing on the relative frequency of specific anatomic causes of death in a given series are commonly reported without reference to such important factors as age distribution, socioeconomic population breakdown and relative frequency of various types of circumstances in which burn injuries occur.

The importance of such considerations is brought out by a comparison of burn cases seen at the Boston City Hospital and at the U.S. Army Surgical Research Unit Burn Center. A high percentage of the burn fatalities occurring at Boston City Hospital is made up of elderly patients, and there is a significant incidence of pre-existing respiratory and cardiovascular disease in these cases. Antecedent genitourinary tract disease is common. Chronic alcoholism is not unusual, and a high percentage of the patients are burned as the result of mattress fires. The inhalation of noxious fumes from the combustion of mattress fillings may lead to a primary respiratory problem that overshadows the gravity of the cutaneous injury. Most injuries occur in conflagrations within closed spaces such as burning buildings. Extensive scald burns are only occasionally seen.

In contrast, of the patients in this series, 39 per cent were children below the age of 10, and most of these were burned either by the direct ignition of clothing without a surrounding conflagration or by scalding. Most of the patients were between the ages of 16 and 40. Only 3 per cent were in the 50 to 60 age group, and an additional 3 per cent were older than 60. Save for the latter group, definite anatomic evidence of antecedent disease was virtually nonexistent. Chronic lung disease, so frequently found in the general autopsy population at Boston City Hospital, was observed in only one case in the Surgical Research Unit series. Burn injuries most often occurred under conditions which precluded significant inhalation of noxious fumes. Chronic alcoholics with nutritional disease were rarely a problem, and burns resulting from mattress fires were unusual.

It is thus inevitable that a comparison of a series of burn cases from these two institutions with regard to discerning the frequency of various pathogenetic factors contributing to death might yield a significantly different over-all picture.

THE FREQUENCY OF SIGNIFICANTLY CONTRIBUTORY PATHOGENETIC FACTORS IN FATAL BURN INJURY

Since the pathologist cannot state conclusively what a patient dies *from* but can only indicate what he dies *with*, serious objections may be raised over the use of the phrase "anatomic causes of death." This is especially true when there is more than one important pathogenetic factor contributory to death—as is almost always the case in fatal burn injury. In Table 3, the classically employed enumeration of anatomic causes of death expressed in percentile is purposely avoided. Instead, percentile figures have been listed which indicate the number of cases showing a given pathologic finding that was considered as a factor contributing to death. Since multiple factors were often present in a single case, the sum of the listed percentages necessarily exceeds 100.

The relative importance of a specific pathogenetic factor in a given case with regard to its role in a fatal outcome cannot possibly be quantitatively expressed. There was obviously a wide spectrum of severity for each

Table 3. MAJOR CONTRIBUTORY PATHOGENETIC FACTORS FOUND
IN 88 CASES OF FATAL BURN INJURY
(U.S. ARMY SURGICAL RESEARCH UNIT 1961–63)

PATHOGENETIC FACTOR	INCIDENCE
Sepsis (type not specified)	93
Burn wound sepsis (flora not specified)	74
Burn wound sepsis by *Pseudomonas*	39
Infected cutdown with septic emboli	7
Bronchopneumonia (grossly significant)	13
Pulmonary edema	32
Other mixed pulmonary alterations	20
Tracheostomy complications	7
Cannula-induced necrotizing tracheitis	
Low lying tracheostomies	
Acute renal tubular necrosis	11
Gastroduodenal ulceration	7

pathogenetic factor; this is simply not amenable to statistical evaluation.
It is certain that in many individual cases a pathogenetic factor that was
listed as contributory to death may not have led to a fatal outcome in the
absence of other operative pathophysiologic processes. In the author's
view, this was particularly true for such pathologic processes as pulmonary
edema, other mixed pulmonary alterations and acute renal tubular
necrosis.

The ever increasing success of topical antibacterial treatment of burn
wound sepsis offers promise of a significantly reduced absolute burn
mortality. This would be achieved by the lowering of the percentage
figures expressed in the upper half of Table 3. If so, it may be expected
that the factors listed in the lower half of the table will come to have relatively increased importance in the future.

PATHOLOGY OF THE BURN WOUND

Depth and Other General Characteristics

Irreversible damage to all dermal epithelial elements constitutes a
full-thickness burn. Incomplete involvement of these elements with potential epithelial regenerative capacity constitutes a partial-thickness burn.
Despite the simplicity of these definitions, it is not always a straightforward
task to render an accurate morphologic assessment of the depth of dermal
injury in the first day or so following burn injury. Irreversible nuclear
damage that is characterized by karyolysis or karyorrhexis is easily recognized. Thermally induced necrosis of dermal connective tissue, when evidenced by conspicuous fusion of collagen fibers and associated loss of

affinity for acid dyes, is likewise readily diagnosed. Heat coagulation of epithelium, however, sometimes constitutes a form (albeit, a crude one) of histologic fixation. Thus, the nuclei of epithelial cells may retain a cytologic appearance that is not conspicuously altered for several days after the burn.

A further complicating factor is the fact that histologic sections through a burn wound, with their elements of markedly varying consistency, will not infrequently show some degree of microtomy compression artifact. Under such circumstances, the nuclei of viable epithelium may assume a compressed, elongated and hyperchromatic appearance that resembles the distorted, elongated and pyknotic characteristics sometimes found in irreversibly thermally damaged cells. Finally, the classically described homogenization, loss of eosinophilia and increased refractivity of dermal collagen fibers are sometimes not very conspicuous in the early postburn period. Special histochemical stains (e.g. orange G and aniline blue) that have been employed to bring out the qualitative changes in thermally damaged dermal collagen produce clear-cut results only when the extent and depth of damage can be appreciated by careful examination of routine histologic preparations. Unfortunately, biopsies of burn wounds are all too often taken during the early postburn period, when the aforementioned diagnostic difficulties may render definitive evaluation impossible.

Even when both clinical and histologic studies of a burned area suggest the presence of partial-thickness injury in the early postburn period, full-thickness injury may subsequently develop at the site. Microcirculatory stasis and vascular alterations incident to burn injury that do not produce outright coagulation necrosis have been demonstrated by light microscope and electron microscope studies. Marginal thermal vascular damage may be due to direct, instantaneous injury and perhaps to an indirect-delayed response. Thermally induced dermal microcirculatory insufficiency leading to delayed ischemic degeneration of deep epithelial appendages may play an important role in the conversion of partial- to full-thickness injury. Furthermore, the injurious effects of bacteria and bacterial toxins on the microcirculation have been studied, and it is quite probable that both bacterial invasion into subjacent viable tissue and the diffusion of bacterial products from the colonized burn wound into the subjacent viable microcirculatory bed account for the well documented full-thickness conversion seen in both human and animal wounds. The finding at autopsy of a necrotic dermis with completely devitalized epithelial appendages does not constitute evidence that full-thickness damage occurred at the time of thermal injury. For a comprehensive, thoughtful and detailed discussion of the pathogenesis of thermal cutaneous injury, the reader is referred to Sevitt's classic monograph on this subject.

In older burn wounds, the routine hematoxylin-eosin histologic examination renders little information of practical value, save that it indicates to what extent granulation tissue has developed beneath the now easily discernible necrotic dermis or hypodermis.

Evaluation of Bacterial Involvement of the Burn Wound

Without a thorough morphologic-bacteriologic study of the burn wound to evaluate the presence or absence of infection, the burn autopsy cannot render an adequate appraisal of burn death. There is now irrefutable evidence based on prospective quantitative bacteriologic-morphologic autopsy studies on humans and confirmatory studies on experimental animals that indicates that the elucidation of burn death frequently lies in the demonstration of significant bacterial invasion of the previously viable tissue subjacent to the colonized burn eschar.

At this point it seems appropriate to define the types of bacterial involvement that one may find in the burn wound. The growth of bacterial colonies on the surface of the burn wound is properly termed *supra-eschar bacterial colonization* (Fig. 15). In both man and experimental animals, supra-eschar colonization is followed by *intrafollicular colonization* within the pits of destroyed hair follicles (Fig. 16). Bacteria then readily penetrate through the eschar, which includes the heat-coagulated dermis and subjacent hypodermal fat in deeper burns (Figs. 15 and 17). Such bacterial infiltration of thermally coagulated tissue is properly termed *intra-eschar colonization* (Figs. 15 and 17). It is only when bacterial infiltration of the subjacent viable tissue can be demonstrated that the term *invasion, burn wound sepsis*, or *burn wound infection*, is justified (Fig. 18).

Mechanisms of Bacterial Wound Colonization

For a short period post burn, the surface of the wound is generally sterile. Within 48 hours, however, bacteria appear to contaminate the surface of the wound and then with the passage of time colonize the depths of the eschar. The source of the contaminating bacteria is not generally agreed upon. With specific reference to *Pseudomonas aeruginosa*, the innumerable phage types of this microorganism that may involve the wounds of different patients on the same ward and the constant change of phage types of *Pseudomonas* found on the ward with the admission of new cases strongly suggest that this microorganism may constitute a part of a given patient's normal skin or colonic flora prior to burn injury. Thus, the role of self-contamination in the pathogenesis of burn wound colonization is presently under serious consideration. While epidemics by the same strain of *Pseudomonas* or staphylococci have been observed on burn wards, the failure to prevent bacterial colonization of wounds under the most aseptic ward precautions may well lie in the problem of self-contamination of wounds by the patient's own cutaneous or fecal flora. Failure to detect nonfastidious and ubiquitous *Pseudomonas* organisms as part of the normal skin or fecal flora of some patients may be the result of the lack of sensitivity of routine bacteriologic swab cultures to detect the very low numbers of bacteria that may be present. The presence of bacteria within the hair follicles may also prevent their detection on swab cultures of the skin

Figure 15   Figure 16

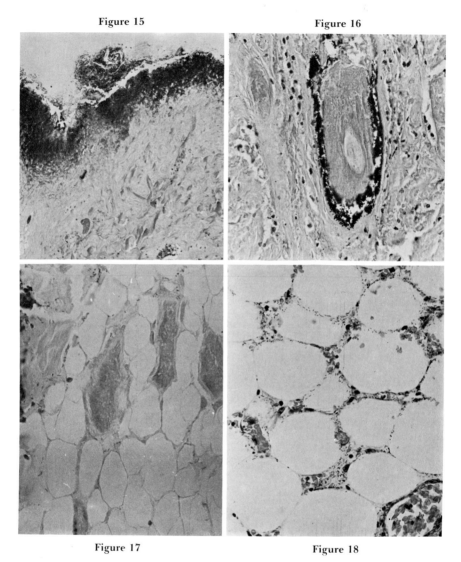

Figure 17   Figure 18

Figure 15. Burn wound 5 days after 87 per cent surface injury. Massive supra-eschar and superficial intra-eschar, gram-negative bacillary colonization produced the dark (deeply basophilic) zone of staining. Quantitative bacteriologic counts: 1.7×10^5 per cm.^{3}. Flora: *Aerobacter, Pseudomonas.* Burn wound elsewhere showed superficial bacillary invasion of subjacent viable hypodermal tissue. Quantitative bacteriologic counts on liver and spleen: 10^5 per cm.^{3}. Flora: *Aerobacter.* Patient died with gram-negative sepsis with endotoxemic shock. Giemsa stain, 75×.

Figure 16. Burn wound 5 days after burn in a 3-year-old child. Staphylococcal colonization around necrotic hair shaft is present. Quantitative bacteriologic counts: 9.0×10^6 per cm.^{3}. Flora: *Staphylococcus* (predominating), *Aerobacter, Pseudomonas,* alpha streptococcus. Giemsa stain, 400×.

Figure 17. Burn wound 96 hours after 86 per cent surface injury in a 19-year-old man. Patient died with renal failure and hyperkalemia. Gram-negative bacilli are infiltrating from the deep dermis (upper left) down through thermally coagulated hypodermal fat. Note co-

surface (Fig. 16). Finally, the possible role of nonculturable protoplasts must be considered.

Quantitative bacteriologic studies performed at the Surgical Research Unit on burn wounds excised during the early postburn period, as well as on the burn wounds from cadavers of patients who died during the same time period, indicate bacterial colony counts generally greater than 10^5 bacteria per gm. of eschar tissue after the fourth or fifth postburn day (Figs. 15, 16, 17 and 19).

Any general statement concerning the bacteriologic flora of burn wounds can only have relative and temporal meaning. Recently, reports emanating from large university hospital centers in the United States indicate that *Ps. aeruginosa* has been recognized with increasing frequency as the most prevalent colonizer and deadly invader of the burn wound. Staphylococci and certainly streptococci no longer occupy the positions of importance that they formerly held in relation to the establishment of fatal infection. With the continuing evolution of improved and effective antibacterial topical therapy, the relative pathogenetic importance of various microorganisms may be expected to change. Between 1961 and 1965 at the Surgical Research Unit, other gram-negative bacilli, such as *Proteus vulgaris*, Providence group. *Aerobacter (Klebsiella)*, *E. coli*, *E. freundii and Mima*, were frequent colonizers of burn wounds. *Proteus* and the Providence group were conspicuously prevalent during this period. The ability of these organisms to invade the underlying subcutaneous tissue has in many instances been clearly documented in quantitative bacteriologic-morphologic studies of the subcutaneous tissue underlying colonized burns (Figs. 20 and 34). Like *Pseudomonas*, *Proteus* causes fatal experimental burn wound sepsis in rats. Fungi, particularly *Candida*, are frequently found as both supra- and intra-eschar colonizers (Fig. 19). Systemic infection by *Candida* and *Mucor* has been documented but is exceedingly rare. It is difficult to foretell what role such microorganisms might have if effective bacterial suppression in the burn wound is achieved in the future.

The unquestioned importance of diffuse and massive bacterial colonization of the eschar lies in the fact that the patient is faced with an ever potential invasive onslaught by these bacterial hordes into the underlying

---

Figure 17. *Continued.*
agulated red cells in necrotic vessels and the absence of viable capillary bed. In contrast to the basophilic interstitial staining which results from bacterial invasion of viable hypodermis, the eosinophilic staining of thermally coagulated hypodermis is preserved even after secondary bacterial infiltration. The picture is, therefore, one of deep intra-eschar (hypodermal) bacterial colonization rather than one of true invasion of viable tissue. Quantitative bacteriologic counts: 1×10^8 per cm.^{3}. Flora: *Aerobacter, Pseudomonas*, alpha streptococcus.

Figure 18.   Subcutaneous fat of 3-year-old child who died 17 days after a 58 per cent burn. Massive burn wound sepsis is present. Gram-negative bacilli invade the interstitium between fat cells. Pyknotic nuclei of sparse necrotic neutrophils are present. Note viable capillaries and venules at bottom. Unlike bacterial colonization of eosinophilic thermally coagulated fat, invasion of viable tissue induces varying degrees of homogeneous interstitial basophilia (slight in this case). The sharply outlined basophilic rods are superimposed on this background tinctorial change. Quantitative bacteriologic counts: 2.7×10^8 per cm.^{3}. Flora: *Pseudomonas, Proteus, Mima, Staphylococcus.*

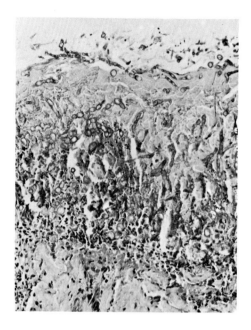

Figure 19. Supra- and intra-eschar colonization by pleomorphic fungal hyphae in burn wound of a child who died 5 days after burn. Quantitative bacteriologic counts: 1.0×10^6 per $cm.^3$. Flora: *Candida* (predominating), *Staphylococcus*, *Pseudomonas*, *Aerobacter*. Degenerating leukocytes are present within the eschar. Giemsa stain, 300×.

viable tissue. Thus, bacterial colonization of the eschar holds the same predisposing relationship to invasion of the subjacent viable hypodermis that bacteriuria in the genitourinary tract holds to invasion of the renal parenchyma (pyelonephritis). This comparison seems even more justifiable when one realizes that the bacterial colony counts of 1-gm. segments of homogenized burn eschar generally contain from 10^5 to 10^9 bacteria, which is the range of colony counts characteristic of colonized urine (bacteriuria). The burn wound is an excellent bacteriologic medium, regardless of whether the wound is treated by exposure for increased dryness or by occlusive dressings for maceration and rapid slough. This is attested to by the fact that the bacterial colony counts found in either type of wound are comparable to those present in overnight trypticase soy broth cultures of the same microorganisms.

Thus, the extensively burned patient is a unique phenomenon in the realm of infectious disease when it is considered that he has as much as 40 per cent or more of his total body surface acting as a bacteriologic medium that may support the rapid growth of millions of bacteria per gram of tissue.

Although it seems reasonable to assume that diffusion of toxic bacterial products through the depths of the eschar into the subjacent viable tissue and capillary bed may occur, no definite studies have documented the role of bacterial wound colonization in the pathogenesis of thermal burn illness. Diffusion of such toxic products could conceivably affect circulatory, metabolic, host defense and other functions of both local and systemic tissues and thus upset the host-parasite balance in favor of the colonizing bacteria. Such postulated altered conditions may then set the stage for rampant invasion of the underlying viable tissue.

The Relationship of Burn Wound Properties, Bacterial Colonization and the Success of Topical Therapy

The success or failure of topical antibacterial agents is in great part a reflection of one or more of the following anatomic or biochemical properties of the colonized burn wound.

1. Bacterial colonization not only occurs in supra-eschar location but also rapidly develops within hair follicles and within the depths of the eschar itself (Figs. 15, 16 and 17). Immediately after burn, viable bacteria may be harbored in the pits of hair follicles (Fig. 16). A topical agent must therefore have the capacity to penetrate rapidly and in high concentration the eschar. Many antibacterial agents are inactivated and bound by tissue protein, and thus they are rendered ineffective at a level beneath the surface of the eschar.

2. Topical antibacterial agents generally have not had a wide enough spectrum to suppress the variegated flora capable of colonizing the burn wound. Selective suppression of one group of microorganisms may be followed by overgrowth of resistant strains.

At this time, the apparent success of Sulfamylon at the Surgical Research Unit would appear to be based on its efficacy in overcoming the aforementioned factors.

BURN WOUND SEPSIS

Since it has not yet been shown that systemic toxemia can result from intra-eschar bacterial colonization, the pathologic diagnosis of burn wound sepsis or infection should be reserved for the anatomic demonstration of bacterial invasion into underlying unburned tissue. The degree of bacterial invasion may range from small foci of superficial microscopic invasion at the junction of dead eschar and underlying tissue all the way to massive diffuse bacillary infiltration of the subcutaneous tissue down to fascia (Figs. 20 and 21). Examples of this latter type of fulminant invasion with involvement of as much as 2000 cm.[3] of previously viable subcutaneous tissue have been noted in cases of *Pseudomonas* burn wound sepsis.

In such instances, the magnitude of invasion is equivalent to seven times the amount of tissue involved in diffuse, massive bilateral pyelonephritis. Most cases of burn wound sepsis lie somewhere between these extremes in terms of extent and depth of invasion. When infection of the subcutaneous tissue is widespread and diffuse, the condition is designated diffuse burn wound sepsis. In the series of 88 autopsies, 39 per cent of the cases showed diffuse burn wound sepsis in which *Pseudomonas* was the predominant organism. In these, between 200 and 2000 cm.[3] of subcutaneous

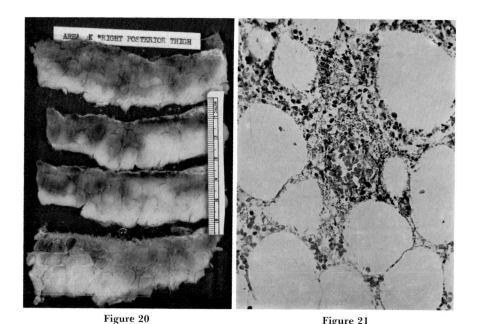

Figure 20   **Figure 21**

Figure 20. Multiple cross sections (sagittal) of eschar and underlying subcutaneous tissue excised at autopsy from the body of a 29-year-old woman who died 33 days after a 40 per cent burn. Eschar is at top and fascial plane is at bottom of each segment. The pink-rose discoloration (dark areas) of the subcutaneous fat which was present is one characteristic gross pattern of gram-negative burn wound infection. Quantitative bacteriologic counts of deep subcutaneous tissue: 1.5×10^8 per cm.[3]. Flora: *Pseudomonas*, Providence group.

Figure 21. Microscopic section of subcutaneous tissue shown in Figure 20. There is massive gram-negative bacillary invasion of interstitium between fat cells. Note viable capillary bed with focal early hemorrhage in lower area. Necrotic neutrophils are scattered sparsely among numerous rods. Giemsa stain, 600×. (For bacteriologic counts and flora, see Fig. 20.)

fat showed massive bacillary invasion. Bacterial colony counts obtained from homogenized 1 cm.[3] of infected subcutaneous tissue are shown in Table 4. The mean bacterial count per cm.[3] was 10^7.

Cases of diffuse burn wound sepsis in which other gram-negative organisms predominated were not infrequently encountered.

Cases of burn wound sepsis in which massive subcutaneous invasion was limited to one area of the burn wound have been observed. In one documented instance, the burn wound showed no bacterial invasion, as evidenced by normal subcutaneous tissue throughout most of the incised burn wound. However, an area of the buttock measuring 5 by 4 cm. and showing no unusual superficial surface characteristics revealed massive trans-subcutaneous bacillary infiltration for a depth of 5 cm. Although the surface area involved was quite small, the calculated quantity of invaded tissue amounted to 100 cm.[3], which is equivalent to the degree of infection present in a case of massive unilateral pyelonephritis.

Table 4.   Burn Wound Sepsis by Pseudomonas in 34 Cases,
Log Distribution of Wound, and
Bacterial Colony Counts (Total 100)

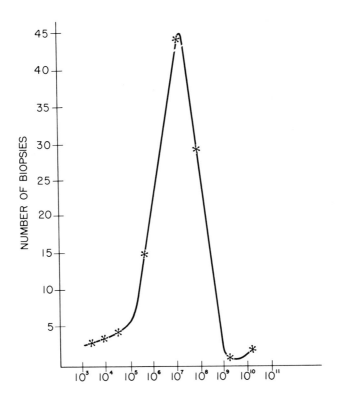

Widespread, multicentric, small foci of invasion were also found, and such cases were especially characteristic of staphylococcal burn wound sepsis.

The Anatomic Recognition of Burn Wound Infection: Technical Aspects of the Wound Examination

Since hematoxylin has replaced methylene blue as the basic dye of the routine histopathologic stain in many laboratories, the tissue demonstration of individually dispersed bacteria, especially gram-negative bacilli, has become exceedingly difficult unless special bacterial stains are utilized. The pathologist has thus come to equate unhesitantly a neutrophilic tissue reaction, especially when seen in pulmonary alveoli and renal tubules, with bacterial infection, even when the causative microorganisms are not morphologically identified. Bacterial stains are unfortunately no longer utilized by many pathologists for the histopathologic confirmation of infection. It is therefore easy to understand that the

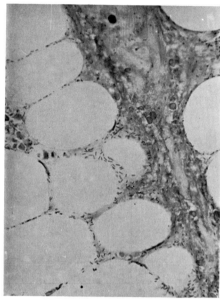

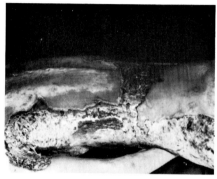

Figure 22   **Figure 23**

Figure 22.   Burn wound sepsis by *Pseudomonas.* Bacilli invade the subcutaneous fat as well as the fibrous lobular septa at right. There is invasion of viable capillaries at left. Neutrophilic reaction is absent. Section removed 15 minutes after death. Bacterial count: 7×10^6 per cm.[3]. Flora: *Pseudomonas.* Giemsa stain, 500×.

Figure 23.   Wound in a 49-year-old woman who died 37 days after a 45 per cent burn. Surface of wound is characterized by extensive suppuration, greenish yellow discoloration, and maceration (clinically thought to indicate infection). Bacterial count at autopsy: 1×10^8 per cm.[3]. Flora: *Proteus, Pseudomonas,* alpha streptococcus; *Achromobacter.* Microscopic examination revealed intra-eschar colonization with conspicuous leukocytic response in eschar but without bacterial invasion of subjacent viable subcutaneous tissue.

general pathologist might utilize marked neutrophilic response as the critical criterion for the diagnosis of burn wound infection. Furthermore, microscopic neutrophilic suppuration is the histologic counterpart of grossly purulent change and it is this latter criterion that has long been used by both surgeons and pathologists in making a clinical or gross diagnosis of wound infection. Although deep colonization of the wound, as well as invasion of subjacent tissue by gram-positive cocci, is associated with a classically suppurative reaction, it is not well enough known that massive invasion of subcutaneous tissue by some gram-negative bacilli — especially *Ps. aeruginosa* — is accompanied by either a very sparse or no neutrophilic tissue response (Fig. 22). It is therefore ironic that the green pus usually associated with wound infection by *Pseudomonas* is, in the case of the extensively burned patient, a favorable indication of a leukocytic reaction either to colonization by *Pseudomonas* or to a minimal, superficial, well controlled infection (Fig. 23). In the 34 cases of diffuse burn wound sepsis by *Pseudomonas*, the gross and microscopic absence of suppuration

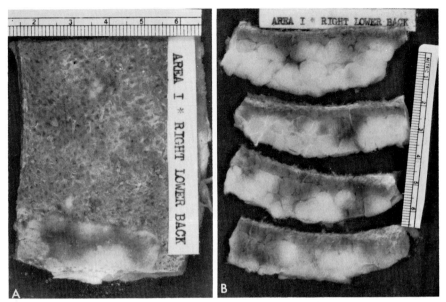

Figure 24. *A*, Surface view of burn wound segment excised at autopsy from 29-year-old woman who died 33 days after burn. Note the bland, nonsuppurative, uninfected appearance. At the junction of normal skin and the edge of the wound there is a serpentine, irregular dark rim which is slightly raised and violaceous. This latter finding, when present, is a diagnostic feature of burn wound infection by *Pseudomonas*. *B*, The excised block of burn wound in *A* has been rephotographed after transection into four equal parts, which are shown in cross sectional view (eschar at top and fascial plane at bottom). There is characteristic discoloration of the subcutaneous fat, which is indicative of gross bacillary invasion. This extends down for 2 cm. in some areas. Bacterial counts on deep tissue: 2×10^7 per cm.^{3}. Flora: *Pseudomonas*, Providence group. Microscopic examination revealed massive diffuse bacillary invasion. The wound depicted is representative of the entire 40 per cent surface injury. Pathologic diagnosis: diffuse burn wound sepsis by *Pseudomonas*.

was characteristic and constant. Although some cases of burn wound sepsis by *Pseudomonas* were associated with a rapid, violaceous darkening of the burn wound surface prior to death, a great many showed massive invasion of the subcutaneous tissue with what appeared to be a completely bland, nonsuppurative, nondiscolored eschar as viewed from the surface by surgeon and pathologist (Figs. 24 and 25). In some cases, the only suggestion of underlying massive invasion was the development of a fairly well circumscribed violaceous, serpentine, slightly raised rim at the junction of the burn and the contiguous normal skin (Fig. 24A). The development of classic ecthyma gangrenosum (hemorrhagic satellite cutaneous lesions) in 30 per cent of the cases was also found (Fig. 26). At the present time, however, aside from the changes which have just been described, there are no consistently adequate clinical criteria for making the diagnosis of burn wound sepsis, inasmuch as massive invasion of the subcutaneous

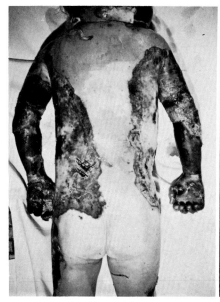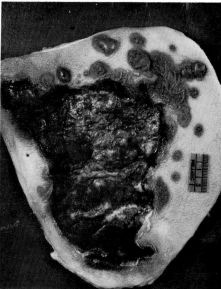

Figure 25   **Figure 26**

Figure 25.   A 4-year-old girl who died 7 days after a 63 per cent burn. Pathologic diagnosis: diffuse burn wound sepsis by *Pseudomonas.* Clinically, there was a rapid red black darkening of areas of the wound during the days prior to death. This change, when it occurs, is
characteristic of burn wound sepsis by *Pseudomonas.* Note the dark serpentine rim between
the burn wound and surrounding normal skin. There are numerous small, dark hemorrhagic
nodules approximately 1 to 2 cm. from the border of the wound. These are satellite ecthyma
gangrenosa, which are pathognomonic of burn wound sepsis by *Pseudomonas.*

Figure 26.   Excised segment of skin showing central patch of burn wound with burn
wound infection by *Pseudomonas.* Note the numerous papular and pustular hemorrhagic satellite ecthyma gangrenosa.

tissue is often not reflected by telltale surface changes. It cannot be too
strongly emphasized that the pathologist's gross and microscopic examination of the burn wound should not necessarily be guided by the superficial appearance of the wound.

GROSS EXAMINATION OF THE BURN WOUND

If proper special consent has been obtained for examination of the
burn wound, long, closely spaced (2 cm. apart) parallel incisions should
be made over the entire wound to expose the underlying subcutaneous
tissue. The posterior aspects of the wound should also be incised in a
similar manner. Infection is more likely to involve the posterior portion,
which is generally more macerated than the anterior aspects.

The uninfected burn wound in the early postburn period generally
shows a sharp demarcation with straight borders between the heat-coagu-

lated tissue (eschar) and the subjacent viable fat. There is usually a thin border of congestion between the zones. With the passage of time, the line of demarcation is apt to be less well delineated and more ragged in its appearance because of the dissolution and irregular shedding of the eschar.

Staphylococcal infection is characterized by suppuration of the subcutaneous fat that generally does not extend down for more than a few millimeters or a centimeter beneath the plane of heat-coagulated tissue. The changes in mixed gram-negative bacillary burn wound sepsis and particularly burn wound sepsis by *Pseudomonas* may vary in appearance from very conspicuous, well circumscribed, firm, nonsuppurative hemorrhagic necrosis to subtle changes characterized simply by a loss of normal luster by the subcutaneous fat and a slight tannish hue. Most cases of extensive burn wound sepsis by *Pseudomonas* were characterized by poorly circumscribed, irregular areas of pink, rose or tan nonsuppurative discoloration of the subcutaneous fat of diffuse extent and varying depth (Figs. 20 and 24B). Not rarely, gross discoloration indicative of invasion was so massive that all fat down to fascia was diffusely involved.

Once the subcutaneous bed of the wound is exposed by the incisions, microscopic sections should be selected from areas which are grossly typical or arouse suspicion of infection. The number of sections taken in a given case will depend upon the size of the wound and the nature of the gross findings. No burn wound can be overstudied, although they may be shamefully understudied. Sections of the burn wound often rendered more information relative to the pathogenesis of burn death than all of the visceral sections.

An accurate description of the extent and depth of subcutaneous invasion must be documented (Fig. 27), and all microscopic sections must be labeled as to the specific site from which they were taken. Cultures of the infected tissue should be routinely submitted. Although there is a close relation between the surface burn wound flora and the invasive flora, it is by no means a one-to-one association. It is therefore necessary that the cultures come from the invaded subcutaneous tissue.

To obtain cultures reflective of invasive flora, the following procedure is recommended (Fig. 28). A cube of deeply situated subcutaneous fat showing changes characteristic of invasion is excised with a scalpel and forceps. The tissue cube is immersed in 95 or 100 per cent alcohol, quickly withdrawn, and ignited. The outer surface of the tissue is allowed to flame for approximately 5 seconds. The flame is extinguished by rapid wrist shaking of the forceps. The procedure is then repeated. Experience has indicated that a cold alcohol flame coagulates approximately 100 micra of surface tissue and thus kills all bacteria on the surface and within the crevices of the tissue cube. The more central portions of the tissue, however, are not affected by the procedure. If contamination of the cube inadvertently occurs, the flaming procedure may be repeated. The tissue is then placed on a sterile surface (Petri dish), and after sterilization of the scalpel blade by alcohol flaming, the tissue is transected. Cultures are

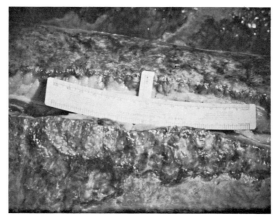

Figure 27.   Wound in a 10-year-old girl who died 38 days after a 70 per cent burn. A long incision has been made through burn wound and subjacent fat down to fascia in order to make an estimation of the extent and depth of burn wound infection. Surface bacterial flora: pure culture of *Ps. aeruginosa*. Bacterial counts from deep infected subcutaneous tissue: 6×10^6 per cm.[3] (see Fig. 28).

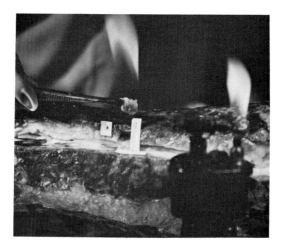

Figure 28.   Procedure used by author for obtaining cube of infected deep subcutaneous tissue for quantitative and differential bacteriologic analysis. The method eliminates contamination by colonizing flora and thus gives a true reflection of the deeply invasive flora. The excised cube of deep subcutaneous fat is being flamed for 5 seconds after having been immersed in 95 per cent alcohol. The instrument at the right is an alcohol lamp with a squirter jet flame device. See text for detailed description.

then taken from the cut surface. If quantitative bacteriologic facilities are available, most information is obtained by submitting the entire cube for homogenization and bacterial colony counts.

Microscopic sections should be taken from the segment of subcutaneous tissue immediately contiguous to the site cultured. In this way only can precise morphologic-bacteriologic correlations be made.

MICROSCOPIC EXAMINATION

Hematoxylin-eosin stain is worthless for the evaluation of burn wound sepsis (Fig. 29). Giemsa stain is excellent for the demonstration of bacteria, particularly individually dispersed gram-negative organisms, and also provides the familiar general basophilic-eosinophilic cytologic effect, which is most suitable for comprehensive interpretation of general histopathologic changes (Fig. 30). The best staining of both burn wounds and viscera is obtained by the use of a modified single-step phosphate-buffered Giemsa stain, which can be used on as many as 40 sections at one time without the usual requirement of differentiation by acetic acid. Subcutaneous tissue showing massive bacillary invasion is deeply basophilic when the slide is grossly transilluminated (Fig. 31). On low power examination, one should search for areas of basophilia in the subcutaneous fat. Bacteria are readily observed under the 40× objective. If they are not demonstrable at this magnification, time need not be wasted utilizing a 100× oil immersion lens. The number of bacilli generally seen is inversely proportional to the degree of local tissue neutrophilia. In cases of fulminant invasion by *Pseudomonas*, the neutrophilic response is sparse or absent, and massive accumulations of bacilli are found in the interstitium between fat cells. Bacillary invasion of fibrous areolar septa between fat lobules may be conspicuous (Figs. 22 and 31). Marked peribacillary cuffing (Fig. 32) or massive bacillary replacement of vessel walls in the absence of neutrophilic response (Figs. 30 and 33) is pathognomonic of invasion by *Pseudomonas*. Perineural bacillary permeation may be seen (Fig. 34).

When gram-positive coccal or mixed gram-negative infection is present, suppuration may obscure the presence of identifiable bacteria. As in bacterial bronchopneumonia or pyelonephritis, failure to identify bacteria by special stains does not rule out infection but, rather, implies that tissue bacteria have been obscured or suppressed below quantitatively detectable morphologic levels by the presence of the numerous leukocytes. On the other hand, the finding of massive infiltration of subcutaneous tissue in the total absence of neutrophilic response in burn wound sepsis by *Pseudomonas* should not lead one to infer that the bacterial growth occurred in the postmortem state. In cases of fatal sepsis involving *Pseudomonas*, many sections of skin that were removed from the wound 5 to

Figure 29   Figure 30

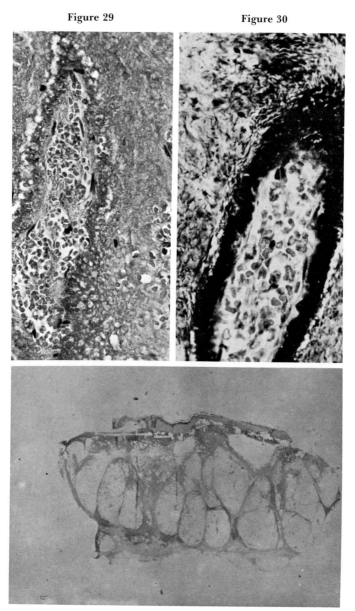

Figure 31

Figure 29.   Section of wound from case of burn wound sepsis by *Pseudomonas* stained with hematoxylin and eosin (H & E). The artery and surrounding soft tissue show a dull homogeneous basophilic hue, but no bacterial rods can be identified. Routine stains which do not contain methylene blue are worthless for the evaluation of burn wounds. 500× (see Fig. 30).

Figure 30.   Giemsa stain of tissue section from case of burn wound sepsis by *Pseudomonas.* The artery shows deep intramural basophilia due to massive confluent infiltration by pseu-
Legend continues on opposite page.

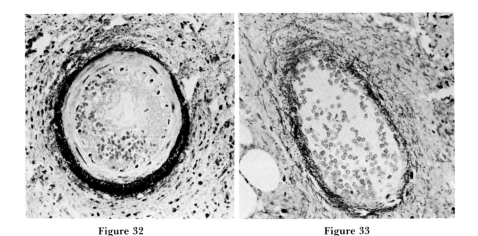

Figure 32   Figure 33

Figure 32. Burn wound sepsis by *Pseudomonas.* An artery shows dense circumferential cuffing by closely packed, deeply basophilic pseudomonads. There are individually dispersed bacilli and a sparse necrotic neutrophilic infiltrate in the surrounding tissue. Perivascular invasion is a feature of tissue invasion by *Pseudomonas.* Giemsa stain, 300×.

Figure 33. Burn wound sepsis by *Pseudomonas.* A vein in the deep subcutaneous tissue shows massive invasion by pleomorphic pseudomonads. The surrounding tissue is also invaded by dispersed pleomorphic bacterial rods. Note the paucity of necrotic neutrophils in the surrounding tissue. (*Pseudomonas* vasculitis.) The absence of vascular thrombosis is noteworthy and is a common feature of *Pseudomonas* vasculitis. Giemsa stain 600×.

Figure 30. *Continued.*

domonads. Note the discretely outlined pleomorphic pseudomonads in the surrounding tissue. Massive bacillary intramural invasion of vessels in the absence of associated neutrophilic response is pathognomonic of infection by *Pseudomonas* (so-called *Pseudomonas* vasculitis). 500×.

Figure 31. Transilluminated, magnified microscopic section of eschar and subjacent subcutaneous tissue from case of diffuse burn wound sepsis by *Pseudomonas.* The interlobular subcutaneous fibrous septa are prominent because of the marked basophilia created by massive bacillary invasion along these pathways. Close inspection reveals many intervening fat lobules with fine dark streaks. These are due to the marked interstitial basophilia induced by subcutaneous bacillary invasion. Infection has extended to the lower edge of the section. The thin eosinophilic eschar of coagulated dermis is hanging loosely at the surface. Giemsa stain, 4×.

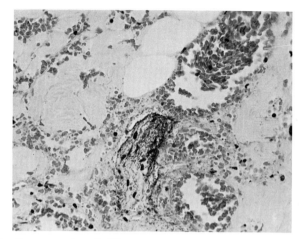

Figure 34. Burn wound sepsis. The structure in midcenter is a nerve showing perineural bacillary spread. No invasion of contiguous viable fat and blood vessels has yet begun. Bacterial counts of contiguous fat: 2×10^7 per cm.^{3}. Flora: *P. vulgaris* (pure culture). Giemsa stain, 300×.

30 minutes after death showed this histologic picture. The identical histopathologic changes are found in tissues of rats dying from experimental burn wound sepsis by *Pseudomonas*, even when the tissue is removed prior to death.

OTHER HISTOLOGIC CONSIDERATIONS OF THE BURN WOUND

Descriptions of extent and quantity of granulation tissue in the wound bed are of interest to the surgeon. Although wound granulations may appear within the week following a burn, it is quite common that granulation tissue response is quite minimal or even absent after a period of as long as 3 weeks post burn. This conspicuously diminished granulation response is more commonly seen in septic cases.

Grafted areas should be examined, particularly when grafts are loose and have not taken (Fig. 35A). In areas in which the changes have been interpreted as early homograft rejection or poor autograft take, bacterial invasion may often be histologically demonstrated as the mechanism for graft slough (Fig. 35B).

VISCERAL MANIFESTATIONS OF SEPSIS (SO-CALLED SEPTICEMIA)

In the clinical literature, the unqualified use of the term septicemia in relation to extensively burned patients has been widely employed. When used in this fashion, septicemia connotes that there is a systemic dissemination of bacteria that is responsible for the toxemic clinical picture and death. It is generally accepted practice in the field of infectious disease to define sepsis in relation to the primary site of infection whenever possible. Thus, one speaks of acute pyelonephritis or lobar pneumonia with or without bacteremia (septicemia). This shift of emphasis is more than just semantic, for it directs the focus of clinical attention on the pathogenesis and treatment of the primary site of infection rather than on the documentation and treatment of a positive blood culture. The same thinking should be employed with regard to sepsis resulting from infection of the body's largest organ, the skin. It is the author's belief that the pathologic basis for defining the possible primary sites of infection in burned patients is now sufficiently well described so that the term septicemia should not be used without a qualifying statement concerning the suspected or proven site of primary infection.

Exhaustive quantitative bacteriologic-morphologic studies on the viscera of patients dying with burn wound sepsis by *Pseudomonas* indicate that metastatic visceral infectious lesions are present in only 30 per cent of cases. Bacteriologic evidence of blood-borne bacterial dissemination secondary to massive burn wound sepsis by *Pseudomonas* may be documented in only 30 to 50 per cent of cases, depending upon the extent and care of bacteriologic sampling. When pseudomonads have been cultured from viscera, they have often been present in incredibly small numbers, as evidenced by colony counts in the general range of 1 to 10 bacilli per cm.^{3} of tissue. These postmortem bacteriologic findings correlate well with the frequently sterile antemortem blood cultures taken from cases with massive burn wound sepsis by *Pseudomonas*. When antemortem blood cultures are positive in burn wound sepsis by *Pseudomonas* quantitative bacteriologic studies on such positive blood cultures have rarely indicated colony counts exceeding 1 to 5 microorganisms per ml. of blood. This extraordinary contrast between the massiveness of primary infection and the paucity of circulating microorganisms is often a striking feature of burn wound sepsis by *Pseudomonas* (Fig. 35C, D, and Table 5).

When metastatic visceral lesions were present in burn wound sepsis involving *Pseudomonas*, round, hemorrhagic, infarct-like subpleural nodules were most often found (Fig. 36). These were usually few in number. In 40 per cent of the cases showing metastatic visceral lesions caused by *Pseudomonas*, only five or less small macroscopic foci of pulmonary involvement could be demonstrated (Fig. 37). Such lesions should not be misinterpreted as foci of ordinary bronchopneumonia.

In sharp contrast, cases of staphylococcal burn wound sepsis are invariably associated with widespread dissemination of numerous metastatic visceral lesions (Figs. 38 and 39). High quantitative bacteriologic counts in viscera and blood are a constantly associated finding (Table 6). Thus, staphylococcal burn wound sepsis was invariably associated with antemortem blood cultures yielding high colony counts. Hematogenous

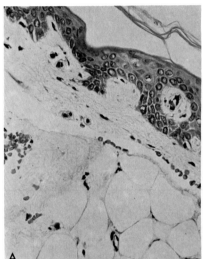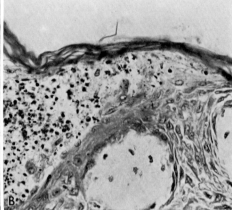

Figure 35. *A*, Section of split-thickness graft and underlying bed 24 hours after graft-ing. The epithelium appears morphologically viable. The graft is not firmly adherent to the underlying bed, and there is an intervening crevice which contains red cells and fibrin. Grafts which do not clinically take often show bacterial invasion. Giemsa stain, 400×.

B, Invasion by *Pseudomonas* of fresh autograft 15 hours after grafting. Bacilli are scat-tered amid the necrotic leukocytes within intra-epithelial bullae. This is the first indication of degeneration. Epithelium at lower right is still morphologically intact. Giemsa stain 400×.

C, Cross sections of burn wound from case of J.R. described in detail in Table 5. Of the 57 per cent full-thickness burn, only a relatively small area on the left anterior thigh showed colonization without subjacent bacillary invasion. The center row shows the cross sections from the uninfected area, with the typically sharp delineation between superficial thermally coagulated hypodermis and subjacent viable subcutaneous fat. Otherwise, the entire burn wound showed diffuse massive invasion down to fascia as evidenced by the marked discolora-tion of fat. Sections labeled right buttock (left column) and right flank (right column) were representative of the degree of invasion seen elsewhere in the burn wound.

D, Transillumination of the microscopic sections obtained from various areas of burn wound (from case J.R. described in Figures 29 *A* and 35 *C* and Table 5). All slides are labeled (A through L), thus indicating the exact site of the burn wound from which they were taken. Sections labeled A and K are from the anterior thigh, which was not infected. Note the thin convex shell of the eschar and the invisible uninfected subjacent subcutaneous fat in those two sections. The characteristic darkened (basophilic) interlobular subcutaneous septa indica-tive of massive bacillary invasion otherwise extends to the depths of other sections. Micro-scopic examination revealed diffuse bacillary invasion of interstitium between fat cells and fibrous septa as depicted in previous photomicrographs. Slide not magnified. Giemsa stain.

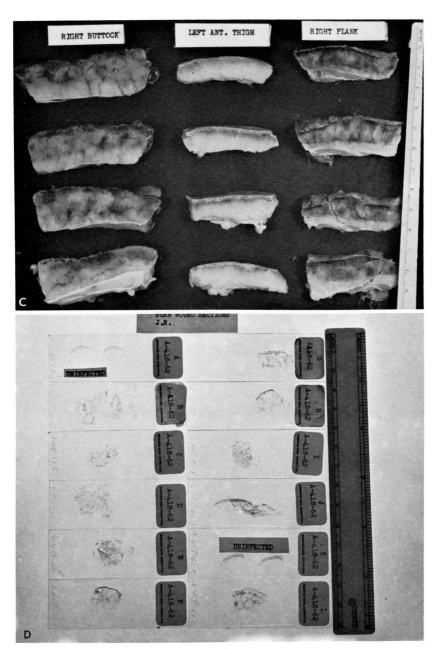

Figure 35C and D. *See legend on opposite page.*

Table 5. Case of Diffuse Burn Wound Sepsis by *Pseudomonas* Showing Dichotomy of (1) Massive Subcutaneous Bacillary Invasion and (2) Sterile Viscera Which are Free of Metastatic Septic Lesions*

SOURCE	ORGANISM (LISTED IN ORDER OF PREDOMINANCE)	FINAL COUNT/CM.^{3}	
		SPECIMEN REMOVED 5–15 MINUTES POST MORTEM	SPECIMEN REMOVED 4 HOURS POST MORTEM
Heart blood	No growth	0	0
Liver	No growth	0	0
Spleen	*Pseudomonas aeruginosa* grew out after 2 days from 15-minute specimen only; 4-hour specimen, no growth	3	0
Kidney	No growth	0	0
Lung	No growth	0	0
Burn wound biopsy site 1 (eschar and superficial subcutaneous tissue)	*Ps. aeruginosa* *Proteus vulgaris* *Aerobacter aerogenes*	2.5×10^8	Not done
Burn wound biopsy site 1 (deep subcutaneous tissue only)	*Ps. aeruginosa* *P. vulgaris*	1.0×10^8	Not done
Burn wound biopsy site 2 (eschar and superficial subcutaneous tissue)	*Ps. aeruginosa* *P. vulgaris* *A. aerogenes*	3.0×10^8	Not done
Burn wound biopsy site 2 (deep subcutaneous tissue only)	*Ps. aeruginosa* *P. vulgaris*	4.0×10^7	Not done

*A 4-year old boy died 25 days after 57 per cent full-thickness body burn. Sodium colistimethate or polymyxin B was not administered. Antemortem blood cultures were negative.

At autopsy, there was diffuse subcutaneous tannish red discoloration down to fascia, except for an area of the left anterior thigh which was uninfected. Microscopic examination showed diffuse massive bacillary subcutaneous invasion. Estimated total amount of infected subcutaneous tissue was 1000 cm.^{3}.

No metastatic (hematogenous) visceral lesions were present. One cm.^{3} of infected burn wound for colony count and sections for microscopic examination were removed 5 minutes after death. Bacterial colony counts were also performed on homogenized 1 cm.^{3} of liver, spleen, kidney and lung. These were performed 15 minutes post mortem after midline abdominal incision. The body was removed to the morgue and a definitive autopsy performed 4 hours post mortem. Quantitative bacteriologic counts were again performed on viscera for comparison with 15-minute specimens.

One cm.^{3} of eschar and superficial subcutaneous tissue were compared with subjacent 1 cm.^{3} of infected deep subcutaneous tissue to differentiate colonizing from invasive flora.

As noted, viscera were sterile at 15 minutes and 4 hours post mortem, except for the spleen, which showed three colonies of Pseudomonas at 15 minutes. These are no longer culturable 4 hours post mortem.

The comparative bacteriology on infected burn wounds with surface eschar taken from two different areas of the body showed *Pseudomonas*, *Proteus* and *Aerobacter*. *Pseudomonas* and *Proteus*, however, were present in the deep infected subcutaneous tissue in both areas. Thus, *Aerobacter* was a colonizer of the wound but was noninvasive. Bacterial counts both on surface and deep infected tissues were virtually identical: 10^8 bacteria per cm.^{3}. Thus, the estimated total number of microorganisms infecting previously viable subcutaneous tissue was 100 billion.

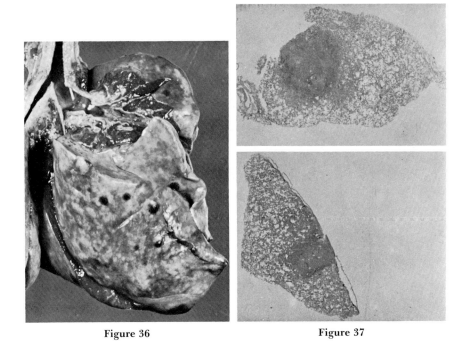

Figure 36   Figure 37

Figure 36. Classic round, hemorrhagic, infarct-like, subpleural nodules, characteristic of *Pseudomonas* metastatic (hematogenous) lesions, in a 4-year-old girl with burn wound sepsis by *Pseudomonas*. Bacteriologic counts on pulmonary septic lesions: 1.0×10^8 per cm.^{3}. Flora: *Pseudomonas* (pure culture).

Figure 37. Transilluminated microscopic sections of metastatic septic lesions in a 28-year-old man with burn wound sepsis by *Pseudomonas*. These were the only two lesions found upon examining the lungs. Note the round, hemorrhagic, well circumscribed nature of the lesions. Such foci are not to be confused with bronchopneumonia. The vessels do not contain septic emboli. Giemsa stain, 4×.

lesions associated with staphylococcal sepsis were always suppurative but sometimes had a superimposed hemorrhagic quality (Figs. 38 and 39).

Gram-negative bacillary burn wound sepsis that did not involve *Pseudomonas* was not uncommonly associated with hematogenous metastatic and visceral lesions. However, in several cases of focal burn wound infection, particularly with *Aerobacter aerogenes*, a rapid endotoxic-like death had occurred, and demonstrable metastatic lesions were not found at postmortem examination. High colony counts of *A. aerogenes* were found in all viscera. Thus the demonstration of endotoxin-producing, gram-negative bacilli (enteric flora) in liver, spleen and heart blood should be considered as strong evidence for an endotoxemic death when the clinical picture of endotoxemic shock is retrospectively present. The level of confidence, however, that one can place on the validity of the finding of enteric endotoxin-producing organisms in viscera is inversely proportional to the death-autopsy interval.

With regard to the pathogenesis of death in cases of burn wound

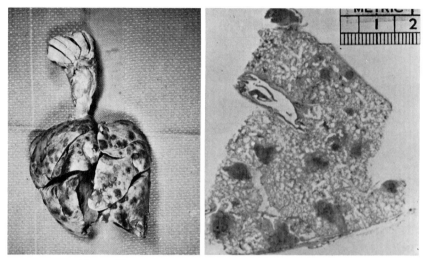

Figure 38   Figure 39

Figure 38. Lungs of 3-year-old girl who died 17 days after a 58 per cent, full-thickness burn. The quantitative bacteriologic aspects of burn wound and visceral examination in this case are depicted in Table 6. Note the numerous metastatic staphylococcal lesions which are suppurative and have a superimposed hemorrhagic quality.

Figure 39. Transilluminated microscopic section from lung in Figure 38. Note widely and evenly dispersed hematogenous staphylococcal lesions. There are pinpoint-size, well circumscribed, dark dots within the centers of some lesions (especially lesion at lower left corner). These are septic staphylococcal emboli within the lumina of pulmonary arteries. Giemsa stain, 4×.

sepsis, the following generalizations appear to be supported by the previous observations. In staphylococcal burn wound sepsis and in focal gram-negative bacillary burn wound sepsis associated with widespread bacterial dissemination and numerous metastatic visceral lesions, the hematogenous-visceral phase of sepsis is of almost certain fundamental importance in the mechanism of death. Contrariwise, in the typical case of burn wound sepsis involving massive invasion of subcutaneous tissue by *Pseudomonas*, the hematogenous-visceral component of the disease is too small to be implicated in the mechanism of death. Observations on experimental burn wound sepsis by *Pseudomonas* in rats indicate that metastatic visceral lesions occur only in the terminal stage of the disease, when the animals are already moribund. It is therefore logical to infer that death in burn wound sepsis involving *Pseudomonas* is most often directly related to the liberation of toxic bacterial products from the site of the primary infection.

Colistimethate sodium and polymyxin B are frequently administered systemically to patients with sepsis by *Pseudomonas* and probably account for the low counts and sterility of the blood and viscera in many of these cases. However, cases of nontreated burn wound sepsis involving *Pseudomonas* have been clearly documented in which circulating pseudomonads prior to death (quantitative blood cultures) as well as quantitative bacterio-

Table 6.   Quantitative Bacteriologic Findings in a Typical Case
of Staphylococcal Burn Wound Sepsis

SOURCE	ORGANISM (LISTED IN ORDER OF PREDOMINANCE)	FINAL COUNT PER CM.^{3}
Heart blood (TSB)	S. aureus	1.6×10^4
	Alpha hem. strep.	
Liver	S. aureus	9.8×10^4
Spleen	S. aureus	4.0×10^5
Kidney (pinhead-size lesions)	S. aureus	8.6×10^6
Renal pelvis (left)	S. aureus	3.5×10^4
Bladder urine	S. aureus	1.9×10^7
	Achromobacter sp.	
Burn wound biopsy 1		
(subcutaneous tissue)	S. aureus	4.3×10^7
	Mima	
Burn wound biopsy 2		
(subcutaneous tissue)	S. aureus	4.6×10^7
	Proteus	
	Mima	
	Pseudomonas	
Burn wound biopsy 3		
(subcutaneous tissue)	S. aureus	2.7×10^8
	Pseudomonas	
	Mima	
Right lung metastatic lesion	S. aureus	2.3×10^8
Left lung metastatic lesion	S. aureus	2.9×10^8

logic counts on viscera after death were in the range of zero to three bacteria per ml. (Table 5). Thus, the low visceral counts are not necessarily a reflection of antibiotic therapy, for they are also a function of the natural course of the disease. Although the above mentioned antibiotics are quite effective *in vitro* against *Pseudomonas* and may sometimes be effective in sterilizing the bloodstream, they are totally ineffective in suppressing the primary infection, as evidenced by uniformly average colony counts of 10^7 bacteria per cm.^{3} in invaded subcutaneous tissue in the face of very high blood levels of these drugs. The failure of colistimethate and polymyxin B to prevent or inhibit subcutaneous invasion by *Pseudomonas* is a problem beyond the scope of this discussion.

The present success of the antibacterial topical approach (e.g. Sulfamylon) has rendered some information that bears on the pathogenesis of burn wound colonization and infection. Wounds effectively treated with Sulfamylon show a multifold log decrease in bacterial counts within eschars. However, sterilization is not achieved. Despite the presence of persistent colonization, invasion of subjacent viable tissue is apparently not found, and patients do not develop the picture of burn wound sepsis. The inference, therefore, is that bacterial colonization is suppressed to a numerical level at which there is a host-parasite relation in favor of the host.

ADDITIONAL PRIMARY SITES OF INFECTION RESPONSIBLE FOR SEPSIS

One of the common sites of infection is the infected cutdown area. Staphylococcal burn wound sepsis may give rise to septic embolization to pulmonary vessels. More frequently, however, septic pulmonary embolization is a manifestation of primary infection of venous cutdown sites (Figs. 40, 41 and 42). As noted in Table 3, morphologically documented infected cutdown sites with subsequent pulmonary septic embolization were a significant contributory factor in the death of 7 per cent of the cases.

Figure 40

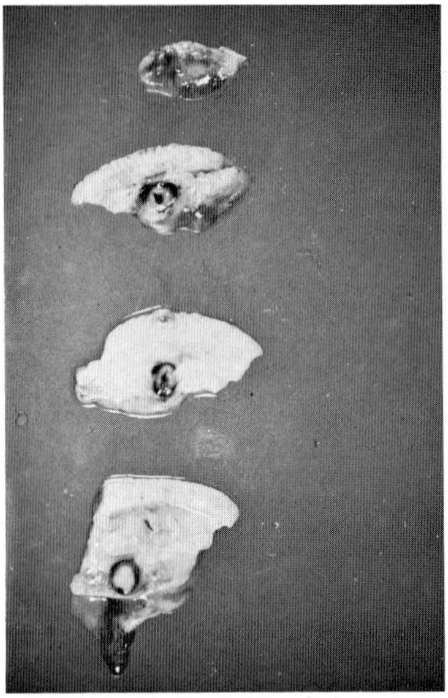

Figure 41

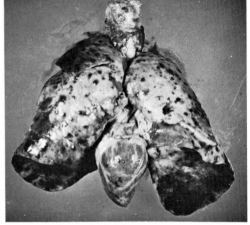

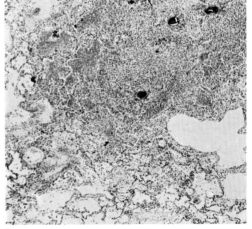

Figure 40. Serial sequential cross sections of greater saphenous vein extending from cutdown site (top) through progressively higher levels of the vein (below). There is a suppurative hemorrhagic thrombophlebitis in this 30-year-old man who died 7 days after a 41 per cent burn. (See Fig. 41.)

Figure 41. Lung of same patient with thrombophlebitis depicted in Figure 40. There is massive involvement of lungs and heart by metastatic staphylococcal lesions.

Figure 42. Microscopic section of lung depicted in Figures 40 and 41. Area of hematogenous pneumonitis at upper right contain many small arteries which are filled with deeply basophilic staphylococcal septic emboli.

Figure 42

Sometimes there is overwhelming infection from areas following primary excision. Multiple staged excisions of burn wounds have not entirely fulfilled their initial theoretical promise. Autopsies performed on patients who died after burn wound excisions have in many instances revealed significant bacterial invasion of the excised bed, even though autografts or homografts have been placed over the area. Occasionally, massive, deep invasion of donor sites has been demonstrated in patients who have died from burn wound sepsis involving *Pseudomonas.*

Pneumonia, infected erosions induced by tracheostomy tube, infected escharotomy sites and the genitourinary tract are other areas sometimes primarily responsible for infection. These are discussed in more detail later in this chapter.

RESPIRATORY TRACT

CLINICOPATHOLOGIC CONSIDERATIONS

Clinical respiratory problems and pathologic changes in the respiratory tract are not uncommon in burned patients. In several retrospective studies of routine autopsy material, respiratory tract alterations have been implicated as the major finding in the consideration of fatal burn injury. In several of these same retrospective studies, the primary role of direct injury at the time of burn has been emphasized as the main pathogenetic consideration for the observed respiratory tract alterations, and severe burns of the respiratory area of the face have been given importance with regard to their association with the observed respiratory problems. In England, there is an apparent infrequency of respiratory tract problems that are attributable to direct damage at the time of thermal burn injury. General discussions on the effect of smoke inhalation without reference to the specific nature of the fumes inhaled are of limited usefulness. The association of respiratory tract damage and the inhalation of specific noxious fumes has been documented. On the other hand, firemen treated for severe bronchopulmonary symptoms following smoke inhalation usually respond dramatically to simple therapeutic measures and are most often discharged within 24 hours without residual symptoms.

Hypoxemia is not uncommonly found in extensively burned patients. It is usually mild. There is difficulty, however, in attributing the observed hypoxemia to either primary pulmonary pathologic alterations or direct respiratory tract injury. Finally, recent studies in which blood lactate and pyruvate levels were performed on extensively burned patients with abnormal pO_2 levels suggest that oxygen delivery at the tissue level was almost always adequate for normal aerobic metabolism.

In this author's series, respiratory tract alterations were commonly observed and considered of sufficient severity to warrant consideration as significant contributory factors in death. Such findings were found in a large percentage of cases (see Table 3). However, the following qualifications should lead to a guarded interpretation of these findings.

1. Severe pulmonary edema and congestion was the most frequently encountered alteration and, on the basis of careful consideration of associated clinical and anatomic findings, was often thought to be a reflection of systemic circulatory dysfunction rather than primary respiratory insult.

2. Gross bronchopneumonia and atelectasis were the two next most commonly observed abnormalities of major importance in this series. However, it is important to note that such pathologic findings are commonly implicated as contributory immediate causes of death in a considerable percentage of nonburned cases in general hospital autopsy series. Thus, the specific relationship of such findings to possible respiratory tract injury at the time of burn is exceedingly difficult to evaluate.

3. When pulmonary alterations were present in a given case in this series, assessment of either their etiology or their possible correlation with clinical respiratory problems was often impossible.

In reports on the frequency of respiratory tract damage in burn cases, perhaps too little consideration has been given to the factor of age distribution in the series studied. The presence of antecedent lung disease is a critical factor that may hamper studies in which the purpose is to define pathophysiologic factors that are inherent to burn injury per se. Furthermore, smoke inhalation of inconsequential significance for a patient with normal lungs might lead to significant respiratory difficulty in one with antecedent chronic bronchitis. In any series of cases that is heavily weighted by an elderly population, it is to be expected that bronchopulmonary problems will occur with greater frequency and severity than in a series with a more evenly balanced age distribution.

At the Boston City Hospital, the high incidence of observed pulmonary disease in burn cases must be evaluated in the context of the large percentage of patients who are elderly and who have antecedent chronic lung disease. There is a very high general incidence of chronic lung disease found at autopsy in this hospital population. Furthermore, chronic alcoholism is relatively common, and a disproportionate number of burns occur when such patients doze off while smoking and inhale the noxious fumes that arise from burning mattress fillings.

In this series of relatively young patients with virtually no evidence of antecedent respiratory disease, respiratory tract problems were observed considerably less frequently than in the Boston series. Table 7 indicates the percentage of cases that showed signs or symptoms that might conceivably be interpreted as a clinical manifestation of a respiratory tract problem.

Cyanosis, tracheobronchial secretions, wheezing, rales, hoarseness, expectoration of carbonized material and abnormal x-ray findings were among the criteria used. In many instances, only one of these criteria was present, and in many the signs or symptoms were not of very great severity.

Table 7. RELATIONSHIP OF RESPIRATORY SIGNS AND SYMPTOMS TO TYPE OF BURN IN 88 AUTOPSY CASES

TIME OF OBSERVED ONSET OF SIGNS AND SYMPTOMS	PER CENT OF TOTAL SERIES WITH OBSERVED SIGNS AND SYMPTOMS	PER CENT OF RESPIRATORY PROBLEM GROUP WITH EXPOSURE TO SMOKE INHALATION OR EXPLOSION	PER CENT OF RESPIRATORY PROBLEM GROUP WITH FULL-THICKNESS BURN OF RESPIRATORY AREA OF FACE	PER CENT OF RESPIRATORY PROBLEM GROUP WITH EXPOSURE TO SMOKE INHALATION OR BURN OF RESPIRATORY AREA OF FACE
Control group without clinical respiratory signs and symptoms (58 cases)	0	27	22	42
Group showing respiratory signs and symptoms observed soon after injury	13	66	55	82
Group showing respiratory signs and symptoms not observed in early period (midonset)	10	66	30	66
Group showing respiratory signs and symptoms late or terminal in onset	11	40	40	60

It is obvious that some percentage of the aforementioned nonspecific findings, which were obtained from the clinical protocols, may have been indicative of systemic circulatory or metabolic pathophysiologic factors rather than of primary respiratory tract alterations. Nevertheless, no attempt was made to differentiate such factors with regard to either severity or etiology. Thus the enumerated percentage figures represent a maximum possible indication of the extent of clinical primary respiratory tract problems in this series. The presence of clinical respiratory problems of early, middle or late onset has been correlated with the possible relationship to conditions at the time of burn that have a known (inhalation and explosion) or possible (burn of the respiratory area of the face) relationship to direct respiratory tract damage. The groups of patients showing clinical respiratory signs and symptoms in the early, middle or late stages of illness are unfortunately too small to give rise to statistically significant correlations. However, the figures do suggest the possibility that there may have been some relationship between exposure to smoke inhalation, explosion or the presence of a full-thickness burn in the respiratory area of the face and the presence of a clinical respiratory problem.

When the author attempted to correlate any of the specific types of pathologic lesions to be discussed later with the presence of respiratory area face burn, smoke inhalation or explosion, few if any correlations could be made.

LESIONS ENCOUNTERED IN FATAL BURN INJURY
(SERIES OF 88 CASES)

UPPER RESPIRATORY TRACT LESIONS

Pharynx

Five per cent of the patients in this series showed focal pharyngeal erosions or necrosis in association with extensive, deep full-thickness burns of the face, including the respiratory area (Fig. 43).

Larynx

Thirteen per cent showed either laryngeal edema, focal erosion, focal laryngitis or necrosis. In a number of instances, the edema was associated with hoarseness and minor symptomatology, but in none of the cases was there clinical or pathologic evidence of obstruction. Because of chance selection in this series of 88 cases, no instances of appreciable laryngeal edema or other significant upper respiratory lesions were found during the first few days following burn, the period when upper respiratory tract damage incident to direct injury is most likely to result in an early obstructive respiratory death. Seventy-five per cent of the laryngeal lesions were found in patients who had survived at least 3 weeks and 50 per cent in those surviving longer than a month. Most of these cases did not show initial clinical evidence of laryngeal damage. Hoarseness, when present, often occurred late in the hospital course. Suction tube trauma with ensuing infection due to the delivery of a high bacterial inoculum from the colonized face burn wound may possibly have been a contributing factor in the pathogenesis of some of these lesions. It did not appear to be justifiable to implicate direct injury at the time of burn as a probable or definite pathogenetic factor in their development (Fig. 44).

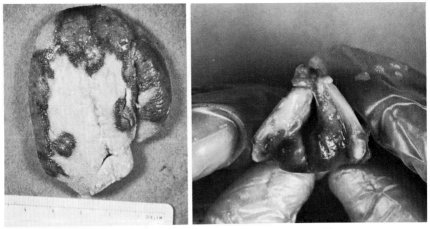

Figure 43   **Figure 44**

Figure 43. Tongue of 11-year-old boy who died 19 days after a 57 per cent burn that was the result of entrapment in a burning vehicle. There were deep burns of the respiratory area of face, and the patient was subjected to fume inhalation. Clinical examination on admission indicated burns of the pharynx and tongue. Severe respiratory symptoms were present. Note the hemorrhagic necrosis with focal serpentine irregular margins. Massive invasion by *Pseudomonas* subsequently occurred at the site of burn wound of the tongue, and there was translingual massive invasion of the hemorrhagic areas by *Pseudomonas.* The patient also had diffuse laryngotracheobronchitis with massive invasion by *Pseudomonas.*

Figure 44. Unopened larynx viewed from above. There is necrotizing, hemorrhagic laryngitis involving corniculate and cuneiform areas. Laryngitis extended down the posterior wall, and there was involvement of the vocal cords. This represents the most severe laryngeal lesion found in this series (88 cases). The 5-year-old girl died 25 days after a 30 per cent burn that was the result of a cotton nightgown being ignited by an open heater. There was no surrounding conflagration and no face burn or possibility of fume inhalation. No respiratory tract signs were present until death. The lesion was considered to be primarily infectious in nature and unrelated to direct initial upper respiratory tract damage at the time of burn injury.

Erosions Induced by Tracheostomy Tube

The most commonly observed lesions in the upper respiratory tract in this series were well circumscribed erosions on the anterior tracheal wall at the abutment site of the tracheostomy cannula tip (Figs. 45 and 46). The erosions became secondarily colonized and then were invaded by the bacterial flora indigenous to the burn wound. In those cases in which bacterial lymphatic dissemination occurred, satellite lesions developed, and there was a resulting severe, focal necrotizing tracheitis (Figs. 47 and 48). The evidence suggests that many of these erosions occurred in the absence of antecedent tracheobronchial damage due to smoke inhalation.

Figure 45   Figure 46

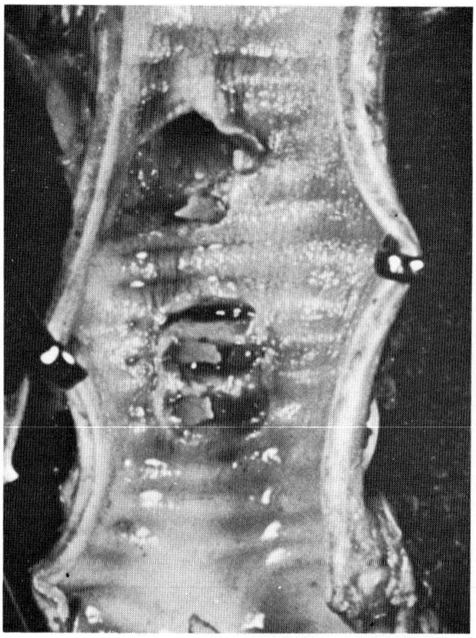

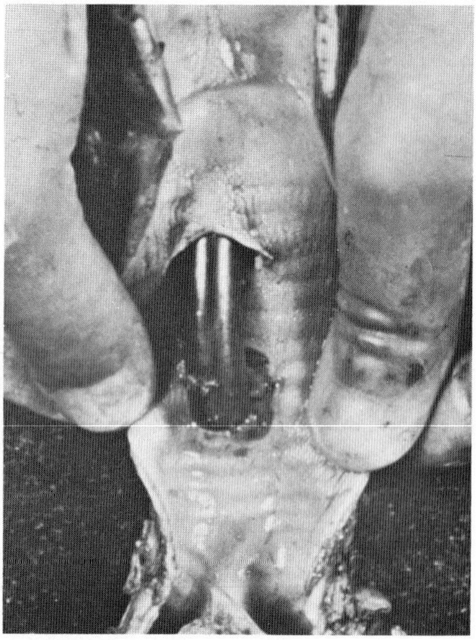

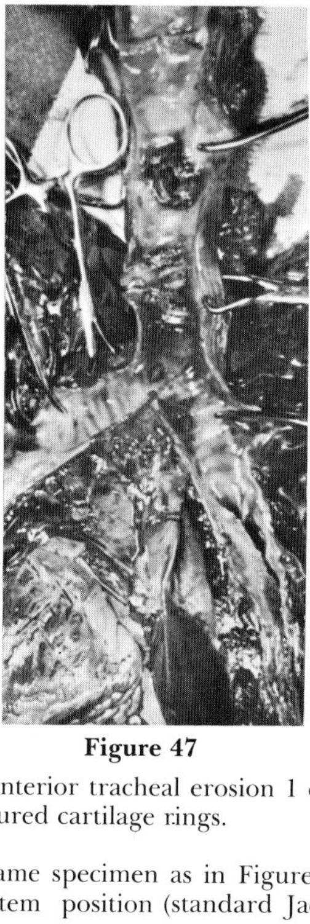

Figure 47 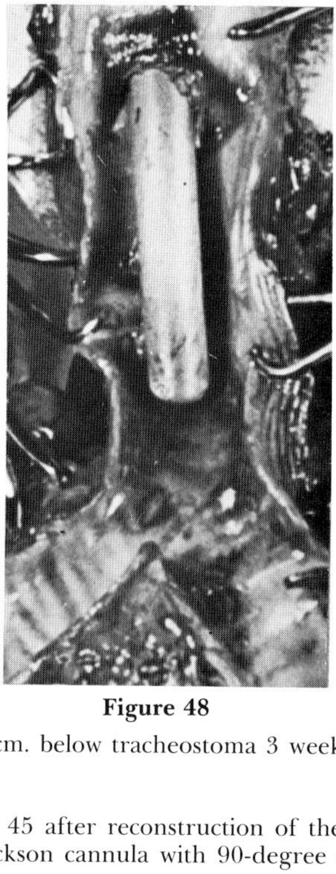   Figure 48

Figure 45. Anterior tracheal erosion 1 cm. below tracheostoma 3 weeks after tracheostomy. Note fractured cartilage rings.

Figure 46. Same specimen as in Figure 45 after reconstruction of the tracheostomy cannula's antemortem position (standard Jackson cannula with 90-degree anterior angulation).

Figure 47. Tracheostomy-induced necrotizing infectious focal tracheitis 7 days after tracheostomy. The tracheostomal margin is infected. Larynx is normal. There is a skip area of normal tracheal epithelium and then a focus of necrotizing tracheitis on the anterior tracheal wall. Microscopic examination revealed massive invasion by *Pseudomonas*, with peri-

Legend continues on opposite page.

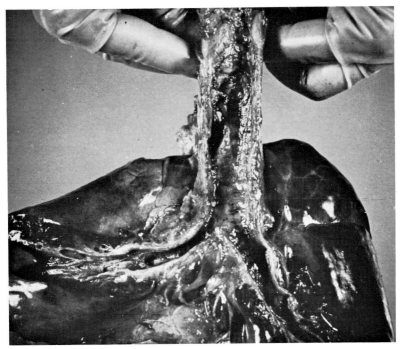

Figure 48A. Diffuse necrotizing pharyngolaryngotracheobronchitis in same patient described in Figure 43. Microscopic examination revealed massive deep gram-negative bacillary invasion with *Pseudomonas aeruginosa* predominating. Necrotizing pneumonia was also present.

Necrotizing, Pseudomembranous or Hemorrhagic Diffuse Tracheitis and Tracheobronchitis

In this series of 88 cases, necrotizing or pseudomembranous tracheitis was rarely observed. There was one case of diffuse necrotizing tracheobronchitis showing massive invasion by *Pseudomonas* (Fig. 48A), and another case that may or may not have been the result of bacillary lymphatic extension from a tracheostomy-induced focal tracheitis. In both instances, death occurred weeks after the initial burn injury, and therefore, these could not be classified with those cases which have been classically implicated as primary causes of death within the first few days following burn. A case of severe tracheitis involving the superior segment and contiguous larynx was also observed in a patient who died several weeks after a burn and

---

Figure 47. *Continued.*
neural lymphatic spread. The smaller lesions beneath the infratracheostomy tracheitis are satellite lymphatic lesions.

Figure 48. Same as in Figure 47 after reconstruction of the cannula as it existed during life. The anterior cervical tissues, including the tracheostomy cutaneous stoma, were placed *in situ* before insertion of the cannula. Note abutment of the cannula in the center of the focus of infratracheostomy tracheitis.

who had not initially shown respiratory difficulty. In several additional instances, tracheobronchial congestion was present. The lack of classically described pseudomembranous tracheitis in this series is probably a result of chance population selection. Although it is probable that the general incidence of such lesions is higher than found in this series, evidence from other autopsy series supports the view that pseudomembranous tracheitis is not a very common entity in thermal burn injury. It is probably not so generally prevalent as might be suggested by reports in which there appears to have been a factor of population selection along the lines previously described.

Pathology of Low Tracheostomy Syndrome in Children

As the result of low tracheostomy in young children, the abutment of a low lying tracheal cannula on the carina or right mainstem bronchus may result in varying degrees of bronchospastic respiratory obstruction. A serious bronchopulmonary syndrome may develop. This is characterized by signs of carinal or bronchial foreign body irritation and hypoxemia. Of 10 seriously burned children from the ages of two to six who as part of their initial resuscitation at other hospitals had undergone tracheostomy, five of those who eventually died showed autopsy evidence of a low tracheal incision (eighth cartilage ring or lower) that had resulted in a carinal or

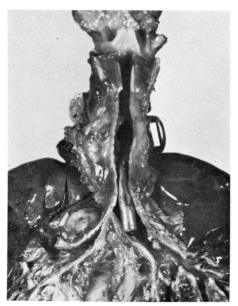

Figure 49. A 4-year-old girl with low lying tracheostomy (tracheostoma at seventh to ninth cartilage ring). After reconstruction of antemortem position of the tracheal cannula with anterior cervical tissue *in situ,* the tube ends in right mainstem bronchus. Note the deep color of the lung parenchyma. This indicates atelectasis.

infracarinal abutment of the tracheostomy cannula (Fig. 49). All these patients had experienced severe bronchospasm and other bronchopulmonary symptoms subsequent to the tracheostomy.

PULMONARY PATHOLOGY

Pulmonary Edema and Congestion

Although it has been stated that severe pulmonary edema during and after resuscitation is uncommonly seen in England, it has been generally recognized as a common occurrence in the United States. Edema with congestion of significant proportions was the most common pulmonary alteration in this series.

Degrees of pulmonary edema were judged on a 1+ to 4+ basis. A 4+ grade designated massive edema characterized by lungs that weighed 2000 gm. or more and, when incised, showed spontaneous transudation of edema fluid. The 3+ grade was defined as lungs weighing 1500 to 2000 gm. with the same gross anatomic findings. Grades 3+ and 4+ were classified together as severe pulmonary edema and congestion. Although grades 1+ and 2+ were commonly found, the discussion to follow pertains only to those cases considered as severe. This finding was presented in 100 per cent of cases in which the patient died within 48 hours following burn and in all but one who died on the third day. Of all patients who died after the third postburn day, 30 to 40 per cent had this finding, irrespective of the time interval following burn. In 32 per cent of the cases, pulmonary edema with congestion was considered as a contributing factor in death. However, in many instances, sepsis and other significant pathogenetic factors were also present so that death might have occurred even in the absence of pulmonary edema. Furthermore, the concomitant pathogenetic factors may have been etiologically responsible for the lung edema.

Although markedly increased permeability of pulmonary septal capillaries may result from the inhalation of certain gases, steam or perhaps very hot air, the classification of the pulmonary edema and congestion generally seen in burns as a primary pulmonary disorder is subject to debate. This finding is probably more often a reflection of circulatory imbalance than of primary pulmonary injury. This point is an important pathophysiologic consideration, since the frequently observed mild hypoxemia in extensively burned patients may be due in part to primary circulatory rather than primary pulmonary dysfunction.

Atelectasis

The incidence of gross atelectasis was 30 per cent; 43 per cent of these had a basal distribution of the type seen in any general autopsy population. Lobar atelectasis was found in association with low tracheostomy and intrabronchial cannula placement in children.

A peculiar atelectatic pattern characterized by fairly well circumscribed, patchy areas of parenchymal collapse that were diffusely scattered throughout the entire lung field was found in 30 per cent of the observed cases of atelectasis. This pattern was conspicuously different from the ordinary basal and segmental varieties of pulmonary atelectasis and warranted special consideration. There were neither gross nor microscopic associated bronchial or bronchiolar obstructive mucinous plugs. Often there was associated severe pulmonary congestion that resulted in the gross picture of so-called congestive atelectasis (Fig. 50). In such lungs the atelectatic areas were dark red and distinctly less violaceous than usual. The areas were full and not depressed below the pleural surface, and thus they resembled foci of consolidation (Fig. 51). Congestive atelectasis was most frequently found in children. Of the eight observed cases, five had tight, constrictive, circumferential, full-thickness burns of the chest. Four were children under 8 years of age. The possibility of mechanical restriction of thoracic expansion must therefore be raised as one possible cause of the apparent difficulty in normal alveolar inflation.

Particular attention was given to the relationship of atelectasis to bronchial or bronchiolar alterations because atelectasis occurring in burn injury has been attributed to such changes. Tracheobronchial damage with slough of epithelium was not found in any of the cases studied.

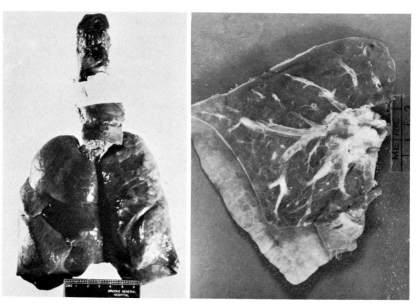

Figure 50.   Classic case of so-called congestive atelectasis involving the lung focally but diffusely. Note fairly well circumscribed areas of dark parenchyma. These are full rather than depressed as in the usual case of atelectasis.

Figure 51.   Lung. Cut surface of area of congestive atelectasis shown in Figure 50. There is fullness and absence of the usual atelectatic dark coloration. The area resembles the consolidation of pneumonia. Microscopic examination revealed complete alveolar collapse with marked septal capillary congestion. Note normal mucosal surfaces of bronchi.

Bronchi and Bronchioles

Bronchial and bronchiolar alterations, including obstructive mucoid and mucopurulent plugs, have been reported as frequent and severe complications of patients dying with thermal burn injury. In the author's series, the incidence of the usually mild acute and chronic bronchitis or bronchiolitis that was observed was 7 per cent. Obliterative organizing bronchiolitis was found in only one patient, who had been treated with intermittent positive pressure for several weeks because of respiratory difficulties. Twelve per cent of the cases showed varying degrees of bronchial congestion without inflammation, but some of these had associated severe pulmonary congestion.

Mucus or mucopurulent secretions and plugs within bronchi or bronchioles were extensive, severe and possibly obstructive in only 4.5 per cent of the cases. All these patients had incurred burns as the result of explosions.

Fifteen per cent showed occasional or rare mucous or mucopurulent microscopic secretions of insignificant terminal proportions found so often in general autopsy populations.

With respect to clinicopathologic correlation, of the 16 patients in this series who were in an enclosed space with burning objects where smoke inhalation was a possible occurrence, 37 per cent had mucinous secretions of the type considered to be of minor importance. Only one showed severe tracheobronchial mucinous plugs of probable pathophysiologic importance.

Pulmonary Emphysema

Pulmonary emphysema was grossly recognized in only two cases. These were old adults. The absence of significant emphysema in this relatively young group of patients suggests that it has an antecedent origin when found in older patients dying with thermal burn injury.

Patchy alveolar dilatation (focal microscopic emphysema) was present in 28 per cent of the cases. This change was not considered to be of definite pathophysiologic significance but was nevertheless of pathogenetic interest. Focal microscopic emphysema was often associated with marked pulmonary edema and congestion. This suggested that terminal hyperpnea may have been a possible causal factor. It was also found alternating with atelectatic areas. In only a very few cases did focal emphysema associated with the presence of even occasional mucinous plugs exist to suggest incomplete obstruction as a pathogenetic factor. Some of the patients had manifested bronchospasm during life; this might have resulted in focal alveolar overdistention.

Thromboemboli

It is generally thought that the burned patient is an ideal candidate for thromboembolic complications, but pulmonary thromboembolism has not been an important finding in published reports of autopsy findings. In this series, macroscopic thromboembolism was exceedingly rare, and only one in the 88 cases had a few scattered gross pulmonary arterial thromboemboli. Perhaps the younger age distribution accounted for this curious absence of a finding that is ordinarily so common in general autopsy populations. Microscopic vascular thromboemboli are not rare in the lungs of patients dying with fatal burn injury. In this series they were predominantly fibrin in composition and occurred in small arteries and venules. The incidence was 16 per cent. In the majority (10 per cent), the microscopic thromboemboli were quite rare and were of the extent and size that are commonly found (in at least 10 per cent) in general autopsy populations when the smallest pulmonary vessels are thoroughly examined. In the remaining 6 per cent, the small microscopic thromboemboli were not difficult to find but were still insufficiently extensive to be implicated by this author as an important pathophysiologic finding. In no instance were microscopic thromboemboli extensive. In three of the 88 cases, small, rare foci of pulmonary infarction were found in relation to vascular occlusion of small arteries.

Septic Emboli

Septic emboli were frequently found within the pulmonary microcirculation (Fig. 42). Small arteries and dilated septal capillaries were involved. In 50 per cent of the cases, staphylococci were implicated. The remainder showed mixed gram-negative flora including *Aerobacter* and *Pseudomonas.* Twenty-five per cent showed associated small foci of septic infarction. In 65 per cent of the cases showing septic pulmonary embolization, associated peripheral septic thrombophlebitis was demonstrated (Fig. 40). Infected veins were most often in relation to cutdowns that had been performed through burn wounds of the lower extremities.

Septic Hematogenous Lesions

Metastatic pulmonary septic lesions without associated septic arterial embolization were one of the most commonly encountered pulmonary lesions and were invariably associated with burn wound sepsis. See section on visceral manifestations of septicemia (Figs. 36 to 39).

Pulmonary Megakaryocytosis

In 12 per cent of the cases, there was a very conspicuous number of megakaryocytes trapped within pulmonary septal capillaries. All but one of these cases were associated with severe sepsis, and therefore, in this series of burns, severe pulmonary capillary megakaryocytosis was a suggestive though nonspecific feature of fatal infection.

Focal Gross Nonspecific Hemorrhage

Well circumscribed, 0.3 to 1.0 cm. round, firm, subpleural hemorrhagic areas containing no bacteria or inflammation were found in 32 per cent of the cases. They were often identical in appearance to the metastatic septic lesions seen in burn wound sepsis involving *Pseudomonas*. Gross focal pulmonary hemorrhage has been found to be an excellent reflection of severe sepsis.

Intra-alveolar Hemorrhage

Minimal focal intra-alveolar extravasation of red cells was present in a fair number of cases but was not considered to be significant. Diffuse intra-alveolar extravasation of red cells of at least moderate severity and extent had an incidence of 11 per cent. Seventy per cent of these cases were associated with severe pulmonary edema and congestion and thus could be attributed to severe septal capillary congestive distention with focal disruption. The remaining 30 per cent were associated with sepsis, and thus capillary damage due to toxemia was a theoretical pathogenetic consideration. Primary inhalation injury could not be ruled out, but there was little evidence to support this possibility in this particular series.

Intra-alveolar Macrophages

In many cases, focal accumulations of intra-alveolar macrophages were found, but in many, they were no more severe than those commonly seen in nonburned patients dying from a great variety of diseases. In 10 per cent of the cases in this series, moderate to severe diffuse accumulations of intra-alveolar macrophages were conspicuous. The macrophages were almost always pigment laden. Although in some cases the macrophages stained positively, for hemosiderin, the pigment was most often anthracotic in nature. The magnitude of intra-alveolar macrophage infiltration was marked enough in some cases so that it was considered to be of possible pathophysiologic significance in relation to capillary alveolar gaseous diffusion. Quite aside from the theoretical physiologic effects of their physical presence, the possible importance of these macrophages as a manifestation of direct pulmonary damage at the time of burn was evaluated. Eighty per cent of the cases with significant, diffuse intra-alveolar macrophage deposition were burned either in an enclosed space or in an explosion. Only 20 per cent of these patients had a third-degree burn of the respiratory area of the face. This was less than the general frequency in the entire series. Forty per cent of these cases had recognized clinical respiratory signs or symptoms in the early or middle part of the course. An additional 20 per cent with this finding showed some evidence of respiratory difficulty in the terminal stages of illness. Thus, clinical signs and symptoms were not universal in this group but were of significantly high incidence and occurred frequently enough after exposure to possible fume inhalation to suggest that diffuse, severe, intra-alveolar macrophage deposition was the single most consistent morphologic pulmonary finding that might reflect some degree of direct pulmonary injury at the time of burn. However, some cases incurring neither face burn nor possible fume inhalation showed severe degrees of this finding.

Bronchopneumonia

The incidence of acute bronchopneumonia was 40 per cent. Although this might sound like an extraordinarily high figure, 27 per cent of the total cases in the series (or 68 per cent of the cases with bronchopneumonia) were examples of microscopic, focal, slight, intra-alveolar, neutrophilic infiltration of terminal and inconsequential proportions. It is this type of bronchopneumonia that is ubiquitous among cases in any general autopsy population and should not be misinterpreted when one retrospectively notes its inscription in the final anatomic diagnosis of routine autopsy protocols.

In 13 per cent of the cases, gross bronchopneumonia was present. In some, bronchopneumonia was present along with classic metastatic focal septic lesions (Fig. 52). It could not, therefore, be determined whether these two infectious processes, when present together, were pathogenetically independent. The extent of bronchopneumonia varied from small, patchy areas to massive, necrotizing pneumonia involving entire bronchopulmonary segments. The extent of bronchopneumonia in this series was sometimes overshadowed by the massive degree of burn wound sepsis, and

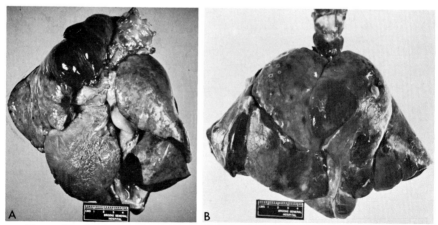

Figure 52. Lungs. Hemorrhagic, necrotizing pneumonia of extensive degree in two cases. In *A* there is associated pericarditis. In both *A* and *B* there are small round subpleural hemorrhagic nodules characteristic of metastatic septic lesions. In both instances there was also severe burn wound sepsis. The pathogenetic relationship, if any, between the confluent pneumonia and the hematogenous septic lesions is doubtful.

thus it was difficult to assess the respective roles of these two conditions in the depression of defense mechanisms. The continued finding of significant bronchopneumonia during a period (1965) when the problem of burn wound sepsis had been considerably decreased by Sulfamylon treatment at the Surgical Research Unit retrospectively suggests that the observed cases of gross bronchopneumonia in this series would have occurred even in the absence of burn wound sepsis.

Fifty-three per cent of the total patients in this series had tracheostomies, and 80 per cent of these were performed through burn wounds which, as previously noted, were colonized by a mixed bacterial flora with counts averaging 10^7 bacteria per cm.^{3}. The huge bacterial inoculum contaminating the tracheobronchial tree might have been expected to cause a higher incidence of significant bronchopneumonia. The frequency in this series was not higher than that found in any general hospital population of patients dying with a variety of serious underlying diseases other than burns.

Fat Embolization

Although fat embolization of slight degree has been described in burns, it was not observed in this series.

General Conclusions on Pulmonary
Changes in Fatal Burn Injury

A variety of pathologic alterations are found in the lungs of burned patients. Except perhaps for the entities of (1) diffuse, severe, intraalveolar macrophage deposition, and (2) so-called congestive atelectasis found in this series, as well as (3) pseudomembranous tracheobronchitis and bronchiolitis, which have been described in other reports, the pulmonary findings in cases of fatal burn injury are nonspecific and are of the type commonly found in general hospital autopsy populations. The very high incidence of metastatic visceral septic lesions and septic pulmonary embolization may be considered a singular expression of the frequency of wound sepsis and infected cutdown sites in burned patients.

Pulmonary findings were considered contributory factors in death (Table 3) in a considerable percentage of cases. The percentages are (1) pulmonary edema and congestion, 32 per cent; (2) bronchopneumonia, 13 per cent; (3) tracheostomy complications, 7 per cent; and (4) miscellaneous primary alterations in which any combination of the previously described pathologic entities was found together in varying and perhaps significant degrees, 20 per cent.

Most of the cases so listed had concomitant severe sepsis, and in a great percentage of cases, it was thought that because of its severity the burn wound infection was primarily responsible for death. Expressing autopsy findings in terms of primary causes of death, however, is strictly a judgment that cannot be scientifically assessed or proven. Until such time when burn wound sepsis and pulmonary edema and congestion incident to circulatory imbalance are eliminated as problems in the management of burn cases, the potential lethality of pulmonary alterations in burns will be difficult to evaluate. It is the author's opinion that, although some reports have overemphasized the general prevalence and severity of pulmonary problems in burns, there is nevertheless a significant pulmonary component in the pathogenesis of burn illness and death. Further elucidation of the pathogenesis and importance of these changes is necessary to provide a scientific basis for a logical therapeutic approach. If this is to be achieved, the attempt must be made to determine the relative importance of (1) primary pulmonary damage incident to direct thermal or fume inhalation injury, (2) primary circulatory and metabolic dysfunctions which indirectly are manifested by respiratory symptomatology, (3) pulmonary problems resulting from antecedent chronic lung disease and (4) nonspecific pulmonary conditions, such as bronchopneumonia, which may be expected to occur with relatively high frequency in any group of patients who have serious underlying disease without implicating any pathogenetic factor peculiar to burn injury as a predisposing condition.

HEART

Despite the serious circulatory problems that occur in burned patients, no specific or significant primary cardiac lesions were identified in either gross or light microscopic examination. Metastatic myocardial septic foci were seen in association with widespread metastatic visceral lesions, but these were of a terminal, inconsequential nature. Staphylococcal bacterial endocarditis, which was not rare between 1959 and 1961 at the Surgical Research Unit, was absent in this series.

In nine cases (8.8 per cent), myocardial foci were noted that showed increased numbers of Anitschkow's myocytes, slight interstitial edema and minimal myocardial fiber fragmentation (Fig. 53). Less occasionally, macrophages and minimal numbers of neutrophils were also present in these foci. Such changes may or may not be designated as minimal focal interstitial myocarditis, depending upon the whim and diagnostic threshold level of the individual pathologist. The extent and severity of these myocardial changes were no greater than those which are frequently seen and disregarded in hearts of unburned patients succumbing to pneumonia, pyelonephritis or other septic processes. Indeed, all of the cases in this series showing these mycardial changes were septic deaths.

No other morphologic myocardial changes including fatty degeneration, were found in this relatively young group of patients. Thus, when cardiac alterations are found in older burned patients, they are probably manifestations of antecedent disease unless proven otherwise.

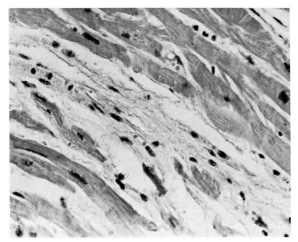

Figure 53. Heart. Microscopic myocardial focus showing increased numbers of Anitschkow's myocytes, interstitial edema and minimal myocardial fiber fragmentation in patient dying with sepsis. Giemsa stain, 300×.

LIVER

Fatty Metamorphosis

In 35 per cent of the cases, fatty metamorphosis of the liver was noted; in only one case was the change moderately severe. There was one instance of early fatty nutritional cirrhosis in a chronic alcoholic. Except in three cases in which the fat had a periportal distribution, the fatty change was predominantly centrilobular. This finding was nonspecific and slight and a probable reflection of suboptimal nutrition.

Hepatic Necrosis

The incidence of varying degrees of hepatic necrosis was 12 per cent. Most cases were limited to insignificant degrees of focal nonspecific necrosis of the type seen in sepsis or shock. One-third of the cases were of centrilobular hemorrhagic necrosis in association with congestion. Marked centrilobular necrosis of the type seen in prolonged shock and hypoxemia occurred in a patient who died 24 hours after a 95 per cent body surface burn. One other case of massive hepatic necrosis was found in a patient dying with shock and circulatory failure following gastrectomy. Focal periportal necrosis similar to that seen in eclampsia was noted in one instance. The patient was a septic child who showed widespread focal visceral necrosis with associated fibrin thrombi in capillaries and sinusoids, including the adrenals. The picture was suggestive of a generalized Shwartzman-type reaction. This has rarely been seen in endotoxemia.

Hepatic Congestion

Fifty per cent of the cases in this series died with some degree of hepatic congestion. It was generally acute, slight and centrilobular.

Unexplained Hepatomegaly

Hepatomegaly without gross or histologic alteration was not rare. Typically, the liver weighed from 2500 to 3100 gm. In one case, hepatic incision performed 15 minutes post mortem resulted in a considerable transudation of serous fluid. Microscopic examination revealed no evidence of detectable interstitial edema. All cases of idiopathic hepatomegaly had severe hypoalbuminemia in the range of 1.6 gm. per 100 ml. It is therefore probable that, in burned patients who have unexplained hepatomegaly in association with marked hypoalbuminemia, hepatic enlargement is the result of decreased plasma osmolarity and resultant edema formation.

The absence of metastatic hepatic septic lesions in cases of fulminant sepsis in which virtually every other organ was involved is noteworthy.

SPLEEN

No pathologic alterations that were of great significance in relation to burn death were found in the spleen. However, interesting alterations reflecting systemic pathophysiologic processes were evident.

Splenic Arteriolar Amyloid-like Material

Twenty per cent of the cases in this series showed subintimal deposits of a slightly eosinophilic, homogeneous material in splenic arterioles. The suspicion that the material was not ordinary splenic arteriolar hyaline was based on its frequent presence in very young children, in whom hyaline arteriolar sclerosis is not normally present. Furthermore, the pale tinctorial qualities of the material were sufficiently different from the usually more dense hyaline to warrant histochemical evaluation. The arteriolar deposits were thioflavine T- and P.A.S.-positive. They showed metachromasia with crystal violet but a negative congo red reaction. They contained no gamma globulin as evidenced by immunofluorescent studies.

The material appeared to be a mucopolysaccharide-protein complex with properties similar but not identical to amyloid. Since one-third of the patients showing this finding died within the first week following burn injury, it was inferred that the material in question was probably deposited during the early resuscitative period. The combination of possibly altered permeability of splenic arteriolar endothelium and the circulation of infused serum protein and colloids was considered a possible pathogenetic factor.

Plasma Cell (Immune) Response

Although the various complex modalities of host defense in burned patients are poorly understood, it is pertinent to describe the plasma cell response found in spleens, which is a direct indication of serum antibody production. Eighteen per cent of the cases showed only very occasional plasma cells per high power field. This is normal in healthy patients who have not been subjected to antigenic stimulation. Of the 16 patients involved, 15 died within 6 days following burn injury. The sixteenth patient died 11 days after burn injury. Thus, absence of plasma cell response was found during that postburn time period before which an antibody response could possibly have been expected. Every other patient in the series showed a definite degree of plasma cell hyperplasia. This was graded as either slight, moderate or marked. Cases of marked plasma cell hyperplasia of the spleen accounted for 34 per cent of the total series. Most of these patients died after the second postburn week. Nineteen per cent showed what was considered moderate plasma cell hyperplasia. The remainder showed slight hyperplasia. Immunofluorescent studies in which rabbit antihuman gamma globulin was used showed bright, specific fluorescence of plasma cell cytoplasm. This indicated active antibody formation. Thus, there can be little doubt that the severely burned patient is quite capable of excellent antibody response.

Infarcts

Splenic infarcts occurred in six cases (7 per cent). Fibrin thrombi were found in small splenic veins in one case. There were associated renal microscopic infarcts without identifiable thrombosis in either kidney or spleen in another case. Although most of the cases were associated with sepsis, circulatory collapse without sepsis was evident in two. As is true in general nonburn autopsy populations, splenic infarction was usually of unexplained etiology.

Acute Splenitis

A marked increase in splenic pulp neutrophils in association with splenic enlargement and softening is commonly referred to as acute splenitis. Although it is considered a criterion for sepsis, in this series acute splenitis was rarely seen in spite of the high incidence of massive sepsis.

Other Splenic Alterations

Splenic eosinopenia, which has been used by Sevitt as a reflection of adrenal hyperactivity in burns, was evaluated in all cases. The presence or absence of splenic eosinopenia could not be correlated with any definite clinical or pathological finding of interest, so it was of no morphologic usefulness in this series. In the series of cases of Curling's ulcer, where stress is thought to play a contributory role, 27 per cent of the cases showed a slight to moderate increase in the number of splenic pulp eosinophils.

Lymphonecrosis (necrosis of follicular centers) of the type described by Sevitt as occurring in the spleens of children dying within the first few days after burn was not seen, inasmuch as there were no early deaths among children in this series. Normal follicles with what appeared to be reactive centers (without mitotic figures) were found in approximately half the children in this series, and in almost every instance the child expired prior to the third week following burn injury. Hypoplastic lymphoid follicles were otherwise found in both children and adults.

Despite the numerous transfusions that many of these patients received, especially those who had undergone staged wound excisions in which replacement of more than the normal body blood volume was necessary, increase in the normal stores of splenic hemosiderin was not observed. No other pathologic alteration of the spleen was identified.

GASTROINTESTINAL TRACT

Acute Gastric and Duodenal Ulcers (Curling's Ulcers)

Perhaps it is the widespread usage and curious appeal of the qualifying name Curling that has seemingly endowed the ulcers found in burn injury with an air of uniqueness. Acute gastric and duodenal ulcers found in association with burn injury, however, are morphologically identical in every detail to the acute stress ulcers found in general hospital autopsy populations. Although Curling restricted his description of cases to the duodenal ulcer, acute stress ulcers found at autopsy in patients with and without burns have a predominantly gastric distribution.

The incidence of gastroduodenal ulceration in this series was 47 per cent. This figure is more than twice that previously reported on the basis of retrospective routine autopsy analysis. The discrepancy is based in part on a semantic consideration. Ulcerations that do not penetrate the muscularis mucosa are commonly referred to as erosions and therefore are not ordinarily called ulcers. The multiple acute ulcers found together in the stomach of a patient or an experimental animal following burn injury often show depths of penetration ranging from autodigestion of the uppermost portion of the mucosa to transmural penetration. Thus, the differentiation of ulceration from erosion in burn cases on the simple basis of depth would appear to be artifactual from the pathogenetic viewpoint. Nevertheless, for the sake of comparison with what has been reported in other series, 54 per cent of the cases with ulcers showed at least one lesion that had penetrated through the muscularis mucosa.

Acute stress ulcers were not rare in burns involving as little as 20 to 30 per cent of the total body surface. They were not found in seven patients who died before the third postburn day.

No age group was spared. The youngest patient was 9 months old. The incidence of gastroduodenal ulceration in children from the 9-month to 5-year age group was 43 per cent (12 of 28 patients).

There was a slight female predominance in contrast to the usual male predominance in peptic ulcer.

In 54 per cent of the cases, ulcers were found in the stomach alone. In 24 per cent, they were present in both stomach and duodenum, and in 22 per cent, they involved the duodenum alone.

Their specific anatomic localization within the stomach or duodenum was distinctive when compared to the classic localization of peptic ulcers. Whereas over 90 per cent of gastric peptic ulcers are located within pyloric (histologic) mucosa, 78 per cent of the ulcers in this series were found within fundic-type mucosa containing parietal and pepsin-producing cells. This differential distribution is not widely realized, and its implication with regard to the independent etiologies of stress and peptic ulcer is important. Eighty-eight per cent of the duodenal ulcers were posterior. This contrasted with the more equal or frequent anterior location of peptic duodenal ulcers.

Whereas peptic ulcers are most often solitary, multiple ulcers were found in 78 per cent of the involved stomachs in this series. Twenty-five per cent of the involved stomachs showed five or more ulcers. In one young girl, more than 200 discrete ulcerations were found by transillumination of the gastric wall (Fig. 54). When duodenal ulcers were concomitantly associated with gastric ulcers, multiplicity at both sites was common, but when only duodenal ulcers were involved, they were always solitary.

With regard to size, gastric ulcers were generally smaller than duodenal ulcers. Seventy-two per cent of the former were less than 0.5 cm. in diameter. Many of the gastric ulcers were no larger than 2 or 3 mm. In two cases, however, the minute gastric ulcers were of sufficient depth to cause massive bleeding (Fig. 55). The difficulty in locating such minute, acute gastric ulcers during exploratory gastrotomy and even at autopsy is noteworthy. In contrast, 81 per cent of the duodenal ulcers were over 0.5 cm. in size, and 31 per cent were larger than 1 cm.

The gross anatomic appearance of these acute ulcers was quite different from the usual peptic variety. In the stomach they were well circumscribed and punched out. They showed no surrounding or underlying induration, edema or injection. Most were round or oval, but some showed irregular, stellate or serpentine configurations. They occasionally had an elongated, narrow contour which aligned the base of rugae and were easily overlooked unless all rugae were carefully pushed aside (Fig. 56).

Ulcers of the duodenum were generally round or oval, and because of their larger size and greater depth, they more closely resembled the usual variety of peptic ulcer. The absence of induration, edema and injection served to differentiate them grossly from the chronic duodenal ulcer.

In 46 per cent of the involved stomachs, the deepest ulcer had not penetrated through the muscularis mucosa. In 22 per cent, there was

Figure 54

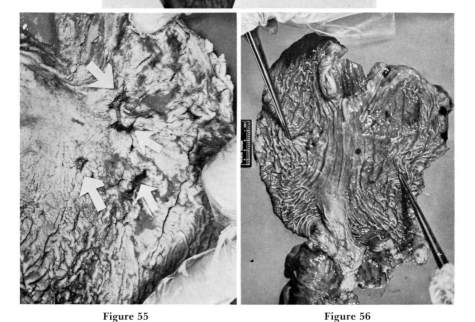

Figure 55   **Figure 56**

Figure 54. Transillumination of markedly dilated stomach showing over 200 tiny acute ulcerations. The patient, a young girl, died suddenly while watching television. At autopsy the markedly distended stomach filled much of the abdomen, and death was attributed to a cardiac arrhythmia due to vagus reaction.

Figure 55. Gastrectomy specimen showing multiple, irregular, punched-out, acute gastric ulcers located within body. The ulcers had penetrated into submucosal vessels and led to massive gastrointestinal hemorrhage.

Figure 56. Multiple round and irregularly shaped acute stress ulcers involving the body of the stomach. The smallest ulcers are easily overlooked unless the rugae are spread apart.

penetration through muscularis mucosa, in 14 per cent through sub-mucosa, in 11 per cent through inner muscularis and in 7 per cent there was transmural penetration with perforation. The duodenal ulcers were generally of relatively greater depth. Six per cent involved the mucosa alone, 12 per cent extended into the muscularis mucosa, 35 per cent penetrated to the inner muscularis and 29 per cent extended to the outer muscularis. Perforation occurred in two instances.

A remarkable feature of stress ulcers was the frequent lack of inflammatory response. Of the gastric ulcerations, 50 per cent showed virtually no inflammatory response, 23 per cent showed minimal neutrophilic reaction, 13 per cent showed what was considered to be slight inflammation and only 10 per cent showed moderately severe inflammation. Ulcers of the duodenum showed approximately the same percentage distribution in occurrence and severity of inflammation. In ulcers from surgical specimens or from autopsies of patients with severe hemorrhage, neutrophilic response was generally greater than in ulcers which were incidental findings. This suggested in part that the absence of inflammation was due to the development of many of these ulcers in the terminal stage of the patient's illness. However, occasional ulcers in gastrectomy specimens were noted which showed almost no neutrophilic response (Fig. 57). The variation in severity and the inconstancy of the inflammatory response in these lesions as contrasted to the uniformity of significant leukocytic reactions in peptic ulcer cannot be completely explained.

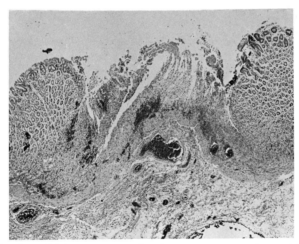

Figure 57. Superficial acute stress ulcer in gastrectomy specimen. Additional ulcers which had penetrated into submucosal vessels were present. The penetration has reached to the muscularis mucosa. There is still residual, degenerating, ghostlike mucosa present within the ulcer crater. The cells scattered in the submucosa are red cells. There was only a very minimal acute inflammatory reaction at the base of the ulcer, despite the fact that the patient was in generally good physical condition at the time of gastrectomy. The lack of inflammatory reaction in acute stress ulcers is often conspicuous. Giemsa stain, 30×.

Although many of the ulcers showed acid hematin within their bases, most did not, and in such cases the microscopic picture differed little from the autodigestion found in postmortem autolysis. In the most superficial ulcerations, the base of the ulcer usually consisted of unsloughed, degenerated epithelium with poorly staining nuclei. This same picture was even seen in superficial ulcers in surgically removed stomachs (Fig. 57). A bland, ghostlike morphology that resembled postmortem autolysis was characteristic of some ulcer beds as deep as the inner muscularis. Although a fibrinoid-like necrosis of the type seen in peptic ulcer was occasionally noted, the bases more frequently showed a bland interface between the autodigested and the underlying viable tissue. It cannot be too strongly emphasized that the lack of inflammation and the histologic postmortem autolytic character of Curling's ulcer were seen in stomachs that were removed within half an hour after death, in stomachs which had been filled with formalin immediately after death and in surgical specimens.

The absence of fibrosis also typified stress ulcers and differentiated them from chronic peptic ulcers.

With regard to the question of hyperacidity in the pathogenesis of acute stress ulcers, it is of interest that 20 per cent of the cases showed gram-negative bacillary colonization or superficial invasion at the surface of gastric ulcerations. This finding was present in stomachs removed within the hour of death. Bacillary invasion was not always an agonal phenomenon, since the stomach that showed most extensive colonization of the ulcer bed was a surgical specimen (Fig. 58). Ten per cent of the ulcers showed monilial colonization or superficial invasion (Fig. 59).

No subjacent identifiable vascular abnormality of any kind was ever present except in occasional vessels in which there was secondary autodigestive damage at the margin of the ulcer base. Vascular congestion and variable submucosal edema were fairly constant findings.

Generalized severe congestion of the stomach was sometimes, but not usually, noted. The stomachs were usually distended if an intubation tube was not in place before death. In the areas not adjacent to the ulcers, histologic abnormality was observed in the gastric mucosa.

Although an association between sepsis and stress ulcers has been suspected, no definite relationship between these two processes could be statistically proven. In no instance was septic embolization to submucosal vessels found in relation to stress ulcers.

A detailed discussion of the pathogenesis of Curling's ulcer is of questionable usefulness at our present state of knowledge. Various specific pathogenetic factors have been implicated on the basis of experimental and theoretical considerations, but the accumulated evidence offers no single theory of pathogenesis that explains all facets of this complex problem. However, certain points that relate to pathogenesis are perhaps worthy of mention. The morphologic similarity of stress and steroid-induced ulcers is considerable. The differences in location, size, multiplicity, sex ratio, inflammatory response and presence of colonizing microorgan-

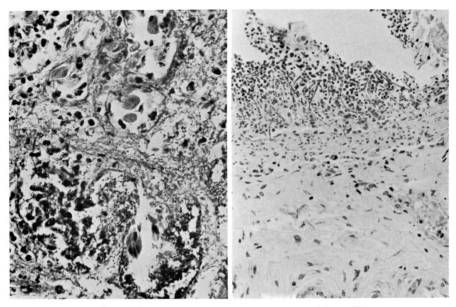

Figure 58   Figure 59

Figure 58. Photomicrograph of degenerating gastric glands at the base of a super-ficial acute stress ulcer found at gastrectomy (same patient described in Figure 57). Note the massive gram-negative bacillary colonization and invasion of the glands at the base of the ulcer. *Aerobactor* was cultured from the ulcer base. There was no evidence of hematog-enous metastatic dissemination of these bacteria to the mucosa. This suggests a lack of hyperacidity at the site of acute stress ulcer formation. Giemsa stain, 500×.

Figure 59. Monilial colonization and superficial invasion of an acute gastric stress ulcer. Giemsa stain, 300×.

isms suggest that the pathogenesis of the acute stress ulcer is probably different from the peptic ulcer.

When one assumes a possible difference in the pathogenesis of peptic and stress ulcers, the solitary, acute duodenal or pyloric ulcer seen in some burned patients may not represent a true stress ulcer but may actually be the earliest stage of an ordinary peptic ulcer that has been initiated during a period of great anxiety.

Complications of gastroduodenal ulcers. In seven of the 41 cases, there was severe gastrointestinal bleeding that was considered contributory to death. In six of the seven, duodenal ulcers were present. This pattern conforms to the general experience that acute duodenal ulcers are more apt to be of clinical significance than gastric ulcers. In three cases, perfora-tion was present (one gastric and two duodenal), and in an additional gastric ulcer, only a thin layer of serosa separated the point of deepest penetration from the peritoneal cavity.

Other Gastric Lesions

Although gastric congestion is not an infrequent finding in burn autopsies, it is not nearly so common as has been described in earlier reports. This is probably due to the fact that a much larger percentage of burned patients formerly died during the early resuscitative period, when marked visceral congestion is constantly present. Focal mucosal hemorrhages were commonly found in association with stress ulcers. Their possible pathogenetic relationship to the ulcers is not clear at this time.

Other Gastrointestinal Lesions

No other gastrointestinal lesions were found that were considered to be characteristic of patients with fatal burn injury. Acute esophagitis was commonly present, but no more often than in a series of general autopsy cases. Occasional gastrointestinal septic lesions, usually involving *Pseudomonas*, were found. In some, the pathogenesis was thought to be metastatic; in others, the question of primary focal enteritis accompanying burn wound sepsis involving *Pseudomonas* was entertained. Two patients developed acute cholecystitis. The role of the antecedent bacteremia that was seen in these patients is not certain.

Pancreas

Although acinar luminal dilatation was not infrequently found, no significant pancreatic lesions were observed in this series.

KIDNEY

Acute Renal Insufficiency (Tubular Necrosis)

Despite the adequacy of postadmission resuscitative treatment, nine patients in this series developed signs of acute renal insufficiency with significant azotemia which was progressive until death. In seven of the nine, death occurred within 5 days after burn injury. In only three of these was death directly attributable to the severe hyperkalemia present. In the remaining cases, including two deaths that occurred on the tenth and thirteenth postburn days, death was not primarily or directly attributable to the acute renal insufficiency although renal functional impairment with associated fluid electrolyte imbalance was thought to be contributory to the fatal outcome. There were, however, no patients in this series with acute renal failure who survived the early postburn resuscitative period (fifth postburn day) and subsequently succumbed to uremia in the absence of other potentially lethal factors. Thus, although acute renal tubular necrosis was not uncommonly found in this series, it was rarely a primary clinical problem. In addition to the previously mentioned cases, one patient became anuric following surgery on the tenth postburn day and died 1 day later with clinical evidence of early acute renal failure.

The pathologic term *acute renal tubular necrosis* is best not used out of the context of its clinical counterpart, *acute renal failure.* The morphologic picture of acute renal tubular necrosis (synonyms are, among others, hemoglobinuric nephrosis, lower nephron nephrosis, pigment nephrosis and shock kidney) is relatively variable, and in some cases the histologic alterations may be so subtle that the pathologist's diagnosis must rely heavily on the clinical documentation of renal functional impairment. Lucké, in his classic description of this entity, used the term lower nephron nephrosis to indicate that the light microscopic changes were fairly well confined to the distal convoluted and collecting tubules. The presence of heme casts was the most prominent finding in this and other series (Figs. 60 and 61), and interstitial cellular infiltrate (Fig. 62) with focal tubular disruption just beneath the corticomedullary junction (after the third to fifth day) was also a specific morphologic feature. On the basis of micro-dissection studies, Oliver et al. observed that tubular damage was not restricted to the distal convoluted tubules, but that it occurred in a focal distribution throughout the extent of the nephron. It is the author's experience that the wide acclaim and impact of Oliver's experimental work has

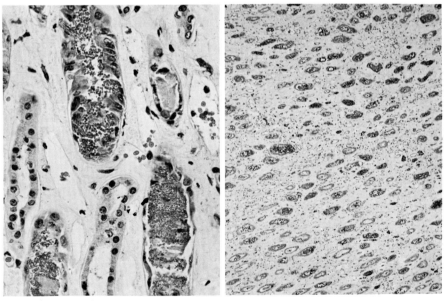

Figure 60   Figure 61

Figure 60.   Kidney. Classic heme casts in medullary collecting tubules. There is an early epithelial reaction in relation to the casts. Giemsa stain, 300×.

Figure 61.   Kidney. Low power photomicrograph of medulla showing numerous collecting tubules filled with heme casts. Patient died with anuria 19 hours after burn. No other histologic alterations were present. Giemsa stain, 60×.

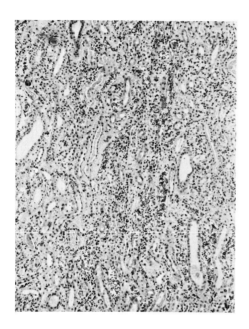

Figure 62. Kidney. Classic interstitial round cell infiltrate between medullary tubules just beneath corticomedullary junction in a case of acute renal tubular necrosis. This change is found only in cases after the third to fifth day postonset period. Giemsa stain, 60×.

led to the misconception that cases of acute renal tubular necrosis due to traumatic shock usually show appreciable *light microscopic evidence* of proximal convoluted tubule change. The absence of this latter finding all too often leads to the conclusion that the anatomic diagnosis of acute renal tubular necrosis is not justifiable.

Although the importance of Oliver's microdissection work in gaining a better understanding of the pathophysiology of acute renal tubular necrosis should not be minimized, it cannot be too strongly emphasized that the microscopic examination of the kidneys of young patients who have died with acute renal failure following burns and hemorrhagic or traumatic shock supports Lucké's light microscopic observations on the usual absence of detectable proximal tubular necrosis. It is usually the elderly patients with advanced arterial and arteriolar renal disease who show significant degrees of cortical proximal tubular necrosis. Conspicuous cortical proximal tubular necrosis as evidenced by light microscopic examination must therefore be considered as a morphologic expression of ischemia beyond that degree necessary to produce lethal tubular dysfunction in the absence of conspicuous morphologic alterations. In this series of young patients, no instance of appreciable proximal convoluted tubular necrosis was noted.

The most consistent morphologic feature of acute tubular necrosis in this burn series was the presence of heme casts in medullary tubules (Figs. 60 and 61). The presence of scattered heme casts in occasional dilated and disrupted distal convoluted tubules was not an infrequent finding in cases that had never shown clinical evidence of acute renal failure. However, when medullary localization of heme casts was found, the patient had always displayed the picture of acute renal failure. In four cases of renal insufficiency in which there were medullary heme casts, no other morphologic findings were microscopically identified save for a slight degree of proximal tubular cloudy swelling. Four additional cases in which medullary heme casts were present showed hyaline droplet formation or fatty degeneration of proximal convoluted tubules. In addition, there were some damaged distal convoluted tubules that showed dilatation, evidence of epithelial thinning or degeneration and hyaline or heme casts within their lumina. The distal convoluted tubular changes were very focal and never extensive. Deposition of pigment casts in medullary tubules is considered by some workers as possibly the most important pathogenetic factor responsible for acute tubular necrosis on the grounds that such casts cause intrarenal obstruction which leads to altered pressure effects, microcirculatory insufficiency and, finally, tubular ischemia. It is, however, pertinent to point out that in only three of the eight cases showing heme casts did the number of plugged collecting tubules appear to be significantly great. In three cases the heme casts were quite occasional, and it required some searching to find them. Finally, two cases in this series with documented acute renal insufficiency showed absolutely no identifiable heme casts in multiple sections. It is of interest that in both these cases the patients did not show severe oliguria during the day immediately following injury; however, it occurred subsequently. It is thus conceivable that the heme casts may have been flushed out of the collecting tubules during the first day. In one of the above cases, the only morphologic alteration was the presence of occasional dilated distal tubules containing hyaline casts. In the remaining case, only slight cloudy swelling was evident. The author has rarely seen other cases of early but well documented acute renal failure following traumatic shock in which there was not the slightest morphologic renal alteration at the light microscopic level, save perhaps for minimal tubular cloudy swelling. These observations on the negative findings in the kidneys of early acute renal failure are emphasized for two reasons: (1) It might appear that the basic lesion in so-called acute renal tubular necrosis may be at an ultrastructural or enzymatic level and thus not always reflected in the light microscopic examination. (2) The absence of light microscopic findings in the kidneys of patients with well documented acute renal failure should not preclude the pathologic diagnosis of acute tubular necrosis.

One other morphologic point of practical interest is the observation that postmortem tubular autolysis appears to proceed more rapidly in the ischemic kidneys of patients dying with acute renal failure. In the usual general hospital autopsy population, where the death-autopsy interval is considerably longer than those cases described in this series, autolysis of proximal convoluted tubules must not be misinterpreted as antemortem proximal convoluted tubular necrosis.

In addition to the above described cases of acute tubular necrosis, five patients in this series showed early oliguria and azotemia which completely receded. However, the patients developed evidence of progressive renal insufficiency in the last few days prior to death. In such kidneys no constant morphologic changes were present save for scattered dilated disrupted distal convoluted tubules that occasionally contained heme or hyaline casts. Varying degrees of fatty degeneration of proximal tubules were also present. These findings suggested the possibility that certain burned patients may develop some degree of initial renal tubular damage in the resuscitative period which may improve sufficiently so that their borderline renal status is not further recognized until there is additional renal insult.

Finally, one of the cases of acute renal insufficiency with progressive azotemia, uremia and hyperkalemia was of the high output type described by Sevitt.

Focal Distal Tubular Alterations

Fourteen per cent of the 88 patients in this series who never showed evidence of clinical renal insufficiency had focal distal tubular renal alterations of the type described above. Sevitt reported similar findings in his series of burn autopsies and concluded that these changes probably represent focal tubular necrosis of insufficient degree to result in renal dysfunction. This explanation appears to be a logical one.

In 25 per cent of the cases, foci of cortical interstitial cellular infiltrate with inconstantly associated interstitial edema were found in patients who had not shown evidence of renal dysfunction. The interstitial cellular population ratio of plasma cells, lymphocytes and eosinophils varied from one case to another. The changes ranged from minute interstitial foci all the way to relatively diffuse changes that warranted the diagnosis of interstitial nephritis. It was impossible to say whether the renal infiltrates were a manifestation of primary renal damage occurring during the resuscitative period or the systemic nonspecific reflection of sepsis that was so ubiquitous in this patient population.

Nephromegaly

Sixty-six per cent of the patients with fatal burn injury showed nephromegaly. Most of these kidneys weighed well over 200 gm. They were generally pale and showed no congestion. In occasional instances when autopsies had been performed almost immediately after death, gross sectioning of the kidneys resulted in transudation of serous fluid. Although microscopic examination frequently failed to reveal evidence of interstitial edema, all of the cases showing renal enlargement had shown hypoalbuminemia in the range of 2 gm. per 100 ml. or less. The nephromegaly was identical to that found in nephrotics and cirrhotics with marked hypoalbuminemia.

GENITOURINARY TRACT

Since indwelling catheters are extensively used during the resuscitative period and bacteriuria is known to ensue frequently under such circumstances, the genitourinary tract has been suspect as a potentially important portal of bacterial entry in burned patients. A prospective quantitative bacteriologic-morphologic study of the genitourinary tract in this series of initially catheterized patients revealed the following: The incidence of bacteriuria at autopsy, based on colony counts of postmortem bladder urine, was 62 per cent. Seventy-six per cent of the bacteriuric cases had indwelling catheters still in place at death, while the remainder had persistent bacteriuria subsequent to catheter removal. In 88 per cent of the abacteriuric cases, the indwelling catheter had been removed. This indicated that their presumptive bacteriuria had cleared after catheter removal.

The flora isolated from bladder urine were, in order of frequency: *Pseudomonas, Aerobacter,* Providence group, *Staphylococcus,* alpha streptococcus and *Proteus.* This bacterial population was identical to the flora colonizing the burn wounds of these patients. Of the cases with bacteriuria, 75 per cent showed morphologic changes of the urinary bladder mucosa. Seventy-five per cent of these alterations consisted of traumatic trigonal mucosal hemorrhage without associated neutrophilic or bacterial infiltration. Nineteen per cent of the bladder lesions showed slight neutrophilic infiltration although in only two instances was superficial mucosal bacterial invasion identified in relation to the observed inflammatory response.

In the abacteriuric group, focal trigonal mucosal hemorrhage due to the initial trauma of the catheter bulb was occasionally noted, but associated inflammation or bacterial invasion was always absent.

Minimal focal acute prostatitis was found in 7.7 per cent of the men in this series.

Routine quantitative bacteriologic cultures were taken from the renal pelvis after the sequence of (1) sterilization of the renal pelvic exterior wall, (2) intraluminal injection of trypticase soy broth, (3) lavage and (4) aspiration of renal pelvic contents. Quantitative cultures were also taken from cubes of renal cortex and medulla. The genitourinary tract bacteriologic findings were correlated with associated bladder and renal lesions as well as with quantitative bacteriologic visceral and heart blood findings. The detailed results of these correlations have been previously reported.

The incidence of acute pyelonephritis in this series was 13 per cent. The focal interstitial and glomerular localization of the lesions was indicative of a hematogenous pathogenesis (Fig. 63). These lesions were identical to those noted in hematogenous pyelonephritis which developed as the result of experimental burn wound sepsis in rats. With the exception of one case, the hematogenous pyelonephritic lesions were very sparsely distributed and therefore inconsequential. Kidneys with the typical morpho-

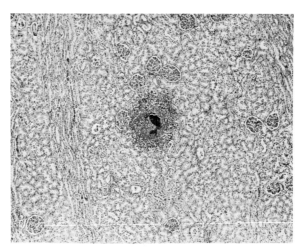

Figure 63. Kidney. Hematogenous pyelonephritis. There is a small microabscess with a colony of staphylococci within the center. The lesions were small, sparsely scattered and inconsequential. Giemsa stain, 30×.

logic characteristics of pyelitis or ascending pyelonephritis were not observed in this series.

Renal pelvic bacteriuria, when found, was highly correlated with the presence of high bacterial counts of the same flora in the renal parenchyma, thus suggesting its relationship to a hematogenous rather than an ascending process.

Thus, in the absence of discernible predisposing functional or anatomic abnormalities of the genitourinary tract in this antibiotic-treated group of relatively young patients, urinary tract infection was infrequent and mild despite the presence of repeated episodes of bacteremia and persistent bacteriuria. As previously noted, the observed focal pyelonephritis was thought to be a reflection of hematogenous bacterial dissemination from infected burn wounds.

Contrariwise, the author has observed massive ascending pyelonephritis in elderly patients at the Boston City Hospital who have sustained fatal burn injury. Thus, in elderly patients who have antecedent anatomic or functional disorders of the genitourinary tract, the potential hazard of the indwelling catheter and the possibility of ascending infection cannot be dismissed lightly.

ADRENALS

The adrenal glands were usually enlarged. Their combined weight was not infrequently 30 to 36 gm. Despite their general increase in size, they usually showed lipid depletion. Unfortunately, no correlation between such anatomic features and physiologic adrenocortical activity could be made. However, the prolonged and significant elevation of urine and blood steroid levels following thermal burn injury is well established.

The most common pathologic finding was marked sinusoidal congestion at the junction of the cortex and medulla. This was seen in 25 per cent of the cases. Generalized adrenal congestion was much less commonly found. In two instances, the marked corticomedullary congestion was associated with focal mild hemorrhage. In rare cases in which the autopsy was performed more than 10 hours post mortem, the marked congestion

Figure 64

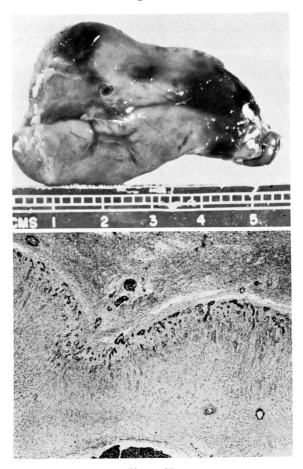

Figure 65

Figure 64. Focal gross cortical hemorrhagic necrosis of the adrenal gland in a child dying with gram-negative sepsis. (See Fig. 65.)

Figure 65. Low power photomicrograph of adrenal gland depicted in Figure 64 shows massive PTAH-positive fibrin deposits within subcapsular sinusoids of the cortical glomerulosa. The changes morphologically suggest a generalized Shwartzman type of reaction. 30×.

in this region, in association with autolysis, produced a picture of what superficially resembled hemorrhage, although close scrutiny indicated that the sinusoidal walls were still intact. Although significant adrenal medullary hemorrhage has been seen occasionally in fatal burn injury, it was not found in this series.

Four cases of bilateral gross cortical hemorrhagic necrosis were observed. In three the changes were focal (Fig. 64), and in one there was massive involvement. All were histologically distinctive and identical with regard to the presence of numerous fibrin thrombi in the sinusoids of the cortical glomerulosa (Fig. 65). The changes were morphologically suggestive of a generalized Shwartzman-type reaction. In one of the cases, fibrin thrombi with associated necrosis were found in other viscera. All four patients had fulminant gram-negative sepsis, and therefore the possibility of a generalized Shwartzman reaction on an endotoxemic basis was considered as an etiologic factor.

Pseudotubular formation in the zona glomerulosa and zona fasciculata has been described by Rich as an indication of sepsis. Sevitt has indicated that such changes are attributable to adrenocortical hyperactivity in the face of hyperemia and edema. Despite the extremely high incidence of sepsis and the documented elevated blood and urine levels of adrenocorticoids in many of these patients, pseudotubular formation was found in only 18 per cent of the cases, and in most of these, the changes were minimal.

CENTRAL NERVOUS SYSTEM

Despite the fact that many patients were in an obtundent or comatose state for varying periods of time prior to death, both gross and histologic examination of the brain generally revealed no abnormalities. In only three of the 88 cases was there gross or microscopic evidence of edema. In two cases, degeneration of cerebellar Purkinje cells was found. One elderly man died with encephalomalacia that was attributed to severe cerebral arteriosclerosis.

Encephalopathy in children was rarely diagnosed clinically, but no C.N.S. findings were present at autopsy. Routine sections taken through thalamus and hypothalamus in patients who had shown profound hypothermia revealed no identifiable histologic abnormality. In cases of staphylococcal burn wound sepsis, microscopic metastatic cerebral abscesses were present. Hematogenous meningitis was rarely found.

INFECTED CUTDOWN SITES

No less than 25 per cent of the patients in this series showed evidence of bacterial invasion of cutdown sites. Venous cutdowns were frequently performed through burn wounds in the lower extremities. The extremely high incidence of septic embolization from infected cutdown sites has been previously discussed.

CHANGES IN BONE MARROW

The marrow of patients dying with burn wound sepsis involving *Pseudomonas* showed myeloid hyperplasia with maturation arrest of the neutrophilic series. This finding was associated with peripheral leukopenia. Otherwise, no specific alteration except marrow hyperplasia in response to infection was noted in this series.

REFERENCES

Altemeier, W.: Discussion of paper by Sandusky, W. R.: Pseudomonas infections. *Ann. Surg.* **153**:996, 1961.

Altemeier, W. A., and MacMillan, B. G.: The dynamics of infection in burns. *In* Artz, C. P. (ed.): *Research in Burns.* Philadelphia, F. A. Davis Company, 1962, p. 203.

Birke, G., Liljedahl, S.-O., and Linderholm, H.: Studies on burns. V. Clinical and patho-physiological aspects on circulation and respiration. *Acta chir. scandinav.* **116**:370, 1958.

Cotran, R. S., and Majno, G: A light and electron microscopic analysis of vascular injury. *Ann. New York Acad. Sc.* **116**:750, 1964.

Curling, T. B.: On acute ulceration of the duodenum in cases of burns. *Med. Chir. Trans. London* **25**:260, 1842.

Elder, J. M., and Miles, A. A.: The action of lethal toxins of gas-gangrene clostridia on capillary permeability. *J. Path. & Bact.* **74**:133, 1957.

Epstein, B. S., Hardy, D. L., Harrison, H. N., Teplitz, C., Villarreal, Y., and Mason, A. D., Jr.: Hypoxemia in the burned patient: a clinical-pathologic study. *Ann. Surg.* **158**:924, 1963.

Epstein, B. S., Rose, L. R., Teplitz, C., and Moncrief, J. A.: Experiences with low tracheostomy in the burned patient. *J.A.M.A.* **183**:966, 1963.

Finland, M.: Respiratory injuries in man resulting from severe burns. National Research Council, Symposium on Burns, 1950, pp. 91–95.

Friesen, S. R.: The genesis of gastroduodenal ulcer following burns. An experimental study. *Surgery* **28**:123, 1950.

Lucké, B.: Lower nephron nephrosis. The renal lesions of the crush syndrome, of burns, transfusions, and other conditions affecting the lower segments of the nephrons. *Mil. Surgeon* **99**:371, 1943.

Mason, A. D., Jr., Alexander, J. W., and Teschan, P. E.: Studies in acute renal failure. I. Development of a reproducible lesion in experimental animals. *J. S. Res.* **3**:430, 1963.

Mason, A. D., Jr., Teschan, P. E., and Muirhead, E. E.: Studies in acute renal failure. III. Renal histologic alterations in acute renal failure in the rat. *J. S. Res.* **3**:450, 1963.

Mallory, T. B., and Brinckley, W. J.: Management of the Cocoanut Grove burns at the Massachusetts General Hospital: pathology with special reference to pulmonary lesions. *Ann. Surg.* **117**:465, 1943.

Moncrief, J. A., Switzer, W. E., and Teplitz, C.: Curling's ulcer. *J. Trauma* **4**:481, 1964.

Moncrief, J. A., and Teplitz, C.: Changing concepts in burn sepsis. *J. Trauma* **4**:233, 1964.

Moritz, A. R., Henriques, R. C., and McLean, R.: The effects of inhaled heat on the air passages and lungs. *Am. J. Path.* **21**:311, 1945.

Nicoloff, D. M., Peter, E. T., Leonard, A. S., and Wangensteen, O. H.: Catecholamines in ulcer provocation. Their possible role in stress ulcer formation. *J.A.M.A.* **191**:383, 1965.

Oliver, J., MacDowell, M., and Tracy, A.: The pathogenesis of acute renal failure associated with traumatic and toxic injury. Renal ischemic, nephrotoxic damage and ischemic syndrome. *J. Clin. Invest.* **30**:1307, 1951.

Order, S. E., Mason, A. D., Jr., Walker, H. L., Lindberg, R. B., Switzer, W. E., and Moncrief, J. A.: The pathogenesis of second and third degree burns and conversion to full thickness injury. *Surg. Gynec. & Obst.* **120**:983, 1965.

Phillips, A. W., and Cope, O.: Burn therapy. II. The revelation of respiratory tract damage as a principal killer of the burned patient. *Ann. Surg.* **155**:1, 1962.

Phillips, A. W., and Cope, O.: Burn therapy. III. Beware the facial burn. *Ann. Surg.* **156**: 759, 1962.

Rabin, E. R., Graber, C. D., Vogel, E. H., Jr., Finkelstein, R. A., and Tumbusch, W. A.: Fatal pseudomonas infection in burned patients. A clinical, bacteriologic and anatomic study. *New England J. Med.* **265**:1225, 1961.

Rabin, E. R., Lundberg, G. D., and Mitchell, E. T.: Mucormycosis in severely burned patients. *New England J. Med.* **264**:1286, 1961.

Report of an Ad Hoc Panel of the Committee on Pathology of the National Research Council on Forty-One Fatal Burn Injuries. Division of Medical Sciences, National Academy of Sciences–National Research Council, Washington 25, D. C.

Sevitt, S.: *Burns — Pathology and Therapeutic Applications.* London, Butterworth & Co., Ltd., 1957.

Sochor, F. M., and Mallory, G. K.: Lung lesions in patients dying of burns. *A.M.A. Arch. Path.* **75**:303, 1963.

Spiro, H. M., and Milles, S. S.: Clinical and physiologic implications of the steroid-induced peptic ulcer. *New England J. Med.* **263**:286, 1960.

Stark, R. B.: Plastic surgery and burns. *Surg. Gynec. & Obst.* **120**:285, 1965.

Stone, H. H., Martin, J. D., Jr., Huger, W. E., and Kolb, L.: Gentamicin sulfate in the treatment of pseudomonas sepsis in burns. *Surg. Gynec. & Obst.* **120**:351, 1965.

Teplitz, C.: Observations on the normal genitourinary tract in bacteriuria and bacteremia. A quantitative bacteriologic and anatomic autopsy study on young fatally burned cases. *U.S. Army Surgical Research Unit Res. Rep.* **288**:43, 1963.

Teplitz, C.: Pathogenesis of pseudomonas vasculitis and septic lesions. *A.M.A. Arch. Path.* **80**:297, 1965.

Teplitz, C., and Davis, D.: Modified buffered Giemsa method: a one step general cytological and bacterial tissue section stain. *U.S. Army Surgical Research Unit Res. Rep.* **288**:54, 1963.

Teplitz, C., Davis, D., Mason, A. D., Jr., and Moncrief, J. A.: Pseudomonas burn wound sepsis. I. Pathogenesis of experimental pseudomonas burn wound sepsis. *J. S. Res.* **4**:200, 1964.

Teplitz, C., Davis, D., Walker, H. L., Raulston, G. L., Mason, A. D., and Moncrief, J. A.: Pseudomonas burn wound sepsis, II. Hematogenous infection at the junction of the burn wound and the unburned hypodermis. *J. S. Res.* **4**:217, 1964.

Teplitz, C., Epstein, B. S., Rose, L. R., and Moncrief, J. A.: Necrotizing tracheitis induced by tracheostomy tube. *A.M.A. Arch. Path.* **77**:14, 1964.

Teplitz, C., Epstein, B. S., Rose, L. R., Switzer, W. E., and Moncrief, J. A.: Pathology of low tracheostomy in children. *Am. J. Clin. Path.* **42**:58, 1964.

Teplitz, C., Raulston, G. L., Walker, H. L., Mason, A. D., and Moncrief, J. A.: Spontaneous hematogenous pseudomonas pyelonephritis in rats. *J. Infect. Dis.* **114**:75, 1964.

Chapter
Three

GENERAL
IMMEDIATE CARE

The care of the burned patient begins at the time of the accident and continues until he has been given maximum rehabilitation so that he is returned to society as a useful citizen and member of his family. Sometimes therapy continues several years after the injury. Early steps in treatment are most important because they frequently are quite significant in the ultimate outcome.

FIRST AID

The first aim in management should be to put out the fire. A person whose clothing is on fire should not run because this only fans the flames. He should not remain standing, because this position may cause him to inhale the flames or cause the hair to be ignited. Falling to the floor and rolling in a blanket or a rug may help put out the fire. Smothering the flames in any expeditious manner is desirable. Coats, towels, or bed clothing may be useful. If no covering material is available, a burned person should lie down and roll over slowly. Water is an effective and comfortable agent for putting out the fire. Dirt and sand should not be used unless nothing else is available. When a small burn on the hand or arm occurs in the kitchen, the affected part may be placed under the cold water tap.

Application of towels soaked in ice water brings almost immediate pain relief; this amount of cold may have some value in arresting the effect of heat on the tissues. The application of cold by any convenient method immediately after the burn is the best known first aid measure.

The wound should be covered as soon as feasible. This minimizes contamination and inhibits pain by preventing air from coming in contact with the injured surface. A clean sheet makes an excellent emergency dressing. Medicaments or home remedies should not be applied. Any burn of more than 2 per cent of the body surface should be seen by a physician. Stimulants must not be used. Burned patients are usually frightened and need to be reassured. Oral intake is avoided.

Chemical burns caused by acid or alkali should be washed immediately with large quantities of water to remove the injurious agent. One should not waste time looking for a specific antidote. All clothing must be removed. If a large quantity of a chemical burning agent has come in contact with the skin, the patient should get into a bathtub or under a shower immediately. The patient suffering from respiratory arrest due to smoke inhalation should receive artificial respiration by positive pressure. The mouth-to-mouth technique should be used.

If the wound is minor it should be cleansed with soap and water and bandaged with some type of greased gauze or anesthetic ointment. Patients with larger burns or burns around critical areas such as the face and hands should be taken to a physician's office or a hospital emergency room. There is absolutely no need to rush. The patient may be taken to the physician at a normal and reasonable speed.

APPRAISAL OF THE SERIOUSNESS
OF A BURN INJURY

It is difficult to make an accurate appraisal of the relative magnitude of different types of mechanical injuries. On the other hand, the severity of the burn injury can be assessed satisfactorily because it depends on only two principal factors—percentage of body surface burned and depth of burn. Additional factors that determine the seriousness of a burn include its location, the age and physical condition of the patient, preexistent disease and the presence of concomitant injury.

Estimate of Percentage of Body Surface Burned

The extent of a burn is usually expressed as a percentage of the total area of body surface that is injured. In 1924, Berkow presented data concerning percentage of surface areas of various parts of the body. Lund and Browder found that Berkow's tables were not applicable to all age groups. They determined the changes in percentage of body surface of various parts that occur during different stages of development from infancy through childhood. The area of the head makes up a relatively large proportion of the total skin area of infants as compared with adults. This disproportion is counterbalanced in infants by the smaller proportionate area of the thighs and legs. The proportion of skin of all other parts is essentially the same for all age groups (Table 8).

The most accurate method for determining percentage of body surface burned is to map out the areas of injury on Lund and Browder charts (Fig. 66). If these charts are not immediately available for an initial estimate, a rapid method of estimating percentage of body surface burned is the use of the Rule of Nines. Information obtained by this simplified rule is sufficiently accurate for clinical purposes. According to the Rule of Nines,

Table 8.   CONTRIBUTION OF VARIOUS BODY AREAS TO TOTAL BODY SURFACE AT DIFFERENT AGES, BY PER CENT*

AREA	BIRTH	1 YEAR	5 YEARS	10 YEARS	15 YEARS	ADULT
Head	19	17	13	11	9	7
Neck	2	2	2	2	2	2
Anterior trunk	13	13	13	13	13	13
Posterior trunk	13	13	13	13	13	13
Buttocks	5	5	5	5	5	5
Genitalia	1	1	1	1	1	1
Upper arms	8	8	8	8	8	8
Forearms	6	6	6	6	6	6
Hands	5	5	5	5	5	5
Thighs	11	13	16	17	18	19
Legs	10	10	11	12	13	14
Feet	7	7	7	7	7	7

*Adapted from Lund and Browder.

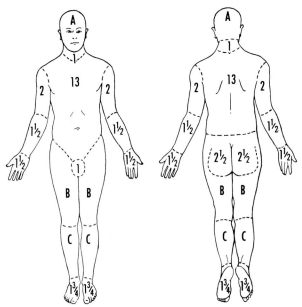

Relative Percentage of Areas Affected by Growth

	Age in Years					
	0	1	5	10	15	Adult
A—½ of head	9½	8½	6½	5½	4½	3½
B—½ of one thigh	2¾	3¼	4	4¼	4½	4¾
C—½ of one leg	2½	2½	2¾	3	3¼	3½

Figure 66.   Lund and Browder charts. These charts permit a rather accurate method for determining percentage of body surface involved.

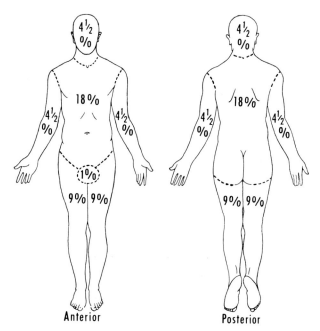

Figure 67. Rule of Nines. A rapid method of estimating percentage of body surface involved.

first devised by E. J. Pulaski and C. W. Tennison, the body surface is divided into areas representing 9 per cent or multiples of 9 per cent: the head and neck 9 per cent; anterior trunk 2 × 9, or 18 per cent; posterior trunk 18 per cent; each lower extremity 18 per cent; each upper extremity 9 per cent; and the perineum 1 per cent (Fig. 67). The Rule of Nines has been widely accepted as a useful guide in estimating percentage of body surface burned. An area equivalent to one side of the hand is about 1 per cent of the body surface.

The extent of a burn is only rarely underestimated. Overestimation is common and frequently results in excessive fluid administration.

Depth of Burn

The seriousness of the injury depends not only upon the percentage of the body surface involved but also upon the volume of tissue destroyed. The depth of burn, therefore, is very important. Obviously, full-thickness burns are more serious than partial-thickness burns. When the injury penetrates the deeper tissues such as muscle and bone, as is so frequent in electrical burns, the seriousness of the injury is much greater.

Although the most experienced observers are often mistaken in their initial judgment of the depth of a burn in a particular area, a fairly accurate over-all estimate of the predominance of one or the other type of injury can be made in most cases. It is difficult to assess the exact relation of sever-

Each per cent of third-degree burn	1 Point
Each per cent of second-degree burn	1/2 Point

Example:

A patient with 20 per cent third-degree plus 20 per cent second-degree burn

Burn	Index
Third-degree - 20%	20
Second-degree - 20%	10
Burn index	30

Figure 68.   The burn index (Surgical Research Unit).

ity of second-degree burn to third-degree burn. Bull and Squire reviewed the case records of 794 patients treated during the years 1945 through 1947 at the Birmingham Accident Hospital in Birmingham, England. The trend of mortality was found to be best expressed in terms of third-degree burn plus one-fourth of the second-degree burn. Thus, area for area, they believed that a deep burn seemed to be four times as serious as a superficial burn. In a study of 323 burned patients who were hospitalized at the Brooke Army Medical Center, Schwartz and co-workers showed that the best correlation between case fatality rate and survival time was obtained when the percentage of second-degree injury was given one-half the weight, area for area, of the percentage of third-degree injury. These authors suggested a burn index based on assessment of one point for each per cent of third-degree injury and one-half point for each per cent of second-degree injury. In a mixed burn of 20 per cent second-degree and 20 per cent third-degree, the index is 20 plus one-half of 20 for a total of 30 (Fig. 68). Such a refinement may be of value in the study of well documented cases. Because the exact diagnosis of burn depth is often difficult and it is subject to revision during the healing stages, most clinicians wisely use the sum of second- and third-degree injury in determining the percentage of burn.

Age of the Patient

The age of the patient plays a very important role in estimating the severity of the injury. Although a 20 per cent third-degree burn in a 60-year-old individual usually results in death, a younger person with the same lesion may be expected to recover without unusual complications in most cases. In burns involving up to 30 per cent of the body surface in patients under the age of 50, the mortality is quite low. As the extent of the body surface involvement increases beyond 30 per cent, the mortality rises in all age groups. But, as the age increases beyond 50, the mortality rises even in burns of less than 30 per cent. In elderly individuals even small third-degree burns have a high mortality. It seems that infants also tolerate burns poorly and the mortality for those younger than one year is quite high. (See Prognosis in Burns, p. 99)

Anatomic Location of Burns

In some parts of the body, burns result in such crippling deformities that they must be regarded as serious even though they are of small extent. Burns in certain areas result in loss of function and disfigurement. The critical anatomic areas are the face, hands, feet, external genitalia, neck and joint surfaces. Respiratory tract injury may be fatal regardless of the amount of surface area involved.

Burns of the upper part of the body, when they include the face and neck, are always much more serious than a similar percentage burn in other areas. The clinician must always beware the patient who has, in addition to other injuries, a deep facial burn. The mortality in such instances is always higher than expected. Sometimes such patients have inhaled noxious agents and have pulmonary damage in addition to the burn.

General Physical Condition of the Patient and Concomitant Injuries

Patients who have pre-existing renal, cardiovascular or pulmonary disease cannot tolerate burns of even moderate extent. In patients with occlusive vascular disease, burns of the lower extremities, especially the feet, are particularly serious. Gangrene requiring amputation is not uncommon after a burn of the foot and lower legs in a patient with peripheral arteriosclerosis of the lower extremities. Associated injuries, such as fractures, soft tissue trauma, intracranial, intrathoracic and intra-abdominal injury, compound the burn insult in accordance with their severity.

DISPOSITION OF BURNED PATIENTS

Any physician who is called upon to treat an open fracture of the femur is aware of the immediate necessity of general supportive care of the patient and transportation to a well equipped hospital that has an experienced staff to care for such an injury. Similar management is required for a severe burn. All too often a physician who sees a patient with a burn of 25 per cent of the body surface believes that he can take care of the patient until it is time for grafting and then refer him to a plastic surgeon. This postponed referral is deplorable. Inadequate management during the initial period is followed by infection, chronic anemia, weight loss, wounds that are not debrided and heaping granulations. As a result, when the patient is referred to the plastic surgeon he is frightened, in chronic pain and demoralized.

CRITICAL BURNS

2° Burns of over 30 %

3° Burns of face, hands, feet or over 10 %

Burns complicated by:

Respiratory tract injury

Major soft tissue injury

Fractures

Electrical burns

General Hospital

MODERATE BURNS

2° of 15 - 30 per cent

3° of less than 10 per cent,

except hands, face,

feet

Community Hospital

MINOR BURNS

2° of less than 15 per cent

3° of less than 2 per cent

Figure 69. An outline for sorting or disposition of burned patients.

It is extremely important to realize that disposition of a burned patient depends on the appraisal of the severity of injury. Three groups of patients may be distinguished: (1) those with critical burns, who must be referred to a well equipped general hospital that has a surgeon experienced in burn care, (2) those with moderate burns, who may be treated in a small community hospital, and (3) those with minor burns, who may be treated on an outpatient basis. (Fig. 69).

Critical Burns

Critical burns include (1) burns complicated by respiratory tract injury, (2) partial-thickness burns of more than 30 per cent of the body

surface, (3) full-thickness burns of more than 10 per cent of the body surface, and burns of the face, hands, feet or genitalia, (4) burns complicated
by fractures or major soft tissue injury, (5) electrical burns and (6) deep
acid burns. In addition, the age and the general physical condition of the
patient may indicate that burns of smaller extent should be considered
critical. In all of these cases, a patient must be sent promptly to an institution at which proper treatment can be given.

Moderate Burns

Moderate burns include (1) partial-thickness burns of 15 to 30 per
cent of the body surface and (2) full-thickness burns of less than 10 per
cent of the body surface, provided that the hands, face, feet or genitalia
are not involved.

Minor Burns

Minor burns include (1) partial-thickness burns of less than 15 per
cent of the body surface and (2) full-thickness burns of less than 2 per cent
of the body surface that may be treated on an outpatient basis until the
patient needs to be hospitalized for minor grafting. Small burns in a child
may be treated in a small community hospital for a few days until the
patient's condition becomes stabilized. The child may then be sent home if
the family can provide intelligent care.

TRANSPORTATION OF BURNED PATIENTS

Transportation from the scene of the accident to a physician's office
or a hospital should be conducted in an orderly and comfortable manner.
It is not necessary to remove all of the patient's burned clothing. If the
hands are burned, rings should be removed. Burned shoes or constricting
clothing should be taken off. The area of injury should be covered with a
clean sheet or bandage. It is unnecessary to rush the patient to the hospital;
in fact, speeding in an automobile or ambulance could result in a greater
injury.

Most burn victims are able to carry on a moderate amount of activity
for the first hour or two after the accident. It is not unusual for a person
with one-third of his body surface burned to drive a car 15 or 20 miles for
help. Because the burn victim remains in relatively good condition for
some time after the accident, the problem of transportation from the scene
of the injury to a hospital is not difficult. If it is a short distance, this can
frequently be accomplished in an automobile. No stimulants or liquids
should be given by mouth. It is important to make sure that the patient
does not have other complicating injuries.

Chemical burns are washed with large quantities of water immediately
after injury and before transportation. All clothing is removed if it is an

extensive chemical burn, and the patient is given a shower before he is taken to the hospital.

When the burn is extensive (involving more than one-third of the body surface) a telephone call should be made to the emergency department of the hospital to notify the personnel that a burned patient is on the way.

The real problems in transportation become evident when a burned patient must be transported from a local physician's office or small community hospital to a larger facility some distance away. The movement over a long distance of a patient with moderately severe burns requires thought and preparation. *It is the referring physician's responsibility to see that the patient arrives at his destination in good condition.* The receiving hospital should be called and arrangements made for admission. The type of transportation, the approximate time of arrival, information concerning those who are to accompany the patient and the medical details of the injury should be given. Because burned patients require large quantities of blood, the referring physician should make every effort to encourage the family to provide blood donors to the receiving hospital.

It is a common misconception to think that a recently burned patient is too sick to be moved. In fact, his chances for survival are much better if he is transported early to an institution having the necessary facilities and trained personnel for definitive care. The best time for transportation is during the first 48 hours after injury. Fluid losses can usually be anticipated. If these are replaced by appropriate therapy as they are lost, the patient usually remains in relatively good condition for the first 24 hours.

All patients are more comfortable after a dressing has been applied. A large, bulky dressing should be applied prior to transport. Morphine given intravenously allays fear and apprehension and alleviates pain. If the transportation will require more than an hour, intravenous fluids should be started so that resuscitative therapy can be administered before and during transportation. The preferred solutions are lactated Ringer's, dextran and plasma. The patient is given nothing by mouth. If movement to the receiving facility will require 3 hours or more, a urinary catheter is inserted. It is often wise to insert a nasogastric tube in patients with more than 30 per cent burn or with deep burns of the face and neck when transportation will take several hours. Unless this precaution is taken, vomiting and aspiration may occur.

Occasionally a tracheostomy is necessary if there has been marked inhalation of smoke or if there is appreciable edema of the neck that might interfere with respiration. Most burned patients, however, can be moved in the first several hours after injury without the aid of a tracheostomy. It is always wise to send a detailed and accurate history of the accident and the type of medication and time at which it was administered. Transportation may be successfully accomplished by car, ambulance or airplane. In some instances, a nurse or physician should accompany the patient. Burned patients tolerate movement by airplane very well, and this is a most expeditious method when long distance is involved.

Table 9.   Bull and Fisher's Grid of Approximate Probabilities for Various Combinations of Age and Area*

PER CENT OF BODY AREA BURNED	AGE (YEARS)																
	0–4	5–9	10–14	15–19	20–24	25–29	30–34	35–39	40–44	45–49	50–54	55–59	60–64	65–69	70–74	75–79	80–84
78 or more	1	1	1	1	1	1	1	1	1	1	1	1	1	1	1	1	1
73–77	.9	.9	.9	.9	.9	.9	1	1	1	1	1	1	1	1	1	1	1
68–72	.9	.9	.9	.9	.9	.9	.9	1	1	1	1	1	1	1	1	1	1
63–67	.8	.8	.8	.9	.9	.9	.9	.9	1	1	1	1	1	1	1	1	1
58–62	.7	.7	.7	.8	.8	.8	.8	.9	.9	1	1	1	1	1	1	1	1
53–57	.6	.6	.6	.7	.7	.7	.8	.8	.9	1	1	1	1	1	1	1	1
48–52	.5	.5	.5	.6	.6	.6	.7	.8	.8	.9	1	1	1	1	1	1	1
43–47	.4	.4	.4	.5	.5	.5	.6	.7	.7	.8	.9	1	1	1	1	1	1
38–42	.3	.3	.3	.4	.4	.4	.5	.6	.6	.7	.9	.9	1	1	1	1	1
33–37	.2	.2	.2	.3	.3	.3	.4	.5	.5	.6	.8	.9	.9	1	1	1	1
28–32	.1	.1	.1	.2	.2	.2	.3	.4	.4	.5	.6	.8	.9	1	1	1	1
23–27	.1	.1	.1	.1	.1	.1	.2	.3	.3	.4	.4	.6	.8	.9	1	1	1
18–22	0	0	0	0	0	0	.1	.2	.2	.3	.3	.4	.6	.8	.9	1	1
13–17	0	0	0	0	0	0	0	.1	.1	.2	.2	.3	.4	.6	.7	.8	.9
8–12	0	0	0	0	0	0	0	0	0	.1	.1	.1	.2	.4	.5	.6	.7
3–7	0	0	0	0	0	0	0	0	0	0	0	0	.1	.2	.3	.4	.5
0–2	0	0	0	0	0	0	0	0	0	0	0	0	0	.1	.1	.2	.3

*The figures are proportional mortalities approximated to a single decimal point. Thus, 0.5 is equivalent to 50 per cent mortality, and 1.0 means most probably a death.

PROGNOSIS IN BURNS

It is extremely difficult to determine prognosis with any degree of accuracy in any specific burn. Mortality increases with the severity of burn and with advancing age. At one time, few patients survived burns involving more than one-third of their body surface, but this is no longer true. For example, with modern treatment many patients with burns involving up to 50 to 60 per cent of the body surface survive, and the outlook for those more extensively burned is not entirely hopeless. The prognosis of the burned patient should be guarded if the percentage of second- and third-degree burn is more than 40. It may be several days or weeks before the ultimate outcome can be predicted. Frequently, extensively burned patients survive the initial few weeks after the injury, only to succumb later to complications. In severe injuries, prediction of survival should be withheld until approximately 30 days after the burn.

The use of probit analysis in consideration of burn mortality was introduced in 1949 by Bull and Squire of Birmingham, England. Bull and Fisher have updated the Birmingham information and prepared a grid of approximate mortality probabilities for various combinations of age and body surface area (Table 9). Using similar computation of probit analysis, two other investigators have made excellent reports on burn mortality in recent years. Barnes summarized the mortality observed at the Massachusetts General Hospital in 785 burned patients over a 15-year period. Pruitt and others in 1964 published an excellent study of 1100 burns treated at the Surgical Research Unit at the Brooke Army Medical Center from 1950 to 1960.

In preparing these analyses the authors took into consideration the percentage of body surface burned and age of the patient. From the data in this series it is possible to obtain the LA_{50} (that percentage body surface

Table 10. SUMMARY OF LA_{50} BY VARIOUS BURN SERIES*

AUTHOR	CHILDREN	ADULTS	ELDERLY
Bull and Fisher Birmingham Accident Hospital 1942–1952 2807 patients	0 to 14 years, 49	15 to 44 years, 46 45 to 64 years, 27	65 and over, 10
Barnes Massachusetts General Hospital 1939–1954 785 patients	0 to 15 years, 39	16 to 35 years, 65 36 to 55 years, 39	56 and over, 26
Pruitt et al. Surgical Research Unit 1950–1960 1100 patients	0 to 14 years, 48.5	15 to 49 years, 55.8	50 and over, 29

*LA_{50} is that percentage of body surface area of second- and third-degree burn which will result in the death of 50 per cent of those incurring such injury.

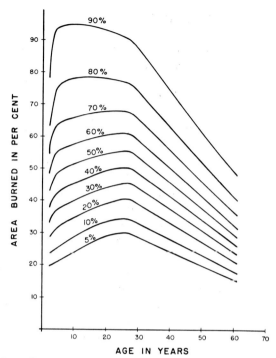

Figure 70. Mortality contours on 1100 burns treated at the U. S. Army Surgical Research Unit, 1950–60. (After Pruitt et al.: Mortality in 1,100 consecutive burns treated at a burns unit. Ann. Surg. **159**: 396, 1964.)

area of second- and third-degree burn which resulted in the death of 50 per cent of those incurring that injury) according to various age groups. A summary of the findings of these three authors is shown in Table 10. Pruitt constructed a mortality contour plot from the data in their series for ease in approximating expected mortality. This graphic illustration of mortality trends according to age and per cent of burn is reproduced in Figure 70.

INITIAL HOSPITAL PROCEDURES

The emergency room care of the patient with a major burn should be the orderly execution of several established routine procedures (Table 11). If two or more physicians can attend the patient, immediate care may be given with greater dispatch. One physician can plan and direct while the other performs technical procedures. Attendants should put on caps and masks. The patient's clothing should be removed as soon as he is admitted and all burned areas completely exposed for evaluation.

The place of initial care depends upon the facilities of the institution. In some hospitals a well equipped dressing room is the preferred place

Table 11. OUTLINE OF IMMEDIATE HOSPITAL PROCEDURES

 1. Obtain a history.
 2. Give intravenous morphine.
 3. Determine need for tracheostomy.
 4. Perform initial venipuncture.
 5. Insert indwelling urinary catheter.
 6. Establish a reliable intravenous portal.
 7. Initiate local care.
 8. Estimate extent of injury; weigh and photograph patient.
 9. Give tetanus prophylaxis.
10. Give antibiotics when indicated.
11. Plan replacement therapy.
12. Consider special nurses, critical list and blood donors; and make worksheet.

for initial care; in others, the emergency room or the operating room, according to the severity of the injury, is preferred. Every hospital should be organized so that there is one good place for the initial care of burns. This area should have the necessary facilities and equipment for cleansing, dressing, performing a cutdown, initiating fluid therapy and doing a tracheotomy if indicated.

History

Although a complete history need not be obtained at the time of initial evaluation, certain essential information is required. This should include how, when and where the accident occurred, any complaints the patient has mentioned that would indicate injuries other than the burn, and his age. Information should be obtained regarding any allergies to drugs, his status of tetanus immunization and whether he is currently receiving any medication, particularly insulin, digitalis, diphenylhydantoin, sedatives, narcotics, reserpine or steroids. It is important to know the general status of health prior to the injury. Does the patient have diabetes or cardiovascular, renal or pulmonary disease? What other persons were involved in the accident?

Sedation

Although pain is not a prominent feature of extensive deep burns, a small dose of morphine is beneficial when given intravenously. Morphine eliminates apprehension, makes the patient more comfortable and alleviates the pain associated with cleansing of the burn wound. Sedation in burns must be given intravenously. If a narcotic is given subcutaneously, it is usually not absorbed until the circulatory deficiency is corrected. All too often, patients receive morphine subcutaneously and the drug gives no particular relief. A second and larger dose is given subcutaneously but again without beneficial effect. After replacement therapy has been accomplished, the large load of morphine that was deposited in the subcutaneous tissue is absorbed. As a result, the patient's vital functions become depressed and breathing is slow; the patient may become cyanotic and show other signs of morphine toxicity. In adults, a dose of 8 to 10 mg. of morphine is usually adequate. A small dose of codeine or morphine may be used for children. A good rule of thumb for dosage of morphine in children is 1 mg. for each 10 lb. of body weight. The morphine should be diluted in 3 to 5 ml. of saline and injected intravenously over a period of 1 or 2 minutes.

After the first 24 hours, a narcotic may not be necessary for sedation. A short acting barbiturate is frequently satisfactory to allay apprehension and to provide rest. Two or three small doses of a narcotic during the first 24 hours are not toxic and frequently make the patient more comfortable. Extensively burned patients may have considerable discomfort, and a few doses of a narcotic may be required every day for the first week. Large and frequent doses of a narcotic should be avoided, but an adequate amount of medication should be administered to assure the patient's comfort. Narcotics should be discouraged after the first few days. They cause constipation and hinder the return of appetite. Burned patients become emotionally addicted to a narcotic unless great care is taken to prevent it. After the first week, a narcotic may be required at the time of operative procedures but not at other times. Short acting barbiturates and promazine are usually adequate.

Extreme restlessness in the first few hours after injury is not an indication for a narcotic. Hypovolemia is the most common cause of restlessness and disorientation in the acutely burned patient. If the patient is in peripheral circulatory collapse, cerebral hypoxia leads to extreme uncooperativeness and even mania. It is not uncommon to see an uncontrollable patient become quite docile and cooperative as soon as the hypovolemia is corrected by the appropriate replacement therapy.

A burned patient rests better in a room in which the temperature is 70 to 75° F. In cooler rooms he may feel quite chilly and uncomfortable.

Tracheostomy

A mechanically clear airway must be assured from the beginning. The need for a tracheostomy can usually be determined while the history is being obtained. A tracheotomy must be performed if there is severe respiratory obstruction. It is also indicated in the initial management when respiratory tract injury is suspected. The presence of established pulmonary damage may be diagnosed by hoarseness, coughing, rapid respirations or cyanosis. A history of the patient being burned in a closed space or the appearance of redness in the posterior pharynx may suggest respiratory damage. Singeing of the nasal hairs or stridor or rales in the chest may give indication of pulmonary irritation.

Although some patients with deep burns of the face and neck may require a tracheostomy later, it is usually not indicated in the first 24 hours. Addition of a tracheostomy to the already complicated condition of the burned patient frequently gives rise to many complications. Many patients with burns about the head and neck do very well without a tracheostomy, which is always associated with increases in water loss and infection and requires additional nursing care. Further indications for tracheostomy in the postburn course and tracheostomy care are discussed in Chapter Ten.

Initial Venipuncture

Although all patients with burns of more than 20 per cent of the body surface should have a cutdown cannula inserted, an initial venipuncture is necessary to obtain a laboratory blood sample and provide a route for immediate infusion of replacement therapy. A large bore needle should be inserted into an accessible vein. Blood should be withdrawn for cross matching, hematocrit, base line electrolyte determinations, blood urea nitrogen, blood sugar and any other tests that seem to be indicated. The initial dose of narcotic may be given through this needle and lactated Ringer's solution attached. Replacement therapy can then be accomplished while time is taken to plan a definitive intravenous lifeline.

Indwelling Urinary Catheter

In all patients with burns involving more than 20 per cent of the body surface, an indwelling Foley catheter should be inserted. This provides the only reliable method for accurately measuring urinary output, which is essential as a guide to initial fluid therapy. A urine specimen should be sent to the laboratory for urinalysis, and the urinary output should be recorded hourly. While the catheter is in place, the patient should receive appropriate medication for urinary tract antisepsis.

In burns, prolonged indwelling urinary catheters may be the source of severe sepsis. The catheter should be removed as soon as it is no longer needed as a guide to replacement therapy. Too frequently a urinary catheter is allowed to remain in place for 10 or 12 days because it provides convenience in care. This may lead to serious infection. When an indwelling catheter remains in the bladder more than 5 days, cystitis develops. In most patients, catheters can be removed on the fourth day.

Establishment of a Reliable Intravenous Portal

Because the life of a burned patient depends upon the infusion of replacement solutions, it is wise to plan initially the utilization of various routes of administration. Although a large bore needle, well anchored in a good vein, is satisfactory for patients with small burns, all patients with burns of more than 20 per cent of the body surface require a reliable intravenous lifeline. Patients are often restless and displace apparently well anchored needles. Repeated venipunctures then become necessary during the first few days. Intravenous fluids may have to be used over a long period of time, and blood transfusions are usually required for weeks or months. Not many veins are suitable for the administration of intravenous fluids in extensively burned patients. Gentle care of veins is therefore essential, and veins must not be thrombosed or rendered unsatisfactory by hematomas during early therapy. Also, there is often an excessive delay between the time when subcutaneous infiltration of fluids is noticed and the time when a repeat venipuncture is performed, especially if infiltration occurs at night. During the delay, marked fluid deficits may accrue. For these reasons an intravenous cannula of some type is mandatory for optimal therapy. It is usually best to perform a cutdown and insert a plastic indwelling catheter. The use of an Intra-cath or a Rochester needle may sometimes suffice. In a patient with a very extensive burn, it may be desirable to monitor the venous pressure. In such instances a plastic catheter should be inserted in a large vein and a venous manometer attached (Fig. 71).

Before the site for the intravenous portal is selected, considerable thought should be given to the best utilization of available veins. Veins in burned patients are used primarily for two purposes, intravenous infusions and procurement of blood samples for laboratory determinations. It is desirable to insert the cutdown in the most distal vein of an available

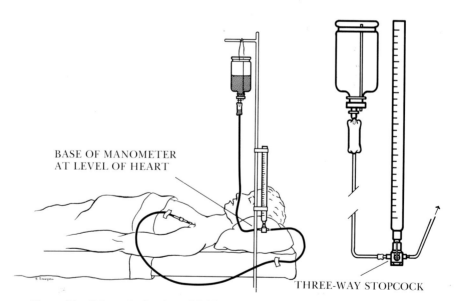

BASE OF MANOMETER
AT LEVEL OF HEART

THREE-WAY STOPCOCK

Figure 71. Schematic drawing of fluid venous pressure manometer in infusion system. This is a convenient method of measuring the venous pressure as an additional guide to fluid therapy. By means of the three-way stopcock it is easy for the surgeon to fill the manometer with a crystalloid solution and then observe the level at which it stabilizes (venous pressure).

extremity because, if thrombosis occurs, the same vein may be used in a more proximal position. Because a cutdown usually remains open longer when placed in the cephalic vein of the upper arm or at the shoulder groove between the deltoid and pectoralis major muscles, this proximal area is sometimes preferred.

In adults it is preferable to use veins of the upper extremities if available because intravenous catheters in the lower extremities lead to more extensive and troublesome thrombotic complications. In infants, however, the most desirable site for a cutdown is the long saphenous vein on the medial aspect of the ankle. After the cannula has been tied in place, venous spasm may occur and retard the rate of flow. In such instances, 2 ml. of a 1 per cent procaine solution may be injected into the cannula. If few peripheral veins are available for sampling, a femoral vein in the inguinal region or the external jugular vein in the neck may be used.

The incidence of septic phlebitis in superficial veins with an indwelling catheter rises markedly after 5 days. When veins are no longer available in any extremity, or if all four extremities are burned, it may be necessary to insert a catheter into the femoral vein. This should be the last place used to establish an intravenous portal. A femoral catheter must not remain in place longer than 5 days, because of the danger of thrombosis and pulmonary embolism. Femoral catheters are convenient, but they carry a high rate of complication.

Local Care

As soon as adequate replacement therapy has been assured, local care of the burn wound should be started. The details of local care are discussed in Chapter Six.

Assessment of Injury

The best time to get an accurate assessment of the injury is after the initial cleansing has been accomplished. It is much easier at this time to determine the percentage of body surface burned and the depth of the burn. The Rule of Nines is a quick and reasonably accurate method of estimating the percentage of body surface burned (Fig. 67). Another method is the use of the Lund and Browder chart. A chart similar to the one shown in Figure 66 should be completed at this time. This gives an estimation of the percentage of burn and a good record of the injury.

A good time to weigh the patient is immediately after cleansing. Too often this is considered time consuming and unnecessary. It is extremely important to have the accurate weight of a patient not only for estimating replacement therapy but also as a later guide to the amount of weight loss the patient sustains. Frequent observations of weight in the early period after injury may prevent overhydration. There must be a 10 per cent increase in total body water before generalized edema is clinically evident.

It is desirable to take photographs at this time. They constitute a valuable part of the record during the course of treatment. It is mandatory to take both color and black and white photographs if there are medico-legal implications associated with the accident.

Tetanus Prophylaxis

Anaerobic microbes frequently colonize the surface of a deep burn. Clinical tetanus has been reported in burns. For this reason, routine tetanus prophylaxis must be given. To patients who have been immunized within the preceding 5 years with tetanus toxoid, 0.5 ml. of toxoid as a booster dose is sufficient. If the patient has not been immunized with toxoid, human immune globulin (human tetanus antitoxin) should be given to provide passive immunization.

Initial Antibiotic Therapy

Although there are differing opinions concerning the use of antibiotics initially in burns, it is doubtful that such therapy is indicated. Some burn surgeons routinely give penicillin and streptomycin to all hospitalized burned patients. Others believe that penicillin therapy for the first 5 days prevents infection by the beta hemolytic streptococcus. It is doubtful that prophylactic antibiotics are necessary in a clean hospital environment. If a streptococcal infection does develop—and this is rare—it is easily abated by the use of penicillin. Routine antibiotic therapy in burns only permits the growth of resistant organisms. Except in certain instances, antibiotics should be withheld until there is some evidence of infection. Then a concentrated effort should be made to determine the offending organism and the appropriate antibiotic administered. When patients have a concomitant disease or injury indicating antibiotics, they should be used.

Almost all seriously burned patients require antibiotics as the burn course progresses. In some patients a peripheral cellulitis may develop. This often responds to penicillin; if not, sodium methicillin is indicated. A discussion of the treatment and control of infection is given in Chapter Fourteen.

Planning Replacement Therapy

As soon as the initial procedures are completed, the physician should methodically plan replacement therapy. The factors to be considered in estimating fluid requirements are the extent of burn, depth of burn and age and general condition of the patient. Vitamin C (1000 to 2000 mg.) and vitamin B complex should be administered intravenously for the first 2 or 3 days and orally thereafter.

Adjunctive Initial Procedures

Consideration should be given to the need for special nurses. Severely burned patients require more than average nursing care. Sometimes this is provided in a special unit or an intensive care unit. If such specialized care is not available, it is usually wise to provide special nurses. When it is indicated, the patient should be placed on the critical list. Because all burned patients require large quantities of blood, plans should be made with the family to provide blood donors. Greater cooperation from donors is received during the first few days after the injury than at any other time during the burn course.

All the initial procedures should be recorded in detail on the patient's chart. Because therapy during the first few days is rather complicated, it is wise to make a comprehensive worksheet. This should include fluid intake, hourly observations of urinary output, record of vital signs and pertinent laboratory data.

Burned patients are usually quite thirsty and demand water. In extensive burns, paralytic ileus and vomiting are common during the first few days. Patients in whom therapy is being given intravenously should have all fluids by mouth withheld for the first 24 to 48 hours. In some patients it may be necessary to insert an indwelling nasogastric tube to alleviate gastric distention, dilatation or vomiting. Gastric dilatation is a frequently unrecognized complication in acute burns.

The initial impression created by the hospital staff is a lasting one in the minds of patients and their families. Every effort must be directed toward making the patient feel that he is cared for by individuals who are genuinely interested in him. A courteous, friendly and informative approach to relatives usually wins their utmost cooperation. A burned patient has many fears. Verbal reassurance can do much to alleviate his anxiety. A family is also more cooperative if it is given an honest appraisal of the patient's condition as well as a clear explanation of the procedures required and the events anticipated in the management of the serious injury. Sympathetic explanations help to establish the patient's and the family's confidence in the physician. Implicit confidence is absolutely essential because of the many uncomfortable procedures that are necessary during the prolonged period of treatment and convalescence.

REFERENCES

Artz, C. P.: The burned patient. *In* Curry, G. J. (ed.): *Immediate Care and Transport of the Injured.* Springfield, Illinois, Charles C Thomas, 1965, pp. 70–79.

Barnes, B. A.: Mortality of burns at the Massachusetts General Hospital, 1939–1954. *Ann. Surg.* **145**:210, 1957.

Berkow, S. G.: A method for estimating the extensiveness of lesions (burns and scalds), based on surface area proportions. *A.M.A. Arch. Surg.* **8**:138, 1924.

Bull, J. P., and Fisher, A. J.: A study of mortality in a burns unit: a revised estimate. *Ann. Surg.* **139**:269, 1954.

Bull, J. P., and Squire, J. R.: A study of mortality in a burns unit: standards for the evaluation of alternative methods of treatment. *Ann. Surg.* **130**:160, 1949.

Lund, C. C., and Browder, N. C.: The estimation of areas of burns. *Surg. Gynec. & Obst.* **79**:352, 1944.

Pruitt, B. A., Jr., Tumbusch, W. T., Mason, A. D., Jr., and Pearson, E.: Mortality in 1,100 consecutive burns treated at a burns unit. *Ann. Surg.* **159**:396, 1964.

Schwartz, M. S., Soroff, H. S., Reiss, E., and Artz, C. P.: An evaluation of the mortality and the relative severity of second- and third-degree injury in burns. U.S. Army Surgical Research Unit Research Report 6-56, August 1956.

Chapter
Four

OFFICE
TREATMENT
OF BURNS

Although a major third-degree burn is a serious and complicated injury, most▸ minor first- and second-degree burns heal in a few days if kept free from infection. The systemic derangements that are so important in extensive burns are of little or no significance in minor burns. The treatment of small burns, therefore, consists primarily of control of pain and local care.

SELECTION OF BURNS FOR OUTPATIENT CARE

All serious burns should be treated in the hospital. One of the most difficult problems in minor burns is the selection of those to be treated on an outpatient basis. Many factors must be considered. These include extent of injury, depth of burn, area of body involved, type of patient, status of patient's home situation and availability of hospitalization.

Almost all persons with first-degree sunburn can be treated at home. There is an occasional individual who injudiciously spends too much time in the bright sunlight on the beach or under a sun lamp, becomes burned over a high percentage of his body surface and, as a result, will require 1 or 2 days in the hospital.

Second-degree burns of less than 15 per cent of the body surface and third-degree burns of less than 2 per cent of the body surface can frequently be treated in the office on an outpatient basis. This is not always true, because some 15 per cent, deep second-degree burns in infants will require hospitalization to provide necessary fluid replacement. Even small third-degree burns of certain critical areas, such as the hands, feet and face, require hospitalization. If a third-degree burn is completely localized to one area on the large, open part of the body, it is probably best to hospitalize the patient, excise the burn immediately and cover it with a skin graft 2 days later.

If it appears that hospitalization is questionable from the nature of the injury, it is usually wise to admit the patient, observe him for 48 to 72 hours and then determine whether or not he can be treated as an out-patient. One must beware the minor burn with respiratory tract damage. Even though the surface injury is very small, if there is any evidence of respiratory tract damage from inhalation of smoke and noxious agents, the patient must be hospitalized. Face burns, especially if there is perior-bital injury, are best treated in the hospital. Special care of the eyes is necessary to prevent infection. Sometimes one may elect to treat a 10 to 15 per cent second-degree burn in a child at home. If it becomes obvious after 24 or 48 hours that the child is becoming dehydrated and not doing well, he must then be hospitalized. Sometimes a hospital bed is not available for a burn of questionable extent. In such instances, the physician may wisely elect to give initial care in his office and treat the patient at home until hospitalization is possible. This is particularly true of third-degree burns of minor extent. It is possible to treat these patients at home by dressings until the area is ready for grafting. When the physician is in doubt, especially in infants and elderly individuals, immediate hospitalization should be elected and the decision to treat on an outpatient basis made after 72 hours of observation.

SUNBURN

Burns from exposure to the sun are usually very superficial. Most sunburns are first-degree burns and heal in a few days. Occasionally a person with very sensitive skin or one who has experienced prolonged exposure may get a second-degree burn with blister formation from the sun or a sun lamp. Obviously the keynote in sunburn is prevention. Early season sunbathers and those with particularly susceptible skin should be advised to use liberal quantities of the many good preparations available for screening out the sun's burning rays.

The treatment of sunburn depends upon its extent and depth. Minor superficial sunburns may be adequately treated by any soothing ointment or lotion. In most instances the burn should be kept exposed and an ointment containing an anesthetic agent such as tetracaine or dibucaine applied to control the burning and stinging pain. Oily sprays containing a local anesthetic agent frequently bring welcome relief in sunburns covering large areas. Soaking in a bathtub of warm water sometimes is soothing. Aspirin helps to lessen the discomfort. In the case of a very extensive sunburn, nausea and vomiting may occur. An occasional patient experiences such great fluid loss, both from the burn and the vomiting, that intravenous fluids may be required. Antinausea drugs are sometimes helpful.

INITIAL OFFICE MANAGEMENT

Minor burns are usually treated in a physician's office, an industrial or military dispensary or an emergency room. From the history and examination of the injury, a decision can usually be made rather rapidly concerning the requirement for hospitalization. Even though the injury may appear to be a very minor one, a good written record should be maintained because such injuries may have compensation or medicolegal implications.

Control of Pain

One of the outstanding problems in small superficial burns is pain. The apprehension associated with the burn usually makes it hurt worse. Frequently, pain can be controlled by the application of wet towels soaked in ice water. This may be suggested by telephone as a first aid measure. Such treatment is particularly effective in second-degree burns of the face (Fig. 72). In burns of the hands, soaking the part in cold soapy water not only cleanses the area but also alleviates pain (Fig. 73). Sometimes it may be necessary to give a narcotic. Most of the pain disappears when the wound is covered by a comfortable dressing. If it appears that the patient will need an analgesic to control discomfort at home, aspirin or propoxyphene hydrochloride should be prescribed.

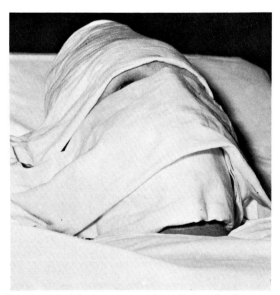

Figure 72. Towels soaked in ice water and applied to the face soon after burn is an effective way to stop pain.

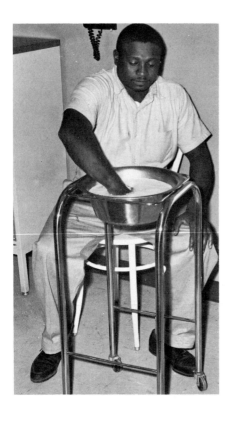

Figure 73. Immediate treatment of a burn of the hand in the emergency room. Soaking in cold soapy water cleanses the area and alleviates pain.

Cleansing the Wound

All burns treated on an outpatient basis should be thoroughly cleansed. This is best accomplished by water and a bland soap. Alcoholic soap solutions sting and should not be used. The application of antiseptics is also contraindicated.

The washing should be gentle so that it will not damage any remaining viable epithelium, but it must also be thorough. Every attempt should be made to remove all dirt and foreign substances. If there is much hair around the burn injury, it should be shaved. Except in instances in which dirt is ground into the burn wound, a brush should not be used.

In general it is best to pull off or cut away any blisters or devitalized epithelium. Minor burns of the hand that involve thick blisters, particularly on the palm, however, do best when the blisters are left unruptured. Although it would appear that the skin of the blister would be the best possible dressing for a wound, this is not always true. Blisters frequently rupture either during the dressing procedure or under the dressing, and the resulting blister fluid and devitalized epithelium only serve as a good pabulum for bacterial growth. If it appears that the blister is a firm one and will not be easily ruptured by cleansing and dressing, it should be left alone.

One of the most difficult injuries to cleanse is the tar burn. A good technique is to apply ice to the area. After a sufficient period of time, the tar usually becomes very hard and can be peeled away from the skin (Fig. 74).

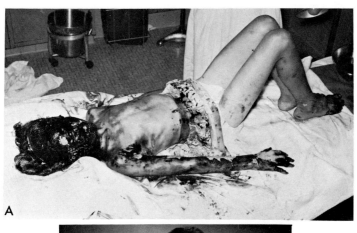

A

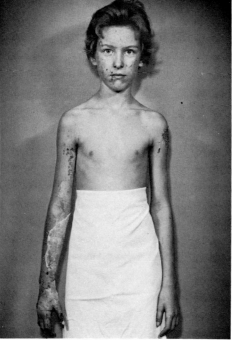

B

Figure 74. *A*, Immediate appearance of young girl who received tar burn of the face. The tar was peeled away with moderate ease after the application of ice packs. The cold packs hardened the tar. *B*, Appearance of tar burn 7 days after injury.

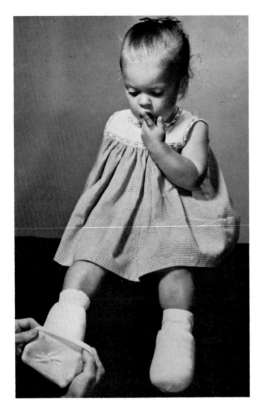

Figure 75. Stockinette with a reverse twist makes an excellent outer dressing for hands and feet.

Dressing the Burn

After the area has been thoroughly cleansed and irrigated with copious quantities of water, a dressing should be applied. Almost all burns treated on an outpatient basis do better when treated by dressings. Superficial burns in small infants and burns of the face probably do better when exposed. A dressing should occlude the entire wound, splint the part, be easily removed and be comfortable. It should also be absorptive because superficial wounds weep serum from the surface, and the aim of a dressing is to absorb this fluid so that the wound surface will be kept as dry as possible. Some type of water soluble ointment or ointment gauze placed next to the wound will usually keep the dressing from sticking. Many preparations are available. It is doubtful that antibiotic ointments are of any particular value. Simple petrolatum gauze, Carbowax gauze, nylon or Owens fabric may be used.

Illustration on opposite page
Figure 76. *A*, Initial step in applying an occlusive dressing to a burned hand. A layer of lightly impregnated gauze is placed over the burned area. The hand and forearm are put on two large abdominal pads. Fluffed gauze is placed on the palm of the hand in such a way that there is dorsiflexion of the wrist and acute flexion of metacarpophalangeal joints. The

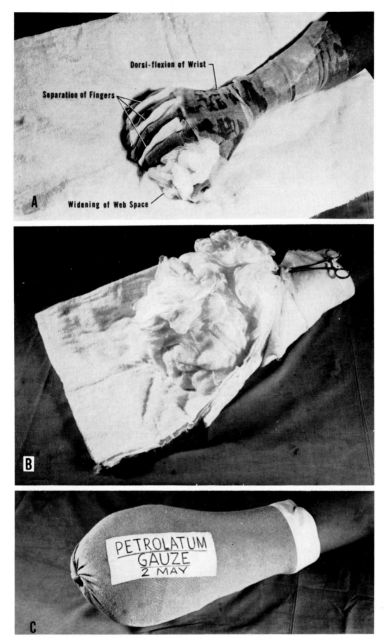

Figure 76. *Continued.*
fingers are separated with gauze and special attention is given to maintaining the width of
the webbed space between the index finger and the thumb.

B, Additional fluffed gauze is placed over the hand to make a large, absorptive dressing.
It may or may not be necessary to put a plaster splint in the dressing to maintain dorsiflexion
of the wrist.

C, The entire dressing is wrapped with even compression by means of an elastic bandage.
Stockinette is placed over the dressing. Then the type of treatment and date applied is noted
on the dressing.

Over the initial gauze layer should be placed an appropriate amount of absorptive material; fluffed 4- by 4-inch or 4- by 8-inch gauze pads make an excellent dressing. This layer should be bulky to provide a splinting effect and to allow the final layer of bandage to be put on with even compression. Most dressings on burns are too thin. Unless a dressing of the extremity is fairly bulky, the outside layer of bandage may become tight in some areas and actually serve as a constricting tourniquet. The best material for an outer layer is a semielastic bandage such as the Kling bandage. Stockinette is a particularly good material for the outer layer of an extremity bandage. It is the best possible covering for dressings of the hands and feet (Fig. 75).

One of the most troublesome injuries to dress is the burn on the bottom of the foot in a child. Unless the dressing is put on with great care, it will come off. Stockinette with the reverse twist, as shown in Figure 75, is the most effective dressing. Hands require a special type of dressing (Fig. 76). They should be dressed in the position of function, with pads separating the fingers.

The dressing should be made to look as neat as possible but, above all, it should be put on in such a way that it will not come off. It is most embarrassing to put a dressing on a child and have the mother call after they return home to say that the dressing has come off. By leaving the tips of the fingers or toes out of the dressing, the circulation can be easily observed. Most dressings need to be fixed in place with adhesive tape. It is convenient to write on this tape the time and date of return for dressing change.

Antibiotics and Tetanus Prophylaxis

Initial systemic antibiotic therapy is not indicated in outpatient burns. Unless there is third-degree injury or an associated injury, no tetanus prophylaxis is necessary.

DRESSING CHANGES

A good dressing will usually remain in place satisfactorily for 5 days. Sometimes if there is a particularly weeping surface the dressing may need to be changed in 2 or 3 days. Removal of the dressing is frequently more painful than the original injury. It is usually wise to remove all the dressing that is not stuck and then either wet the remaining dressing or soak the part in warm water. Gentle removal of the dressing not only prevents pain but also protects any thin viable epithelium. Sometimes if the inner layer of gauze is clean it may be allowed to remain and only the outer dressing need be changed. The wound should be examined for any evidence of infection; a culture should be taken if pus is present. The wound should be irrigated with warm soapy water; it should not be scrubbed. The second dressing should also be occlusive, but it may be a little thinner than the first dressing.

After 5 days a second dressing change will be necessary. Many superficial burns will have healed. If the wound has not yet healed but is obviously healing, another dressing should be applied for a few more days.

INFECTED MINOR BURNS

Should the burn wound become infected, a culture should be taken and the patient placed on appropriate systemic antibiotic therapy. Infection in second-degree burns with *Pseudomonas* will respond very nicely to simple exposure. Sometimes an antibiotic ointment is of value in superficial infections. When there is a moderate amount of suppuration, probably the best method of treating an infected burn wound is by wet soaks or repeated change of wet dressings. If a burn of moderate size is infected, it may be wise to hospitalize the patient.

GRAFTING MINOR WOUNDS

Should it become evident after a few dressing changes that the burn is full thickness, grafting must be considered. Most areas of more than 1 inch square should be grafted. Smaller areas will probably epithelize without too much delay. Very small wounds can sometimes be grafted in the office. A split-thickness skin graft can be taken from an accessible area after the injection of 0.5 per cent procaine. Small sheets of split-thickness skin can be obtained with a razor blade. Patients with larger, granulating wounds, of course, should be hospitalized, and grafting should be done in an operating room.

RECOVERY OF FUNCTION

Assurance of early and complete healing is a most important factor in recovery. Once the wound is healed, however, passive followed by active exercises will produce improvement in function in almost direct proportion to the cooperation exhibited by the individual patient. Burns of the hand should be put in warm water and exercised four times a day as soon as the skin has healed.

When there is injury to the skin overlying a joint, graduated exercises extended to encompass the full normal range of motion must be carefully explained to the patient and insisted upon. In burns of the hand, the use of a sponge rubber ball that fits easily into the palm and is intermittently squeezed has been found to be of value. To carry a ball reminds the patient of the importance of his own repeated efforts. More extensive injury of the hand may require the assistance of a physical therapist for maximum results.

After a second-degree burn has healed, it is probably wise to suggest to the patient that he not expose the injured area to prolonged sunlight until after 2 or 3 months. In burns of the hands, white cotton gloves are very useful.

Chapter
Five

INITIAL
REPLACEMENT
THERAPY

The burn injury calls forth innumerable systemic changes. The most important of these in the early treatment of a burn are the alterations in fluid and electrolyte dynamics. These changes are not unique to burns, but are seen to some degree in all forms of trauma as an integral part of the basic pattern of tissue response to injury. Since the burn is such a large wound, marked fluid shifts occur. If untreated, these lead to burn shock; therefore, initial replacement therapy is extremely important. Under ideal conditions in a well staffed, well equipped hospital, almost all extensively burned patients can be kept alive for 2 or 3 days if current methods of fluid therapy are used. Successful management of the patient in the early period of rapid shifts of water, electrolytes and proteins, however, does not assure ultimate survival. Most extensively burned patients who die do so because of complications other than burn shock. Two decades ago many patients died in the first few days after injury from inadequacy of replacement therapy. This is not true today. Although much remains to be learned about replacement therapy, most deaths that occur should not be due to improper fluid management.

PATHOPHYSIOLOGY OF BURN INJURY

The changes that take place after burn injury have fascinated investigators for many years. Although more research is needed for a precise definition of the pathophysiologic derangements that occur after a burn, much has been learned in this area.

The Burn as a Three-dimensional Wound

Although it is customary to think of a burn as a two-dimensional wound—that is, a wound involving surface area rather than volume—

a burn is really a wound of three dimensions. The area concept is appealing because of the appearance of the burn wound. It is popular to speak of the burn in terms of the percentage of body surface area involved. Depth of tissue injury, which is the third dimension, is difficult to visualize and cannot be measured accurately. Beneath the injured skin, a myriad of changes occur that evoke many systemic derangements. Thus, the third dimension of the burn injury becomes extremely significant from the standpoint of treatment.

Tissue Damage

Studies on the interrelationship between time and temperature exposure were made by Moritz and Henriques in 1947. They emphasized that it was important to know both the intensity and duration of the exposure to characterize any episode of hyperthermia as critical in respect to its capacity to destroy skin. When the temperature of the skin is maintained at 44° C., the rate of the injurious change exceeds that of recovery by so narrow a margin that an exposure of approximately 6 hours is required before real damage is sustained at the basal cell level. At surface temperatures of 70° C., however, less than 1 second is required to cause epidermal necrosis. At surface temperatures between 44° and 51° C., the total exposure time required to destroy the epidermis is essentially identical to the total duration of the steady thermal state within the epidermis, and under these circumstances the rate at which the burn occurs is almost doubled with each additional degree of temperature. The earliest histologic change is a redistribution of chromatin within the nuclei. This occurs first in the intermediate and later in the deep layer of cells of the epidermis. Because of the changes in the basal cells or in the intracellular cement that binds them to the epidermis, an irreversible impairment of the attachment between the epidermis and dermis occurs. This is frequently seen clinically because in many burns the surface of the epidermis is easily peeled off the burned surface. A further rise in temperature causes coagulation, progressive desiccation and finally carbonization.

The type of burn, because of variation in tissue damage, influences replacement therapy. For instance, Fox has pointed out that the amount of replacement solution required for a scald burn (low intensity, long exposure) was considerably greater than the amount necessary for a burn of similar thickness caused by flash (high intensity, short exposure). It is a well documented observation that burns caused by low intensity heat and long exposure are characterized by more severe changes in the deeper tissues. Prolonged exposure to heat increases the thrombosis and capillary permeability of subcutaneous vessels and produces greater edema than high intensity flash burns of short duration.

The destruction of tissue in electrical or chemical injury is entirely different from thermal injury. The differences are discussed in Chapter Nine.

Edema

The most important aspect of the inflammatory reaction following a burn is the development of abnormal capillary permeability, which allows protein-rich fluid to escape into the tissue spaces. This diminishes the colloid osmotic pressure difference between the capillary plasma and the tissue fluid exudate. In addition, a rise of intracapillary pressure associated with capillary dilatation and increased blood flow occurs. Using radioactive colloids, Cope and Moore have shown that the capillaries in the burned skin of dogs become almost as permeable to colloids as normal capillaries are to ions. This increased permeability has been termed sieving of the capillaries. This is a very descriptive term, for it shows exactly what happens in a burn: the capillaries leak fluid into the interstitial space; therefore, the plasma volume is diminished and the interstitial fluid is increased.

Arturson studied sieving characteristics of capillary membranes in burned and unburned areas of the dog, using dextran as the test substance. The local alterations of the sieving characteristics of the blood-lymph barrier in scalded areas were found to be correlated with the severity of the burn. The more severe the burn, the greater was the escape of the larger molecules through the capillary walls. Alterations were also noted in unburned areas. After third-degree burns of 25 per cent or more, an increase in the leakage of the dextran molecules was found in all areas investigated except the blood aqueous humor. It would appear that capillary permeability increases in and around the burned tissue and also in other areas of the body after severe burning.

Another, but yet poorly understood, factor associated with edema concerns changes in the permeability of tissue cells in and around a burned area, which may allow abnormal interchange of water and electrolytes between the cells and the interstitial fluid. The formation of edema is limited primarily by tissue tension. As more and more fluid accumulates in the interstitial spaces, tissue pressure increases. This is an important factor limiting further extravasation of fluid.

Depth of burn is an extremely important factor that affects the volume as well as the composition of fluid losses from the circulation. In a first-degree burn, vasodilatation is the only major change that occurs. Protein losses are insignificant and edema is barely perceptible. A second-degree burn is characterized not only by more severe capillary damage but also by damage involving a larger amount of tissue than a first-degree burn of the same extent. Although the area burned is easily gauged by inspection of the wound, the depth of tissue in which capillaries are functionally deranged is not immediately evident. A large volume of fluid can accumulate beneath the surface of the wound before any visible swelling occurs. The extensive fluid loss caused by a third-degree burn appears to be due to the injury of a large amount of tissue beneath and surrounding the area of full-thickness skin destruction.

Subcutaneous edema can be locally displaced by pressure, will gravitate to dependent parts and is able to spread well beyond the burned area. The rate of formation of edema and the volume present at any one time depend upon the time since the injury, the area burned and the temperature and duration of the burn itself. The location of the injury is of some importance when the fluid losses are considered in burns of the same extent and depth. Burns of highly vascularized areas, such as the face, are generally believed to cause greater losses of fluid than comparable burns in other locations (Fig. 77).

Contrary to popular belief, visible fluid losses of second-degree burns constitute only a small fraction of the total amount of fluid that is functionally lost; the greater fluid losses occur deep in the wound. Even more misleading are third-degree burns that are characterized by a dry surface and a small amount of visible swelling. In such burns, the firm eschar may prevent obvious swelling, but large volumes of fluid extravasate into the deeper tissues. From a clinical point of view, it is extremely difficult to achieve correlation between the amount of fluid lost into an injured area and visible formation of edema. Large quantities of fluid may accumulate in deeply located tissues without any evidence of swelling. In both second-degree and third-degree burns, relatively small changes in a measurable parameter, such as the circumference of a limb, may be associated with a surprisingly large fluid accumulation (Fig. 78).

Cope's exhaustive investigations furnish excellent information as to the rate of fluid loss and edema formation. The losses are incurred most rapidly in the early period after burning. The rate of edema formation and fluid losses decline about 48 hours after the injury, at which time edema is maximal. Loss of fluids continues until (1) the capillary endothelium returns to normal when the permeability effect is reversible, (2) the tissue pressure rises and equals that of the capillary hydrostatic pressure, at which point filtration will cease, or (3) stasis of the capillary blood flow occurs. Observations on increases in weight in severely burned patients have shown that the maximum extent of the edema is about 10 per cent of the body weight, or roughly 50 per cent of the combined extracellular fluid volume.

Resorption of edema fluid seems to occur chiefly by way of lymphatic drainage. In uncomplicated burns of minor extent, the rate at which edema fluid is withdrawn from the wound approximates the rate of its accumulation. In more extensive burns, however, and in those complicated by infection, the wound edema may persist for 2 or 3 weeks. At times, edema about the wound subsides, but the load of fluids given as initial therapy is not excreted through the kidneys or the exudate. Apparently the fluid is lost by evaporation or is translocated to other portions of the body. Of course, this fluid is eventually excreted, but excretion may be delayed for days or weeks after all traces of visible edema have disappeared.

Early Protein Changes

The amount of protein lost from the plasma may vary from one burn to another and also in different parts of the same burn. Most of the

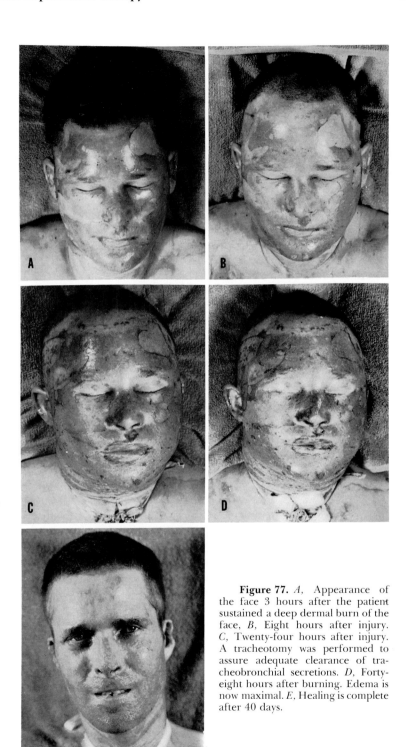

Figure 77. *A*, Appearance of the face 3 hours after the patient sustained a deep dermal burn of the face. *B*, Eight hours after injury. *C*, Twenty-four hours after injury. A tracheotomy was performed to assure adequate clearance of tracheobronchial secretions. *D*, Forty-eight hours after burning. Edema is now maximal. *E*, Healing is complete after 40 days.

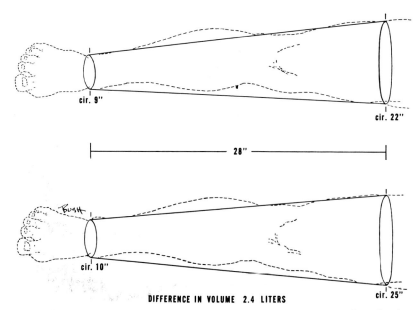

Figure 78. Relatively small changes in the measurable parameter, such as the circumference of an extremity, may be associated with large fluid accumulations. A lower extremity is here considered as the frustrum of a cone with an upper circumference of 22 inches and a lower circumference of 9 inches. A change of 3 inches in the upper circumference and a change of 1 inch in the lower circumference would result in a volume change of 2.4 liters.

data concerning early protein losses in burns were derived from measurements of the composition of blister fluid and lymph drainage from burned areas. In both blister fluid and lymph, the ratio of albumin to globulin is always higher than in the plasma. This phenomenon is explained by the relative size of the protein molecules. The larger globulin molecules appear to have greater difficulty in migrating across the injured capillary membrane. The amount of protein in blister fluid is usually between 4 and 5 gm. per 100 ml. It has been demonstrated that the increased protein content of lymph is a result of capillary damage and not merely a reflection of tissue lysis with the release of plasma proteins. By injecting albumin tagged with certain dyes, it has been shown that the increased lymph protein is undoubtedly derived from the plasma.

One of the immediate changes after thermal injury is an increase in the protein concentration of the plasma. Although proteins are lost from the plasma into the burn wound, water and electrolytes are lost more rapidly. This increases the plasma protein concentration and tends to compensate for the oligemia resulting from fluid losses at the wound site by draining interstitial fluid from unburned tissues into the vascular system. This occurrence probably represents one of the important mechanisms of compensation for the parasitic effects of the wound in untreated patients. With appropriate fluid therapy, the plasma protein concentration falls. As time progresses in the burn course, there is a decrease in plasma proteins; albumin is decreased to a much greater degree than globulin.

The loss of protein-rich fluid from the plasma at the site of the burn is a factor of overriding importance in the causation of the clinical condition of shock in untreated burned patients. The fluid loss results in a fall in plasma volume. The natural defense reaction of the body is to counteract this fall of plasma volume in three ways: (1) by withdrawing fluid from the undamaged part of the extracellular space, (2) by a general constriction of blood vessels in the splanchnic area and the skin (this constriction of vessels reduces the space that the available blood volume has to fill and increases the peripheral resistance so that the blood pressure is maintained and an adequate blood supply to the vital organs is continued) and (3) by ingestion and absorption of fluids from the gut in response to a feeling of thirst. With these mechanisms, the body may be able to compensate adequately for the fluid loss when the rate of loss is not too great. In minor burns, the patient may be able to stay out of shock if provided extra fluids to drink. When the burn is more severe, however, the rate of loss is more rapid, and the plasma volume continues to fall. If the patient remains untreated or inadequate replacement therapy is given, shock ensues.

Electrolyte Shifts

Water and electrolytes freely permeate the normal capillary. Burning affects water and electrolyte shifts directly through increased capillary hydrostatic pressure and indirectly through protein shifts. Injury to tissue cells may be another important factor that influences the movement of water and electrolytes. Fox contributed much to our knowledge of the movement of sodium following a burn by the use of tracer studies with radiosodium. In deep burns in mice, Fox noted the loss of potassium from burned tissues and its apparent uptake in unburned tissues. This loss of potassium was accounted for quantitatively by an increase in sodium in the burned tissues, this increase occurring over and above that expected on the basis of interstitial edema. These data suggest that sodium is lost into burned tissues by the entrance of sodium into injured cells as well as by the accumulation of interstitial edema. Hypo-osmolarity of the extracellular fluid could be a consequence of the sodium shift into injured cells, and water would, therefore, shift into unburned tissues. Thus, a twofold fluid loss may occur—at the site of injury and in unburned tissue cells. From a clinical standpoint, the use of sodium ion in the early management of burns is well established.

Experimental deep burns are characterized by a transient hyperkalemia. This appears to result both from the release of potassium by burned tissue and from hemolysis of erythrocytes (225 ml. of human erythrocytes contain approximately 23 mEq. of potassium). Potassium changes during the first 24 hours are of little clinical significance. Solutions containing potassium in more than minute quantities should certainly not be given during the first 48 hours.

Moore has calculated a first approximation of the magnitude of loss of certain substances into the edema fluid and from the body in a 40 per cent burn during the first 72 hours. These interesting figures are as follows:

Edema water, 6500 ml.	Sodium, 900 mEq.
Cell water, 1000 ml.	Chloride, 600 mEq.
Pulmonary water, 2000 ml.	Bicarbonate, 200 mEq.
Surface water, 1000 ml. or more	Potassium, 250 mEq.
Red blood cells, 250 ml.	Protein, 325 gm.

Loss of Red Blood Cells

In some burns, red blood cells may be lost in sufficient numbers to cause a substantial fall in total red cell volume, and the result of this will be an intensification of the effect of the plasma loss. It has been known for many years that patients with severe burns may show free hemoglobin in the plasma and urine, indicating that red cells have been hemolyzed by heat at the time of injury. In 1945, Evans and Bigger pointed out the rationale of whole blood therapy in severe burns. The loss of red cells is generally associated only with deep burns and not with superficial ones. The magnitude of the red cell loss in third-degree burns has been under study for several years. Improved methods for total red cell volume estimation have shown that the loss of red cells is usually gradual and not so severe as was originally thought. Topley and Jackson measured the red cell volume in major burns during each postburn phase and found that during the period from burn to operation 2 or 3 weeks later, the red cell loss averaged about 45 per cent of the red cell mass. Estimates of red cell loss were found to correspond, in general, with the total amount of third-degree involvement. In a major burn, 12 to 25 per cent of the total red cells may be lost in the first 12 hours after injury. The accumulated losses over the entire burn course were about 185 per cent of the total red cell mass. This means that a severely burned patient will require transfusion equal to about two times his blood volume during his hospital course. Levin has noted that decreased red cell survival time occurs in burns and may be correlated with the severity of the lesion.

The loss of red blood cells during the initial postburn period is due to several factors: (1) Red blood cells in the burned area, at the time of injury, are hemolyzed. These cells are hemolyzed at once and give rise to the hemoglobinemia and hemoglobinuria that are observed during the early period in extensive deep burns. The finding of free circulating hemoglobin in the plasma of a recently burned patient indicates that the injury has been severe. (2) Delayed hemolysis is observed for 24 to 48 hours after burning. It results from lysis of red blood cells that are partially damaged by heat. (3) Thrombosis occurs in the capillaries of burned tissues and contributes to the decrease in red cell mass. (4) The phenomenon of sludging is well demonstrated in burns. The magnitude of its contribution to the functional removal of red cells is not known but it may be considerable.

Insensible Water Loss

Marked insensible water loss in burns occurs by two routes—evaporative loss through the burned tissue and increased loss by the respiratory route. Although increased insensible water loss in burns has been recognized for many years, the magnitude of such loss has not been truly appreciated until recently. As more burns have been treated by the exposure method, attention has been focused upon the loss that occurs from the burned surface. Accurate determinations of insensible water loss have been made possible by the use of a specially designed hydraulic scale capable of measuring changes in weight with an accuracy of ± 3 gm. Roe and Kinney made some very precise measurements of evaporative water loss in two patients during the first few days after injury. One adult male with a 50 per cent deep body surface burn had evaporative water losses of 120 to 350 ml. per hour (normal resting values 35 to 50 ml. per hour). In another patient with a 50 per cent burn, the evaporative water loss varied between 90 and 160 ml. per hour. Moncrief and Mason report evaporative water losses in major burns from 100 to 300 ml. per hour. This same group in a later study reported very detailed studies made on 21 patients—18 adults and three children. Their studies covered the first few days after injury. In summarizing their findings, they calculated total hourly and daily water loss from evaporation, drainage into pads and urinary excretion. From these data they calculated that the total fluid requirements for burns from 8 to 40 per cent ranged from 3.0 to 4.7 liters per day—an average 3.1 gm. per kg. per per cent burn per 24 hours. The larger burns, from 40 to 91 per cent, required 4 to 10 liters per day— 2 gm. per kg. per per cent burn per 24 hours. Evaporative loss constituted about 60 per cent of the total loss. They believe that during the early period

Table 12. DAILY RESPIRATORY WATER LOSS*

ROUTE	VENTILATION (6 LITERS/MIN.)	VENTILATION (18 LITERS/MIN.)	VENTILATION (18 LITERS/MIN. PLUS FEVER 104°F.)
Normal nasopharyngeal	185 ml.	555 ml.	735 ml.
Tracheostomy	280 ml.	840 ml.	990 ml.

*After Roe and Kinney.

Table 13. Predicted Energy Requirements in Kilocalories per
Square Meter per 24 Hours in Burns*

AGE	PER CENT BODY SURFACE BURN			
	0 TO 40 PER CENT		OVER 40 PER CENT	
	MALE	FEMALE	MALE	FEMALE
Children (6 to 10 years)	1450	1350	2050	1950
Adolescents	1300	1200	1850	1675
Adults (20 to 50 years)	1150	1100	1625	1550

*From Harrison et al.: *Surgery* **56**:203, 1964, The C.V. Mosby Company, St. Louis, Missouri.

of the burn, patients with both second- and third-degree burns appear similar in the extent to which they lose water transcutaneously.

Although a moderate insensible water loss from the pulmonary route occurs in all burns, the loss is always greater when a tracheostomy is present. Roe and Kinney have attempted to summarize insensible pulmonary losses under varying conditions. Table 12 is taken from their calculations and points out the increased respiratory water loss when a tracheostomy is present.

In addition to pointing out the large quantities of water required in burns, these studies of evaporative water loss also emphasize the tremendous energy loss. It is generally recognized that each gram of evaporative water removes approximately 0.580 kilocalorie of heat from the body. Moyer has estimated this increased heat must be as high as 3000 kilocalories per day over normal maintenance levels.

Studies based on insensible water loss made at the Surgical Research Unit also predict high energy requirements in burns. A summary of the findings is shown in Table 13.

TREATMENT DURING THE FIRST 48 HOURS

Burns differ from most conditions characterized by losses of water and electrolyte in that the rate, volume and composition of fluid losses can be anticipated. Clinical shock is preventable provided that adequate therapy can be instituted soon after injury. How successful a physician is in preventing shock depends upon how soon after injury he sees the patient and upon his ability to estimate losses before they occur.

A patient's general condition may appear satisfactory in the first 6 hours following injury although only little fluid therapy has been given. Signs of circulatory decompensation often develop slowly; once they occur, treatment may be very difficult. The insidiousness of this development of difficulty must be always kept in mind. It must not be allowed to cause a delay in vigorous therapy.

Clinical Signs and Symptoms of Fluid Deficiency

Thirst. Thirst is usually the first symptom. Frequently it is intense and may not be completely relieved by therapy. In fact, all well treated burned patients are thirsty for the first 48 hours.

The importance of thirst lies in the fact that a patient who is given access to unlimited amounts of water is in danger of developing water intoxication—a serious complication that Moyer has repeatedly emphasized. Water intoxication is caused by intracellular edema resulting from dilution of the extracellular fluid. In a normal subject, osmotic pressure of the extracellular fluid is closely regulated and maintained within a remarkably narrow range by the osmoreceptors. Ingestion of water in the normal subject tends to dilute the extracellular fluid and inhibit secretion of antidiuretic hormone by the posterior pituitary. The result is a prompt renal excretion of water. In a burned patient, renal excretion is altered by the shifts of fluid into the wound and, possibly, by an increased secretion of antidiuretic hormone. With a decrease in osmolarity of the extracellular fluid because of ingestion of water that cannot be excreted, the osmotic balance between the cells and the extracellular fluid is disturbed in such a way that water is shifted from the extracellular fluid into the cells. Water intoxication is characterized clinically by headache, tremor, muscle twitching, blurring of vision, vomiting, diarrhea, disorientation, excessive salivation and mania. Generalized convulsions may occur in advanced cases.

Vomiting. Vomiting may be a sign of circulatory collapse, acute gastric dilatation, paralytic ileus or a nonspecific effect of injury. Vomiting occurs frequently in extensive burns and contraindicates the use of oral fluids soon after injury. Vomiting is usually a sign of difficulty, but it is of little help as a specific sign for fluid deficiency.

Central nervous system. Disturbances in the central nervous system are useful in following the progress of therapy. Restlessness, disorientation and maniacal behavior usually indicate that cerebral hypoxia exists and that fluid replacement should be intensified and the cause of hypoxia, probably inadequate ventilation, corrected.

Restlessness is commonly the first indication that therapy has failed to keep pace with fluid losses. It is a remarkably sensitive and useful sign. Treatment consists of intensifying fluid therapy and administering oxygen. Great caution must be exercised in the use of sedation in restless patients.

Disorientation is more difficult to appraise. If it occurs during the first 24 hours after injury, disorientation generally indicates a need for more intensive therapy. After 48 hours, disorientation is usually associated with emotional factors, such as denial of illness, or it may be a sign of invasive infection.

Mania is a complication indicating serious trouble. It may be caused by severe circulatory collapse, by cerebral hypoxia due to pulmonary damage or by water intoxication. If it is caused by circulatory collapse, vigorous fluid therapy is indicated. Therapy should also include the administration of 100 per cent oxygen by mask and the withholding of all types of sedation.

Pulse rate and blood pressure.   Pulse rate and blood pressure are not as sensitive indices of adequacy of therapy in burns as they are in circulatory collapse due to hemorrhage. A normal pulse rate and normal blood pressure do not indicate the absence of circulatory deficits, for serious fluid deficits may be occurring while these signs are still normal. It is not uncommon, for example, to see a burned patient who is restless and oliguric but who has normal pulse rate and blood pressure. Pulse and blood pressure should be taken and recorded every half hour during the early phase of burn therapy, since serious difficulty is certain when the pulse rate suddenly increases or the blood pressure falls. Usually a diminution in blood pressure is an indication for intensification of therapy with colloids.

Urinary output.   Prior to therapy the urinary output is scanty. If the kidneys are not diseased, the urine will be concentrated and have a high specific gravity. A better guide to the degree of concentration is the osmolarity. Sometimes red blood cells or sugar in the urine cause a falsely high specific gravity. A low urinary volume with high osmolarity and low urinary sodium (under 20 mEq. per liter) is indicative of fluid deficiency in relatively good functioning kidneys.

Fluids During the First 48 Hours

The aim in fluid therapy should be to prevent burn shock with an adequate infusion of replacement solutions without overloading the vascular system or causing excessive edema. All well treated burned patients gain considerable weight during the first 48 hours. This increased weight is caused by expansion of the interstitial space (Fig. 79). As the burn course progresses, this expanded interstitial space returns to normal with diuresis.

Small burns.   In general, intensive intravenous therapy is required in burns involving more than 20 per cent of the body surface. Patients with burns of lesser extent usually do well when permitted to take a normal diet and fluids as desired by mouth. In some instances, an oral replacement solution may be necessary. Haldane's solution, made by dissolving 3 to 4 gm. of salt (one-half teaspoonful) and 1.5 to 2 gm. of bicarbonate of soda (one-half teaspoonful) in a quart of water, is an excellent mixture for oral use (Fig. 80). The solution should be flavored with lemon and thoroughly chilled for optimal patient tolerance. In other small burns, especially if vomiting occurs, lactated Ringer's solution can be given intravenously during the first 24 hours in amounts of about 2 ml. per kg. for each per cent of burn.

In time of disaster, the use of an electrolyte solution orally may be satisfactory for burns involving up to 35 per cent of the body surface. As a palatable and effective oral replacement solution for burns, Lindsey has suggested the following: sodium chloride, 2.0 gm.; sodium gluconate,

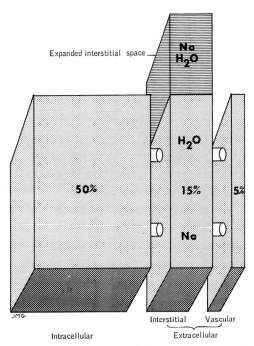

Expanded interstitial space

Na
H₂O

H₂O

50%   15%   5%

Na

JMG

Interstitial   Vascular
Intracellular   Extracellular

Figure 79. Body water compartments and changes that occur after burning. There is a shift of water from the vascular and intracellular spaces into the interstitial space. With additional replacement therapy this interstitial space expands. This expanded interstitial space contains sodium and water. This means that the body of a well treated burned patient has an excess of water and sodium. As the interstitial space returns to normal after 48 hours, the loss of water is relatively greater than the loss of sodium because of the high insensible water loss. During this period the serum sodium concentration is an excellent guide to fluid therapy. A serum sodium level of about 135 mEq. per liter seems to be ideal. (From L. Davis (ed.): *Christopher's Textbook of Surgery.* 9th ed. Philadelphia, W. B. Saunders Company, 1968.)

17.4 gm.; sodium bicarbonate, 2.1 gm.; citric acid, anhydrous, 4.8 gm.; sodium cyclohexylsulfamate, 1.0 gm.; and water q.s., 1000 ml. This solution offers a pleasant taste and attractive fizz in the following ionic composition: sodium, 145 mEq. per liter; chloride, 35; gluconate, 80; bicarbonate (converted to citrate); citrate, 25; citric acid, 47; and cyclohexylsulfamate, 5.

Fluid formulas. In planning fluid therapy, it should be remembered that the rate of loss from the circulation is maximal over the first few hours and gradually declines over the course of the next 2 days. The rate and volume of fluid loss increase with the size of the burned area. Since the amount is determined by the size of the patient and the extent of the injury, the volume and composition of fluid losses can be anticipated. Clinical shock is a preventable syndrome in almost all burns provided that adequate therapy can be initiated soon after injury. Every clinician needs some method for estimating the type and amount of fluid that will be lost so that he can intelligently initiate replacement. Because of this, several formulas have evolved.

It is clear from the discussion of pathologic physiology that fluid requirements are governed by many complex and inadequately explained variables and that it is impossible to express the intricate physiologic phenomena of fluid shifts in burns in simple arithmetic terms. No mathematical formula exists by which all burns can be treated. A given formula should be regarded only as a means of providing the clinician with an order of magnitude of fluid requirement and not as a regimen that must be followed blindly. A burn formula expresses the fluid needs of a patient about as well as the average digitalizing dose expresses digitalis requirements. Just as the internist is guided in the admininstration of digitalis by certain signs and symptoms, the surgeon treating burns varies the fluid requirements predicted by a formula in accordance with the clinical response of the patient. Moore prefers to estimate initial fluid therapy by what he terms "a body weight burn budget." He feels that the term budget is more descriptive than formula. A budget, he states, is a general scheme or forecast plan that must be changed if conditions vary, and according to the needs and circumstances. It is a starting plan, or road map; it is not a precise chemical formula or expression that should be pursued with a compulsive desire to avoid change. It is frequently stated that a burn fluid formula is like a family budget—made to be broken.

THE BROOKE FORMULA. The Brooke formula, published in 1953, is a slight modification of the Evans formula. It estimates the following fluid requirements for the first 24 hours following injury:

Colloids (blood, dextran or plasma): 0.5 ml. per kg. per per cent of body surface burned.

Lactated Ringer's solution: 1.5 ml. per kg. per per cent of body surface burned.

Water requirement (dextrose in water): 2000 ml. for adults, children correspondingly less.

The second 24-hour period requirements for colloids and lactated Ringer's solution are about one-half those for the first 24 hours. In applying this formula to burns larger than 50 per cent, requirements must be calculated as though only 50 per cent had been burned. Usually it is not necessary to give more than 10 liters of fluid during the first 24 hours to any patient regardless of the extent of the burn. If, in a burn of more than 50 per cent in a large patient, fluid therapy based on a 50 per cent restriction fails to prevent signs and symptoms of circulatory failure, therapy must be cautiously increased. One-half of the estimated fluid requirement for the first 24 hours is usually given in the first 8 hours, one-fourth in the second 8 hours and one-fourth in the third 8 hours.

THE EVANS FORMULA. The Evans formula was introduced in 1952. The fluid requirements during the first 24 hours are as follows:

Colloids: 1 ml. per kg. per per cent of body surface burned.

Physiologic saline solution: 1 ml. per kg. per per cent of body surface burned.

Nonelectrolytes: 2000 ml. of 5 per cent dextrose in water, or correspondingly less in children.

Evans recommended one-half these amounts of colloids and electro-lytes during the second 24-hour period. He was the first to warn that in a burn involving more than 50 per cent of the body surface fluid require-ments should be estimated as though only 50 per cent of the body surface had been burned.

MOORE'S BUDGET. The Moore budget consists of giving the patient 10 per cent of his body weight as colloid solution in isotonic electrolytes during the first 48 hours on a descending scale of infusion. The patient is given one-half of this in the first 12 hours, one-fourth in the second 12 and one-fourth in the second 24 hours. One-fourth of the colloid is given as dextran because the low molecular weight component causes a mild diuresis. The remainder is given as virus-free plasma. In addition, the patient should receive 1000 ml. of dextrose in water each day to cover pulmonary losses and 1500 ml. of dextrose in saline solution each day to compensate for his urinary and skin water losses.

THE MGH FORMULA. The Massachusetts General Hospital formula favors a therapeutic approach in which plasma with only a very small amount of added saline is used. In adults, this formula calls for the follow-ing fluids:

For the first 24 hours:

1. *125 ml. plasma per per cent of burn.*
2. *15 ml. saline per per cent of burn.*
3. *2000 ml. 5 per cent dextrose in water.*

For the second 24 hours:

1. *One-half of the first 24-hour requirement of plasma and saline.*
2. *2000 ml. 5 per cent dextrose in water.*

For children, a more precise allowance for surface area is necessary, and it is recommended that 90 ml. of plasma and 10 ml. of saline for each per cent of burn times the surface area in square meters be used to calcu-late the colloid and electrolyte requirements. In addition, an amount of 5 per cent dextrose in water is given according to the calculated normal fluid needs of the child.

THE PARKLAND REGIMEN. Many years ago, at the Parkland Hospital, Moyer initiated a regimen for initial fluid replacement in burns. This regimen consisted entirely of lactated Ringer's solution. Since that time, he has continued to recommend such a program, and those following him at the Parkland Hospital, namely Wilson, Shires and Baxter, have continued their enthusiasm for this regimen. *During the first 24 hours post burn, lactated Ringer's solution is given in the amount of 4 ml. per kg per per cent of body surface burned.*

EIGHT HOUR ATTACH TWO ZEROS RULE. This new formula proposed by Phillips is a very simple rule that was devised primarily as a rapid, simple aid for the determination of fluid therapy in burns in disaster situations. According to this formula, the total fluid requirements for the first 8 hours after injury may be calculated by attaching two zeros to the extent of burn expressed in per cent of body surface involved. Thus, for a 40 per cent burn the total requirement for the first 8 hours would be 4000 ml.

Obviously, this formula lends itself to use in adults only. The same amount of fluid should be repeated between the ninth and twenty-fourth hours and again on the second day. One liter of the amount calculated for the first 8-hour period should be given as 5 per cent dextrose in water, the balance being divided between colloid and electrolyte solutions according to their availability in the area of the disaster.

Selection of a formula. Obviously, there are many ways of calculating initial fluid requirements in burns. It is of interest that all investigators proposing a formula have rather comparable successful results. All methods of calculation seem to give about the same amount of fluids to a burn involving about 40 per cent of the body surface. They vary in amount in small burns and in very extensive ones. The Moore budget and the MGH formula favor larger quantities of colloids and less electrolyte solution. The Parkland regimen uses no colloids and accomplishes the entire replacement therapy with a balanced salt solution.

The Brooke formula is a middle-of-the-road one. At the present time it is the most popular. In 1962, Allgöwer, in letters to more than 40 surgeons who treat an appreciable number of burned patients, made inquiry concerning methods of replacement therapy. He found that most American surgeons follow the Brooke formula. Over the years, the Brooke formula has proved to be quite satisfactory. To bring it into accordance with current knowledge of fluids in burns, however, this formula requires certain specific adjustments. It seems most adequate for a burn of up to 40 per cent in an adult. In more extensive burns, it is probably wise to increase the colloid estimate at the expense of the electrolyte requirement. Certainly in infants, a larger proportion of the replacement solution should be made up of colloids than is estimated in the Brooke formula.

Each individual clinician should use the formula with which he is most familiar. There is an advantage to selecting one method of estimating fluid requirements in burns and gaining as much experience as possible with it.

Colloid solutions. Blood, plasma, Plasmanate, albumin and dextran have been used in colloid therapy in burns. In recent years it has become evident that less blood is required in the first 48 hours than was formerly believed. It is doubtful that any blood should be used in the case of a second-degree burn. Occasionally, in deep burns involving more than 50 per cent of the body surface and in electrical burns, one unit of blood is advisable in the first 48 hours. Thereafter, the blood requirements should be determined by the hematocrit. When the hematocrit falls below 36, blood should be given.

Plasma is the preferred colloid for use in burns. Before it is given, one must be sure that it is free of the virus that transmits homologous serum hepatitis. When plasma is not available, Plasmanate (heat-treated plasma) or albumin may be used. Clinical dextran (average molecular weight 75,000) in saline is an excellent plasma volume expander. It has been used abundantly in the treatment of burns with very rewarding benefits. Because of its protein content, plasma is preferred as a colloid solution by most clinicians.

Gelin has reported that low molecular weight dextran is of value in the early period after burn injury. He believes that this agent is able to increase the fluidity of the blood and decrease the viscosity. He demonstrated that it inhibits intravascular agglutination and prevents capillary stagnation. Further research in the use of this material in burns is necessary before it can be recommended as a routine colloid solution.

Electrolyte solutions. Sodium chloride in 0.9 per cent solution — physiologic or normal saline — is used extensively. It is inexpensive and available in any hospital, but it is far from ideal as an electrolyte replacement solution. Its chief drawback is the excessively high concentration of chloride. The normal concentration of plasma sodium and chloride is approximately 140 and 103 mEq. per liter respectively (Fig. 80). In 0.9 per cent saline solution, the concentration of both sodium and chloride is 155 mEq. per liter, and consequently, such a solution is markedly hypertonic to plasma as regards chloride. Massive infusions of 0.9 per cent saline solution in burned patients are usually associated with hyperchloremia; the plasma chloride concentration may increase to a range of 110 to 120 mEq. per liter. Hyperchloremia, an undesirable and unnecessary complication, is easily prevented by giving a balanced electrolyte solution in place of physiologic saline solution. One of the undesirable effects of hyperchloremia is that it tends to produce acidosis.

A balanced electrolyte solution is preferable. A standard one is lactated Ringer's (Hartmann's) solution. This is not to be confused with plain

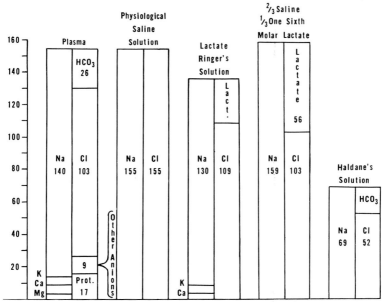

Figure 80. Comparison between the composition of various electrolyte solutions used in the treatment of burns with the composition of normal plasma.

Ringer's solution, which, like saline, contains an excessive concentration of chloride. If lactated Ringer's solution is not available, a solution containing 159 mEq. of sodium and 103 mEq. of chloride per liter can be prepared by mixing 0.9 per cent saline solution and one-sixth molar lactate solution in proportions of two volumes of saline to one volume of one-sixth molar lactate (Fig. 80).

The composition of various electrolyte replacement solutions is shown in Figure 80. The best and most convenient one is lactated Ringer's. In most hospitals, the electrolyte requirement in burns is given with the solution of 5 per cent dextrose in lactated Ringer's solution.

Water requirements. In most burn formulas, the amount of water estimated is usually based upon daily insensible water loss. On the average, this is about 2 liters for an adult. Obviously, in hot climates, in very extensive burns or in patients with high fever, this water requirement is much greater. It is usually administered as 5 per cent dextrose in water.

A rough guide to normal daily water requirements in infants and children is 0 to 2 years, 120 ml. per kg.; 2 to 5 years, 100 ml. per kg.; 5 to 8 years, 80 ml. per kg.; 8 to 12 years, 50 ml. per kg.

Clinical Approach to Therapy

After an approximation of fluid requirements has been made, some thought must be given to the order in which various solutions should be administered. If a patient is seen within 1 or 2 hours after injury, treatment may be initiated with lactated Ringer's solution followed by a colloid solution. The first 8-hour period is the most important because the most rapid fluid losses occur soon after thermal injury. Generally one-half of the first 24-hour fluid requirement is given in the first 8 hours, one-fourth in the second 8-hour period and one-fourth in the third 8-hour period. Fluid therapy so planned should be calculated for the period following injury rather than the period following admission to the hospital. If the patient's treatment has been delayed, initial fluid therapy should be given as colloid. Sometimes it is advisable to give the colloid solution in one vein and lactated Ringer's solution in another. The initial fluid should be given rather rapidly, at least 1 liter during the first hour (faster if seen several hours following burn injury). Thereafter, the rate of administration should be determined by rate of urine flow. At the same time that fluid orders are being written, a detailed worksheet should be made so that there is an accurate and detailed record of intake and output. In addition, all bottles of fluids given during the first 48 hours should be numbered. This simplifies the execution of fluid orders, which may be not only quite complicated but also changed at frequent intervals during the early postburn period. It also enables the physician to note quickly how much fluid has been infused. Unfortunately, there are no laboratory determinations that serve as adequate guides to therapy. Sometimes in the first 48 hours, observations of the hematocrit are helpful. Severe thirst, collapsed veins and hypotension obviously denote a fluid deficiency. The best guide to rate of fluid infusion is the urinary output, which should be measured and recorded hourly. The ideal output in an adult is 30 ml. per hour. The rate of infusion should be increased if the urinary volume falls below 15 ml. per hour and decreased if it exceeds 50 ml. per hour. Excess water and electrolytes in amounts that will produce a urinary output of 50 ml. per hour may lead to overexpansion of the interstitial space. Too often the clinician feels that the patient must be doing well if he is excreting 100 ml. of urine per hour. With such an output, the intake must be more than is necessary, and additional troublesome edema may develop. Excessive fluid administration is a more common error than inadequate fluid therapy. A decreasing blood pressure and decreasing urinary output mean that colloids should be given. A decreasing urinary output with a normal blood pressure indicates that additional electrolyte solution or water is required. Gross hemoglobin in the urine is an indication that the burn is quite deep. In such instances, the kidney tubules should be flushed by forcing a high renal output. This may be accomplished with a high fluid intake; sometimes mannitol is used. This washing out of the hemoglobin in the renal tubules prevents acute renal failure.

Regular auscultation of the lungs and chest roentgenograms to detect the early signs of pulmonary edema should be routine. In patients with burns about the head, cerebral edema may occur during the course of treatment. This is more common in children. It is usually heralded by sudden rise in temperature in a patient who otherwise is doing well. Should the temperature rise to 104° F. in a well hydrated patient, the eyegrounds should be examined. Determination of the venous pressure is one of the best guides in avoiding overinfusion. It should probably be used routinely in all severe burns. It is of little value in determining adequacy of therapy, but when the venous pressure rises above normal, there is positive evidence that fluid therapy should be temporarily curtailed. A venous pressure above normal means that the right side of the heart is being overloaded. Either too much fluid is being given or there is impending heart failure.

It is preferable not to give anything by mouth for the first 48-hour period in extensively burned patients. Vomiting and aspiration may occur. If thirst is severe, and it almost always is, even in well treated burned patients, a few ice cubes may be given by mouth. Frequent examination of the abdomen is desirable. If distention develops, a nasogastric tube must be inserted and then gastrointestinal suction instituted. Acute gastric dilatation is a common complication and may prove fatal unless it is promptly recognized and treated. A record of the pulse and blood pressure should be maintained.

The clinician should plan to evaluate therapy by personal observation every hour. If the patient's progress is satisfactory, it may be sufficient to evaluate his condition every 4 or 5 hours. Such a long interval between bedside observations, however, is permissible only when the nursing staff is trained to recognize danger signs such as oliguria, restlessness and vomiting. One physician must assume complete responsibility for the entire fluid program. If a team of physicians is assisting in the care of the patient, one-man responsibility for fluid therapy is extremely important. This precaution applies particularly in hospitals with a large house staff. Many may advise but only one is in charge. The care of a patient who has sustained a severe burn is a full time task for several persons. Urine must be measured, blood must be drawn, the chest and abdomen must be examined frequently and fluid therapy must be regulated. No formula can provide a substitute for attention to these clinical details.

A real dilemma for the clinician arises when the patient who is seemingly receiving adequate replacement fluids fails to excrete urine. Should this be considered indicative of acute renal failure, or should it be assumed that therapy has not been sufficiently intensive? This is a crucial question, since the accepted method of treatment for acute renal failure is restriction. Fluid restriction leads to almost certain disaster when applied to an inadequately treated patient. Under these circumstances, the best possible course of action is to intensify therapy with whatever fluid appears to have been deficient on the assumption that oliguria is caused by inadequate therapy and that severe organic changes have not yet occurred in the renal tubules. A water or plasma volume expander loading test may be tried. About 1000 ml. of plasma or dextran or 1000 ml. of dextrose in water is given rapidly. The venous pressure is monitored during this period. If the cause of oliguria has been inadequate therapy, this loading test will stimulate the excretion of urine. If the test fails to increase urine flow, acute renal shutdown must be considered. Another aid in such instances is the use of mannitol. This osmotic diuretic is frequently of value in stimulating the excretion of urine in an oliguric patient. The patient with impending acute renal shutdown usually has a low rather than a high urinary osmolarity and a urinary sodium level of more than 20 mEq. per liter. It must be remembered, however, that the most common cause of failure to observe an adequate urinary output is a plugged catheter.

TREATMENT AFTER 48 HOURS

At 48 hours wound edema is maximal, fluid extravasation into the injured tissue has ceased and hypovolemic circulatory collapse is unlikely. In moderate burns, the patient will usually take oral fluids and regulate his own intake. In extensive burns, paralytic ileus may prevent oral fluid administration and necessitate prolonged parenteral therapy.

After 48 hours, most of the fluids should be electrolyte-free water and blood. The most useful laboratory determination after 48 hours is the serum sodium concentration. Hyponatremia is usually present in spite of the large sodium load in the interstitial space. A burned patient who is adequately hydrated has a plasma sodium concentration of 132 to 138 mEq. per liter on the third or fourth postburn day. A low serum sodium in burned patients is associated with a good clinical response and is desirable. The insensible water loss after the first 48 hours may be quite marked—as much as 3000 to 6000 ml. per day in an adult. After the acute stress of the burn injury, the body has a tendency to conserve sodium, and very little is excreted by the kidneys. The loss of water by the insensible route and by the urine will be relatively greater than the loss of sodium. This means that the water load is diminishing more rapidly than the sodium load, and therefore, a rise in serum sodium may occur. The urine volume is not a good guide to therapy after 48 hours. In fact, the urine volume at this stage may be greatly misleading as to the patient's state of hydration (Fig. 81). A urine volume of 1500 ml. has been observed repeatedly despite increasing signs of water deficiency and a rising serum sodium concentration. When the serum sodium rises to 145 mEq. per liter, additional electrolyte-free water must be given. When insufficient water is infused, the serum sodium may rise rapidly. This may lead to a severe hypernatremia. This is a serious complication and is characterized by serum sodium of 170 mEq. per liter, convulsions and petechial hemorrhages in the brain and in the gastrointestinal tract. Should these changes occur because of hypernatremia, they are irreversible and death ensues. Few burned patients with a serum sodium of 170 mEq. per liter survive. Careful observation of the serum sodium is an important requisite of fluid therapy after 48 hours.

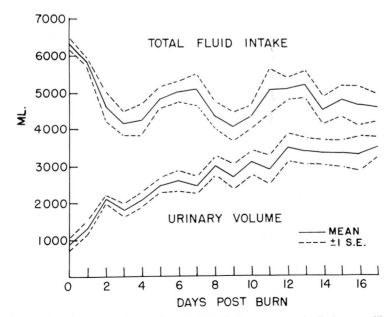

Figure 81. The urine volume characteristically increases gradually but steadily after 48 hours. The data shown in this figure were obtained in 24 severely burned patients.

Sometimes, especially when little sodium has been given initially, the signs and symptoms of salt deficiency develop despite the persistence of edema in the wound and the unburned tissues. These include collapsed veins, poor tissue turgor, a small tongue volume, oliguria and hypotension. It is strange that symptomatic salt depletion occurs in the presence of an increased total body sodium. Under these circumstances, there is no choice but to give fluids containing sodium. The amount to be given depends upon the individual case. The aim of therapy should be to give the smallest sodium load necessary to abolish the signs and symptoms. The plasma sodium concentration is of greater value in regulating the water needs than in regulating the sodium needs.

Although potassium administration must be avoided during the first 48 hours following injury, it is usually indicated after 48 hours. A shift of potassium from the intracellular compartment can be demonstrated within a few days after thermal injury. If the patient can take food and fluids by mouth, parenteral potassium is unnecessary. If, however, the patient must remain on intravenous fluids, 80 to 120 mEq. per day should be given.

In major burns, blood is usually required on the fourth or fifth day. The hematocrit is the best guide to determining the desirability of a blood transfusion in a well hydrated patient. During the first 2 days after burning the hematocrit rises and thereafter begins to fall. Transfusion is indicated when the hematocrit drops to 36.

LABORATORY STUDIES

When a patient is first admitted, a chest roentgenogram and several base line laboratory determinations should be made. These include hemoglobin, hematocrit, blood urea nitrogen, serum protein, A/G ratio, blood glucose, serum sodium, potassium, chloride and carbon dioxide combining power. Electrolyte determinations are of little value in guiding fluid therapy during the initial 48 hours. Hematocrit determinations during this period offer some guide to the clinical evaluation of fluid replacement but should not be the sole determinant for the types and amounts of therapy. After 48 hours, the serum sodium concentration should be obtained each day. In extensively burned patients, a battery of serum electrolyte determinations may be required every other day. When problems exist, these should be done every day along with urine electrolyte determinations. The blood urea nitrogen frequently is a guide to prognosis; few patients survive with a persistent level above 100 mg. per 100 ml. The hematocrit should be determined every other day for the first week and twice weekly thereafter.

REFERENCES

Allgöwer, M.: Blood, plasma or electrolytes in the treatment of burns. *J. Internat. Coll. Surgeons* **38**:421, 1962.

Arturson, G.: Pathophysiological aspects of the burn syndrome with special reference to liver injury and alterations of capillary permeability. *Acta chir. scandinav. Suppl.* 274, 1961.

Brooks, F., Dragstedt, L. R., Warner, L., and Knisely, M. H.: Sludged blood following severe thermal burns. *A.M.A. Arch. Surg.* **61**:387, 1950.

Burke, J. F., and Constable, J. D.: Systemic changes and replacement therapy in burns. *J. Trauma* **5**:242, 1965.

Cope, O., Graham, J. B., Moore, F. D., and Ball, M. R.: The nature of the shift of plasma protein to the extravascular space following thermal trauma. *Ann. Surg.* **128**:1041, 1948.

Cope, O., and Moore, F. D.: The redistribution of body water and fluid therapy of the burned patient. *Ann. Surg.* **126**:1010, 1947.

Evans, E. I., and Bigger, I. A.: The rationale of whole blood therapy in severe burns; a clinical study. *Ann. Surg.* **122**:693, 1945.

Evans, E. I., Purnell, O. J., Robinett, P. W., Batchelor, A., and Martin, M.: Fluid and electrolyte requirements in severe burns. *Ann. Surg.* **135**:804, 1952.

Fox, C. L., Jr., and Baer, H.: Redistribution of potassium, sodium and water in burns and trauma and its relation to the phenomena of shock. *Am. J. Physiol.* **151**:155, 1947.

Fox, C. L., Jr., and Keston, A. S.: The mechanism of shock from burns and trauma traced with radio-sodium. *Surg. Gynec. & Obst.* **80**:561, 1945.

Fox, C. L., Jr., Lasker, S. E., and Winfield, J. M.: Relative lack of efficacy of fluid therapy: comparison of flash burns and scalds in monkeys. *Am. J. Surg.* **99**:690, 1960.

Gelin, L. E.: Local and general effects of injury. *Bull. Soc. Internat. Chir.* **21**:132, 1963.

Harrison, H. N., Moncrief, J. A., Duckett, J. W., Jr., and Mason, A. D., Jr.: The relationship between energy metabolism and water loss from vaporization in severely burned patients. *Surgery* **56**:203, 1964.

Levin, W. C., and Blocker, T. G., Jr.: Studies in burn anemia. Annual Report, U.S. Army Contract DA-49-007-MD-447, 1958.

Lindsey, D.: Effectiveness of gluconate, chloride, and other sodium solutions in treatment of experimental burn shock. *Proc. Soc. Exper. Biol. & Med.* **98**:803, 1958.

Moncrief, J. A., and Mason, A. D., Jr.: Evaporative water loss in the burned patient. *J. Trauma* **4**:180, 1964.

Moore, F. D.: Burns. *In* Warren, R.: *Surgery.* Philadelphia, W. B. Saunders Company, 1963.

Moritz, A. R., and Henriques, F. C., Jr.: Studies of thermal injury; the relative importance of time and surface temperature in the causation of cutaneous burns. *Am. J. Path.* **23**:695, 1947.

Moyer, C. A.: Recent advances in the chemical supportive therapy of thermal injury. *Texas J. Med.* **45**:635, 1949.

Moyer, C. A.: The metabolism of burned mammals and its relationship to vaporizational heat loss and other parameters. *In* Artz, C. P. (ed.): *Research in Burns.* Philadelphia, F. A. Davis Company, 1962, p. 113.

Moyer, C. A., Margraf, H. W., and Monafo, W. W., Jr.: Burn shock and extravascular sodium deficiency; treatment with Ringer's solution with lactate. *A.M.A. Arch. Surg.* **90**:799, 1965.

Reiss, E., Stirman, J. A., Artz, C. P., Davis, J. H., and Amspacher, W. H.: Fluid and electrolyte balance in burns. *J.A.M.A.* **152**:1309, 1953.

Roe, C. F., and Kinney, J. M.: Water and heat exchange in third-degree burns. *Surgery* **56**:212, 1964.

Roe, C. F., and Swersey, B. L.: A hydraulic scale for in-bed weighing of patients. *J. Appl. Physiol.* **19**:820, 1964.

Soroff, H. S., Pearson, E., Reiss, E., and Artz, C. P.: The relationship between plasma sodium concentration and the state of hydration of burned patients. *Surg. Gynec. & Obst.* **102**:472, 1956.

Topley, E., and Jackson, D. M.: The clinical control of red cell loss in burns. *J. Clin. Path.* **10**:1, 1957.

Chapter
Six

INITIAL
LOCAL CARE

The stimulus that provokes the physiologic derangements is the burn wound. The effect of the wound is directly related to the amount of tissue destroyed. Depth of injury, therefore, as well as extent of body surface burn, is important in assessing the magnitude of trauma.

DEPTH OF BURN

The skin is composed primarily of a superficial cellular ectodermal derivative—the epidermis and its appendages (sweat glands, hair follicles and sebaceous glands)—and a mesodermal derivative—the corium, or dermis. These two layers cover a layer of adipose tissue of variable thickness. The skin thickness (epidermis and dermis) varies from 0.5 mm. over the eyelids and the ears to 3 to 6 mm. on the soles and the palms. The entire organ, exclusive of the fat layer, constitutes from 14 to 17 per cent of a lean adult's weight. The thickness of the epidermis, exclusive of that on the palms and the soles, which is very thick (0.5 to 0.8 mm.), varies between 0.06 and 0.12 mm. The area of skin of the body is about 0.25 sq. m. in newborn infants and from 1.5 to 2.2 sq. m. in adults.

Although different classifications have been used to differentiate various depths of burn, it has been common practice to divide burns into three categories: first degree, second degree and third degree. First- and second-degree burns are known collectively as partial-thickness burns; third-degree burns are full-thickness burns. Since the systemic and local changes are directly related to the amount of tissue destroyed, this classification is probably an oversimplification. Greater clarity might result if second-degree burns were further divided into superficial second-degree and deep dermal burns. Third-degree burns should be classified as full-thickness loss and as deep third-degree burns in which the injury involves the underlying subcutaneous tissue, muscle or bone.

142

First-degree Burns

A first-degree burn involves only the epidermis (Fig. 82). It is characterized by erythema that appears after a variable latent period. A first-degree burn may follow prolonged exposure to bright sunlight or instantaneous exposure to more intense heat. Since tissue destruction is so superficial, minimal systemic derangements occur. Pain and a slight amount of edema are the chief problems. The uncomfortable burning sensation and pain usually subside after 48 hours unless the first-degree burn is quite extensive. Since this is only a superficial injury, the capacity of the skin to prevent infection is retained. Healing usually takes place uneventfully. Within 5 to 10 days the epidermis peels off in small scales. There may be residual redness for a few days but no scarring results.

Second-degree Burns

A second-degree burn is a deeper injury than a first-degree burn. It involves all the epidermis and much of the corium (Fig. 82). Most second-degree burns are characterized by blisters. They are usually accompanied by considerable subcutaneous edema. The rate of healing is dependent upon the depth of the skin destruction and on whether or not infection

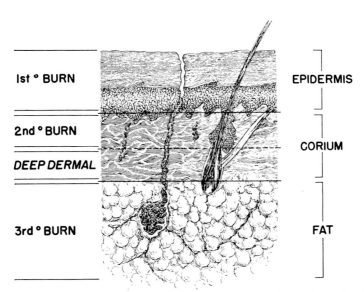

Figure 82. Schematic outline of cross section of skin. First-degree burns involve only the epidermis and heal rapidly. Second-degree burns involve the upper portion of the corium and many islets remain which proliferate to cover the area in about 14 days. Deep dermal burns extend into the corium, and the only epithelium remaining is the lining of the sweat glands and hair follicles. Third-degree burns involve the full thickness of skin and extend down to subcutaneous fat.

occurs. In *superficial partial-thickness burns*, healing usually occurs uneventfully in a period of 10 to 14 days unless infection supervenes.

Deep dermal burns are injuries that extend down deep in the corium (Fig. 82). Epithelial regeneration takes place principally from the epithelial lining of sweat glands and hair follicles. In the event of infection, deep dermal burns are readily converted to full-thickness injury. If the wound is properly protected, however, it will be covered with a thin layer of epithelium in 25 to 35 days. There may be thick scarring. Not infrequently this thin epithelium is injured. This gives rise to denuded areas and further scar formation. When the thin epithelial covering of a deep dermal burn is stretched by motion, blister formation may occur.

The deep dermal burn is of significant clinical importance. It is difficult to diagnose. It causes physiologic derangements that are more severe than those following superficial second-degree injury. It heals spontaneously if kept free from mechanical and bacterial trauma. If infection occurs, it becomes converted into full-thickness injury, and grafting is necessary. Many areas commonly diagnosed as third-degree burns are really only deep dermal burns. By newer methods of local chemotherapy, such as Sulfamylon and silver nitrate, bacterial growth is controlled, and epithelization occurs.

Third-degree Burns

Third-degree burns are a very severe form of injury. The entire dermis down to the subcutaneous fat is destroyed by coagulation necrosis (Fig. 82). Thrombosis occurs in the small vessels of the underlying tissues. Increased capillary permeability and edema are greater than in a second-degree burn. In 2 or 3 weeks, the full-thickness dead skin liquefies, partially by autolysis and partially by leukocytic digestion. This process is usually accompanied by suppuration. Capillary tufts and fibroblasts organized into granulating tissue are found beneath the eschar.

Deep third-degree burns are considerably different from the third-degree burns that involve only full-thickness skin loss. If the burn extends into the subcutaneous fat, liquefaction occurs in that area. Burns deep into the muscle cause increased destruction of red blood cells. The physiologic derangements that occur in deep third-degree burns may be severe even when the injury is of limited extent.

The management of a full-thickness burn consists of the removal of the eschar and the application of a skin graft to cover the wound. If grafting is not performed, a thick layer of granulating tissue will form followed by severe contracture of the area. The only method of epithelization in this type of burn is slow proliferation from the wound edges that occurs at the rate of about one-eighth of an inch per week. The granulations become soft, overgrown and infected, thus hindering epithelization. After months and even years, the wound might heal, but not without considerable scarring and disfigurement.

CLINICAL DIAGNOSIS OF DEPTH OF BURN

Even in the most experienced hands, the diagnosis of the depth of burn is not too accurate, because there are no definite clinical criteria for assessing the depth of burn. This difficulty might be expected because there are various gradations of injury in the extensive burn. In addition, thickness of the skin varies with age and body location. The central area of the burned surface may be full thickness, with a surrounding zone of deep dermal and superficial second-degree burn and first-degree burn at the periphery. One depth of injury seems to fade into the other in such a way that definite demarcation and gradation are almost impossible. There are certain reasonably reliable guides, however, for estimating the depth of the injury (Table 14).

First-degree burns usually occur after gas explosions, brief contact with hot liquids or prolonged exposure to sunlight. They appear as a simple erythematous flush. First-degree burns are dry and quite painful; blistering seldom occurs.

Second-degree burns are caused by short periods of exposure to intense flash heat or contact with hot liquids, or they may form the peripheral zone of a deeper flame burn. They are frequently characterized by the formation of blisters. The surface is mottled red or pink in appearance, and it is usually moist because a plasma-like fluid exudes from the injured area. A second-degree burn is quite painful and sensitive to the air. In a *deep dermal burn* the surface may be moist, but the exudate that forms is not as profuse as in the superficial second-degree burn. The surface has a mottled appearance, with a predominance of white rather than pink or red areas.

Third-degree burns are generally caused by flames or contact with hot objects. Electrical burns are almost invariably third degree. Since the entire layer of the skin is involved in a coagulation necrosis, the third-degree burn is usually dry and dead white or charred in appearance. The skin feels leathery in contrast to the moist, soft surface of a partial-thickness burn. Third-degree burns are not very painful. In fact, the area is almost insensible because the terminal nerve endings are inactivated by the deep injury. The impairment in sensation has been used clinically as a test for depth of skin loss. A hypodermic needle may be used to test pain sensation

Table 14. Characteristics of Various Depths of Burn Injury

DEPTH OF BURN	CAUSE	SURFACE	COLOR	PAIN SENSATION
First degree	Sun or minor flash	Dry, no blisters	Erythematous	Painful
Second degree	Flash or hot liquids	Blisters, moist	Mottled red	Painful
Third degree	Flame	Dry	Pearly white or charred	Little pain, anesthetic

in the injured area. This so-called pin-prick test may show greatly reduced pain sensibility, which is indicative of full-thickness injury. If there is increased sensitivity to pain or only slightly diminished pain sensibility, most likely the burn is partial thickness. One of the best ways of differentiating between second- and third-degree areas is by pulling on a hair. If the hair pulls out easily and painlessly, it is third-degree burn. *Deep third-degree burns* that extend into the other layers beneath the skin are characterized by a charred appearance that is initially sunken and hard.

AIMS OF LOCAL CARE

The primary aims of local care are the prevention and control of infection and the closure of the contaminated wound as soon as possible. Systemic supportive therapy in fluid and electrolyte replacement should be instituted before any attempt is made to care for the burn wound.

There are several principles of local care:

1. Clean the burn wound and remove all pieces of detached epithelium. Dirt and dead tissue remaining on the wound provide an excellent culture medium for bacterial proliferation.

2. Prevent further destruction of the remaining viable epithelium. Mechanical cleansing should be gentle, and irritating local applications must be avoided.

3. Produce an environment on the burned surface that is unfavorable to the growth and multiplication of bacteria.

4. Aid the separation of burn slough, and at the same time, prevent invasive infection and provide a suitable surface for grafting.

5. Apply skin coverage as soon as possible.

6. Secure healing in a minimum period and thereby permit early motion and minimal loss of function.

7. Cause as little pain as possible.

8. Accomplish these objectives without overcommitting the already decreased body reserves. Frequent anesthetics and massive surgery may prevent an optimal systemic response to the effects of the extensive burn wound.

IMMEDIATE CLEANSING OF THE BURN WOUND

After fluid therapy has been instituted, attention may be directed to the definitive care of the wound. If the patient is admitted in poor condition, local therapy must be postponed until adequate resuscitation has been achieved by vigorous fluid therapy.

Every effort should be aimed at minimizing further contamination and achieving a surgically clean wound. All personnel who come in contact with the patient must be masked. The patient is taken to a clean dressing room or operating room. The temperature of the room should be about 80°F., and currents of air should be avoided because they cause increased discomfort. Anesthesia is contraindicated. The cleansing technique produces considerable discomfort but no unusual pain. Intravenous morphine analgesia is usually sufficient.

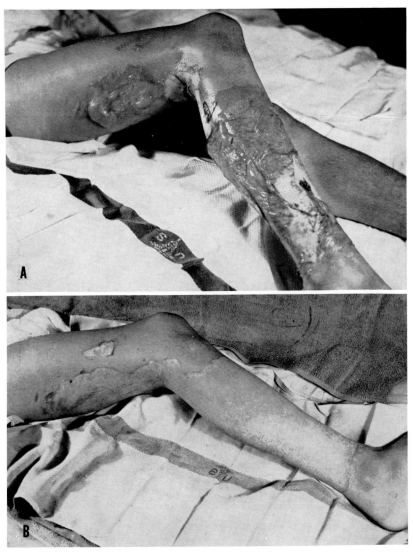

Figure 83. *A*, A partial-thickness burn of the right lower leg sustained by a 9-year-old boy when he was accidentally scalded by hot water. The thin blisters are typical of second-degree burn.

B, The blisters have been broken, and all detached epithelium has been cut away. The area has been cleansed gently with soap and water and care has been taken not to injure remaining viable epithelium. The wound healed uneventfully in 16 days.

The burned areas are cleansed thoroughly. All debris and detached epidermis must be removed (Fig. 83). Greases or ointments that have been applied may be removed with soap. Tars and other oily preparations may be dissolved with benzene. Alcoholic soaps and scrubbing brushes must never be used, because they cause unnecessary trauma to the remaining viable epithelium. The areas are cleansed with bland soap and water at a temperature of 100°F. This soap may be applied with soft, moist gauze pads and removed by irrigation with water.

All blisters are broken, and the devitalized epithelium is cut away with sterile scissors. Some surgeons favor leaving unruptured blisters and blebs because they feel that the epidermal covering provides a good dressing. Most blisters, however, break before complete healing occurs, leaving devitalized tissue on the wound surface where bacteria will proliferate rapidly. Firm, thick blisters that form on the palms of the hands may be left unruptured because they have a tough covering and are not likely to be broken before epithelization occurs.

After all detached epidermis has been removed, the wound is again washed gently with soap and irrigated with copious amounts of warm water. After the area has been rendered as clean as possible, a decision is made as to the type of further local care.

Selection of Method of Local Care

There are many acceptable methods of local care. These may be classified primarily as occlusive dressing, exposure, initial excision, Sulfamylon cream or silver nitrate soaks. Most burn surgeons use all methods. The type selected varies with each patient. In many instances, some areas will be treated by one method and other areas by another in the same patient. Many times, treatment of a burn may be started by one method of local care and then changed to another during the course of therapy. It is impossible to dictate any particular method. All are acceptable and available, and it is up to the physician to select the one most desirable for a particular patient at a particular time. The choice of method is determined by the location of the burn, size of the injury, depth of the burn, type of patient, facilities available and patient's response. Only certain small full-thickness burns lend themselves to initial excision. Most patients treated on an outpatient basis do better when the wounds are dressed. Exposure, Sulfamylon cream and silver nitrate soaks require more nursing care than other methods.

INITIAL EXCISION

Initial excision is a very desirable procedure when it is indicated because it permits removal of all dead tissue and thereby furnishes early coverage of the wound. It is particularly valuable in small full-thickness burns with clearly defined edges. Such a burn is typically found after direct contact with a hot object or in flame burns. Initial excision is indicated in patients with burns not exceeding 15 per cent of the body surface when there is definite evidence that the injury is third degree and the patient is in good physical condition (Fig. 84). Because it is most difficult to determine areas of full-thickness injury on the face, and because of subsequent disfigurement, facial burns should never be excised.

The procedure has two distinct disadvantages: (1) Within a few hours or even days it is difficult to determine accurately the extent of full-thickness burn; (2) the initial injury is compounded by the surgical procedure of excision.

When this technique is elected, excision is usually performed within the first 48 hours after injury. The patient is prepared for surgery after adequate replacement therapy has been given. When areas on the extremities are excised, it may be wise to perform the operation under tourniquet constriction. Under general anethesia, the dead burned skin and subcutaneous tissue are removed down to the underlying fascia. If only the skin is excised, the underlying fatty subcutaneous tissue may slough because of thrombosis of the vessels and leave an inadequate barrier against infection and a poor surface for grafting. Since it is quite difficult to judge viable fatty tissue beneath a full-thickness burn, the safest procedure is to remove all tissue down to the fascia. In addition, bleeding is less troublesome at this level. After careful hemostasis, a large bulky dressing is applied. Skin grafting is done 2 or 3 days later. Some surgeons prefer to apply a skin graft immediately after excision. If the area is very small, this may be desirable, but in most instances, this procedure is not as good as applying a dressing and delaying grafting for a few days. Such a delay gives the surgeon an opportunity for a second look to make sure that all the dead tissue has been removed. If grafting is done immediately after excision, bleeding beneath the grafts may cause a poor take. Delay before coverage also permits the formation of small granulating buds, thereby decreasing the possibility of infection and enhancing the take of the graft.

Immediate excision requires a certain degree of courage and judgment on the part of the surgeon. It is a very excellent method of local care, however, because the patient's rehabilitation can be well under way by the end of the third or fourth week and the period of hospitalization is decreased. One of the pitfalls of immediate excision is the frequent error in judgment concerning the extent of the full-thickness wound. If all the full-thickness burn is not removed, the edges surrounding excision and grafting will become infected and may cause partial loss of the graft. It is advisable to excise generously and to make sure that all the full-thickness burn is removed. Since there are so many advantages to this type of treatment, it might seem that extensive burns could be handled by this method. Unfortunately, this is not true. Even in the most experienced hands, initial excision of burns of more than 15 per cent of the body surface is

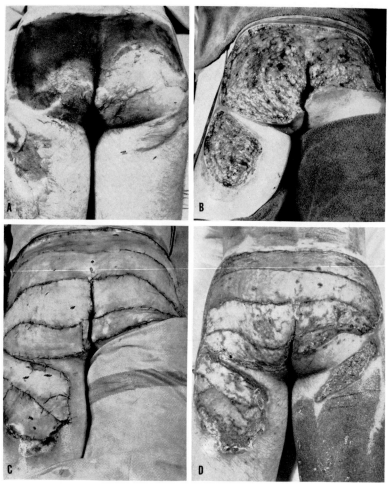

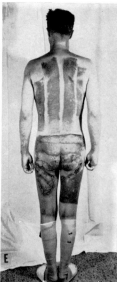

Figure 84. *A,* Deep third-degree burn of buttocks sustained when patient was in an aircraft accident. Area of burn shown in the photograph is only area of injury. Because of patient's excellent condition it was decided to excise all of the burned area soon after admission.

B, Area of third-degree burn has been entirely excised at 26 hours after injury. A large, bulky dressing was applied, and the area was grafted a few days later.

C, The sixth postburn day. Split-thickness grafts taken from the back have been sutured in place. The patient was prepared for this operative procedure with cleansing enemas. He was then given paregoric to prevent bowel movements for 6 days. A large, bulky dressing was applied as a stent dressing and changed on the fifth postoperative day.

D, The thirty-first postburn day. All the grafts have taken and healing is almost complete.

E, The thirty-first postburn day. Patient is ambulatory; the donor sites have healed; and the patient

followed by greater morbidity and higher mortality than other methods of treatment are.

OCCLUSIVE DRESSINGS

The occlusive dressing technique has been popular for many years. For most burns other methods are preferable but dressings can be used advantageously in some hospitals and for certain burns. The aim of a good dressing is that it cover the wound by the best available means in order to protect it from the constant danger of reinfection. Therefore, it must extend 3 or 4 inches beyond all margins of the burn. It should be absorptive to keep the wound surface dry and thereby inhibit the growth of bacteria. The dressing must be bulky to provide a splinting effect and assist immobilization. It must be put on with even, resilient compression so that it eliminates dead space and supports the lymphatic and vascular systems.

The material placed next to the wound should not macerate the tissue or damage the remaining viable epithelium. Because of the tendency of the dressing to stick to burn wounds, and because of the pain and tissue trauma associated with the removal of the dressing, many preparations have been suggested to provide an inner nonadherent layer of dressing material. No preparation seems perfect. Nylon and other finely woven materials have been used as an initial layer in the hope that they would not stick to the injured surface. The disadvantage of these finely woven materials is that the minute interstices become filled with dry exudate and prevent the absorption of fluid from the wound surface by the bulky part of the dressing. Thus, a moist surface is obtained and bacteria can multiply rapidly, forming abundant purulent exudate that is held to the wound. A lightly impregnated water-miscible ointment gauze or dry fine-mesh gauze seems to be the most satisfactory. The ointment gauze can be made easily by placing a roll of fine-mesh gauze bandage in a jar and then adding the ointment and 2 ml. of water (Fig. 85). The preparation is then placed in the autoclave. An excessive amount of ointment does not adhere to the fine-mesh gauze, and the roll is easy to handle. The common ointments used are Carbowax, because it is water soluble, and Furacin ointment. It is doubtful that Furacin has any great advantage in preventing infection, but this ointment does have a pleasant base. Commercial preparations of roll gauze are now available and are very easy to use.

A very absorptive, bulky layer of fluffed gauze should be placed next to the initial layer. Some hospitals prepare thick, one-piece dressings of various sizes. Such burn pads are very convenient, as they save a great deal of time during dressing changes. These are not prepared com-

---

Figure 84. *Continued.*

is almost ready for discharge from the hospital. Ace bandages have been applied to the legs to protect the thin epithelium covering donor sites.

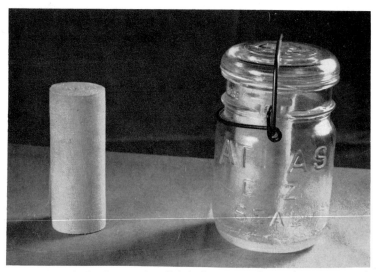

Figure 85. Method of preparing lightly impregnated petrolatum gauze. A 3-inch gauze roller bandage is placed in a jar; white petrolatum and 2 ml. of water are added before autoclaving. An excessive amount of petrolatum does not adhere to the fine-mesh gauze. The roll is easy to handle.

mercially and therefore must be homemade. The Brooke Burn Dressing, which is a mass of fluffed gauze sandwiched between two layers of cotton, has been very useful. In the military service, a one-piece burn pad known as the Universal Protective Dressing is available. This large, one-piece dressing is packed with two rolls of conforming cotton bandage. It has been standardized as a field gauze compress for use by the U.S. Armed Forces and stockpiled for disaster.

The dressing should be fixed in place with semielastic bandage, Ace bandage or stockinette. This must be applied in such a way as to create even, resilient compression on the part (Fig. 86). Avoiding areas of constriction is an important aspect in the application of a dressing. If there is adequate bulk to the dressing and the outer bandage is carefully applied, this will not occur. Too often the patient complains of pain beneath the dressing, and this is treated with a narcotic rather than by adjustment of

---

Illustration on opposite page
Figure 86. *A,* Technique of application of an occlusive dressing. After initial cleansing and removal of all debris and detached epithelium, the surface should be covered with fine-mesh gauze. In this instance, lightly impregnated petrolatum roller gauze was used. Individual strips were applied in a circular fashion. When a continuous circular bandage is used, it does not conform evenly to the part and may become constrictive if excessive edema occurs. It is important that this first layer be applied smoothly and without wrinkles.

B, Large abdominal pads have been placed beneath the leg. The petrolatum-impregnated gauze has been fixed in place with a single layer of dry 4- by 8-inch gauze pads, and a large layer of fluffed gauze is being placed over the extremity.

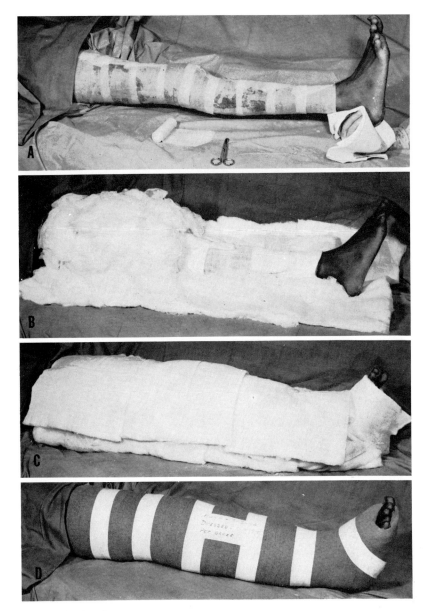

Figure 86. *Continued.*

C, A final layer of large abdominal pads is placed over the bulky layer of fluffed gauze. Although the foot was not involved, the dressing extends down over the foot. When the terminal portion of the extremity is not incorporated in the bandage, there is a tendency for excessive edema formation.

D, The occlusive dressing has been completed by an outer layer of conforming bandage. This bandage has been applied in such a way that there is even, resilient compression over all areas. A bulky dressing of this type immobilizes the extremity, and a splint is unnecessary. Adhesive tape has been used to anchor the dressing in place. By labeling the dressing, information is always readily available as to the time of burn, time of application of the dressing, and the type of immediate covering of the wound.

the bandage. The dressing may become tight after edema occurs. After the dressing has been applied, the part should be elevated to hasten resolution of edema.

Dressings are preferable for outpatients. They provide a great deal of comfort and prevent the danger of additional contamination when used in the patient who must be transported for a long distance. They permit good immobilization and provide probably the most comfortable method of local care. Since eschar separation is enhanced by active bacterial autolysis, third-degree burns are usually ready for grafting a little earlier when treated by dressings. This increased growth of bacteria under a dressing enhances the loosening of the burn eschar. In a second- or third-degree burn of 10 to 15 per cent of the body surface, a dressing is a comfortable method of management and permits the area to be ready for grafting earlier than other methods. In burns of greater extent, local burn wound sepsis may become life threatening; therefore, other techniques that aid in the prevention of infection are preferred. Dressings may be advantageous when it seems wise to discontinue other methods.

A distinct disadvantage of dressings is that they must be changed, and frequently this procedure is painful. Hyperpyrexia is more common with dressings. Their use is usually associated with offensive odors. The chief disadvantage of dressings is that there is less control of infection than there is in other methods.

Subsequent Dressing Changes

The time for subsequent dressing changes is regulated by the necessity for keeping the wound as clean as possible. The dressings must be changed when it is believed that the burned surface has become unduly moist and may allow bacterial proliferation. They should be changed whenever the bandage is stained because a soaked bandage provides an excellent tract for the entry of microorganisms. The first dressing change may have to be accomplished by the second or third day but thereafter only about every 5 days. The dressings should be changed under as sterile conditions as possible. It must be done slowly and painstakingly in an effort to be as gentle as possible. If the dressing is moistened before the innermost layers are removed, there is less pain and trauma to the area. Anesthesia should be avoided, but this is not always possible.

Functional Positioning

It is essential to position injured parts properly to gain the best possible recovery of range of motion of joints after prolonged periods of immobilization. Proper positioning must be started immediately after injury and maintained until skin coverage is nearly complete. Because of contracture, certain positions of immobilization seem best for burned patients. In many instances, these are not necessarily the same as those described by the orthopedic surgeon as ideal for ankylosis.

The neck is kept in as extended a position as possible without undue discomfort. The trunk and hips are maintained in an anatomic position. Almost complete extension is advised for the knees, regardless of the location of the burn. The ankles are positioned in 90-degree flexion to prevent shortening of the Achilles tendon. The shoulders must be kept in an anatomic position, except in burns of the axilla, which require immobilization with the arm in 90-degree abduction. A position of about 140 degrees of flexion is suggested for the elbow. If there is a burn of the antecubital fossa in which there is danger of contracture in partial flexion, complete extension of the elbow is indicated.

The metacarpal, phalangeal and interphalangeal joints of the thumbs are kept in approximately 15-degree flexion. The thumbs are abducted to maintain the breadth of the web space.

The metacarpophalangeal joints of the fingers must be immobilized in almost 90 degrees of flexion. This prevents contracture of the collateral ligaments and skin over the dorsal surface of the joint. The proximal interphalangeal joints of the fingers are immobilized in 30 to 45 degrees of flexion. The wrist is extended.

THE EXPOSURE METHOD

The accepted technique for the exposure method includes initial cleansing of the burn wound and placing the patient in bed on clean sheets in the most comfortable position that best exposes the affected areas. Sterile sheets are unnecessary. The exudate of a partial-thickness burn dries in 48 to 72 hours and forms a hard crust that serves as a natural protective cover for the wound. Epithelial regeneration proceeds beneath this crust unless impeded by infection. In 14 to 21 days, the crust falls off spontaneously, leaving an unscarred, well healed surface (Fig. 87).

The evolution of a full-thickness burn treated by exposure is different. Surface exudation is minimal and crust formation does not occur. The dead skin of the full-thickness burn becomes dehydrated, and it is converted to a thick, tough eschar after about 72 hours of exposure. This eschar serves as a temporary cover until liquefaction occurs beneath it in 12 to 21 days. The term eschar refers to dead tissue of a full-thickness burn; the term crust should be reserved to designate the firm cover over an exposed partial-thickness burn, which is composed principally of dried exudate.

Since crusts are formed of drying exudate, they tend to be elevated above the intact skin. Deep dermal burns, in which exudate is characteristically scanty, form smooth crusts that are level with the intact skin. Eschars shrink because of dehydration and, as a consequence, are de-

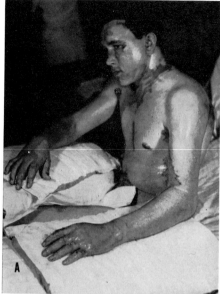

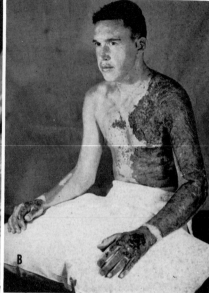

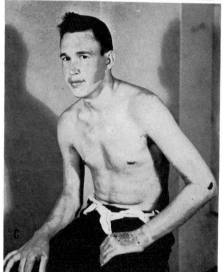

Figure 87. *A*, Second-degree burn treated by exposure. This patient was burned when a gas stove exploded. The second-degree burned areas over the left shoulder, arm and left side of the chest have been cleansed and all detached epidermis has been removed. A plasma-like exudate is exuding from the injured surface.

B, The ninth postburn day. A firm, natural protective covering of the wound has formed from the drying of the exudate. Some of the superficial areas on the left side of the face and front of the chest have completely epithelized. The band of normal skin on the left forearm was uninjured because of protection from a wrist watch. With a burn on only one side of the body, this patient was ideal for treatment by exposure.

C, The nineteenth postburn day. The entire crust has desquamated, leaving a well epithelized surface. There is reddening and diminution of pigment over the burned areas on the face, left arm and left chest; but there is no evidence of scarring.

pressed below the intact skin. The temperature and humidity of the environment influence considerably the rate of crust or eschar formation. A dry environment hastens the development of the protective cover.

The crust over a superficial second-degree burn desquamates in 10 to 20 days, the time depending upon the depth of the injury. In deep dermal burns, the crust tends to be thicker and to remain adherent for 25 to 30 days. In third-degree burns, liquefaction of the dead tissue occurs beneath the eschar. This process is hastened by infection. The depth of the third-degree burn influences the time at which the eschar loosens. In particularly deep burns—those that extend into the subcutaneous tissue— liquefaction beneath the dead skin occurs at the end of the second week. When there is little bacterial growth beneath the eschar, it remains adherent for a longer period of time.

Rationale of Exposure

In contradistinction to mechanical wounds, the local injury of the burn is primarily a wound of area and extent rather than of depth. This may explain the effectiveness of the exposure treatment. Free drainage is always present in partial-thickness burns unless it is blocked mechanically. The excellent drainage of such a burn cannot be duplicated in any other wound. Because of this drainage, only a thin layer of exudate can cover the large surface at any one time. As a result, much of the exudate is exposed to the air. Evaporation and drying are thus promoted.

It is not known how crust formation occurs without infection. When bacteria are transplanted to a new environment, there is a preliminary period in which certain bacteria die off and others fail to multiply. In their effort to adjust metabolically to a new environment, bacteria are thwarted by what happens on an exposed burned surface; the exudate dries and the bacteria are subjected to an environment that is cooler than body temperature. Drying is a deterrent to bacterial reproduction. Although contaminating microorganisms may be present in abundance on the burned surface, their proliferation is hindered, and the dry cover prevents the invasion of bacteria.

The eschar of a full-thickness burn is composed of dehydrated dead skin. As long as it remains dry, it appears to be an effective barrier against the invasion of microorganisms. Bacteria are around the hair follicles and in the sweat glands of all full-thickness burns. These organisms multiply rapidly beneath the eschar. Thus, all full-thickness burns become infected. It is the degree of infection that becomes important.

Technique of Exposure

The technique of exposure may be different in every patient because different configurations of the burned surface pose individual problems. Much of the success of exposure depends upon the ingenuity of the surgeon and nursing staff in achieving a good protective cover. This protec-

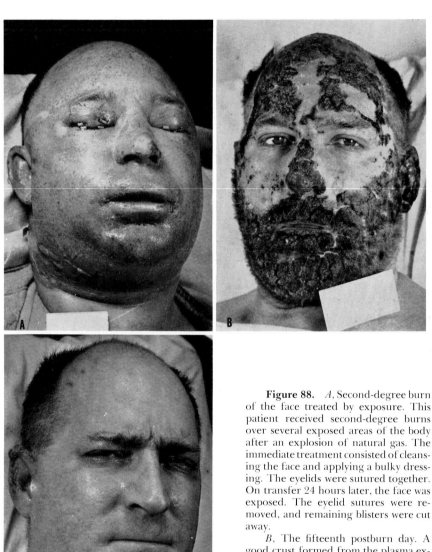

Figure 88. *A*, Second-degree burn of the face treated by exposure. This patient received second-degree burns over several exposed areas of the body after an explosion of natural gas. The immediate treatment consisted of cleansing the face and applying a bulky dressing. The eyelids were sutured together. On transfer 24 hours later, the face was exposed. The eyelid sutures were removed, and remaining blisters were cut away.

B, The fifteenth postburn day. A good crust formed from the plasma exudate, and in the more superficial portions of the injury over the forehead, part of it has desquamated. The remainder of the burn crust is beginning to loosen as epithelization occurs beneath it. All of the initial edema of the face has disappeared.

C, The thirty-fifth postburn day. At this time, the patient was discharged with complete epithelization of the face and no evidence of scarring. A few small crusts from deeper burns remain on the right ear.

tive cover must be managed in such a way as to minimize softening, maceration and cracking.

Burns of the face are easily exposed (Fig. 88). Because of the good vascularity of the face, rapid healing of partial-thickness burns occurs, and eschars sequestrate early. In full-thickness burns, removal of eschar may be hastened by application of saline soaks beginning on the eighth to the tenth day. In burns of the anterior aspect of the neck, the neck should be in extension. This minimizes maceration. In almost every instance, cracks will occur in the region of the thyroid cartilage because of deglutition. Fortunately these cracks are rarely troublesome because the excellent blood supply of the neck promotes rapid healing.

Burns that are circumferential are more difficult to position. In a circumferential burn of the upper extremity, the part may be tied to a standard. This provides elevation and reasonably comfortable exposure. Circumferential burns of other areas of the body must be exposed on one side, then turned and exposed on the other. This is usually accomplished by the use of a turning frame, probably the best is the circular electric bed. If the patient is turned every 4 hours, a fairly good protective covering will form.

One of the chief problems in exposure of circumferential burns is the adherence of the bed clothing or a dressing to an exposed area. It is always painful when the patient is turned because he is stuck to the dressing. Only recently has a truly nonstick, comfortable dressing been devised. The nonadherent plastic dressing (Microdon) is most advantageous in the exposure method of treating burns (Fig. 89). This smooth material does not adhere to the wound surface and is easily pulled away when the patient is turned. Thus, in exposing a circumferential burn the nonexposed burned areas are placed on this nonstick dressing. Should a crust develop to make the dressing adhere, a small amount of water is placed on the back of the dressing, and it immediately and painlessly slides away from the wound surface. Burns of the perineum are difficult to expose properly and drying is rarely seen. Some suppuration is almost inevitable; but fortunately, the skin of the perineum possesses a great capacity for regeneration, and spontaneous healing occurs even in the presence of minimal infection. Eschars in this area become moist and must be removed as early as possible.

Clinically, all patients that are exposed complain of being cold. This is especially true on a cold ward or in an air-conditioned room. Drafts of air make the patient particularly uncomfortable. It is common to hear patients complain of chilliness as a nurse whisks past the bed in her freshly starched uniform. Some type of tent made by sheets and blankets should be placed over the exposed burned patient. In an ordinary hospital bed, a cradle may be used. Children's cribs can be covered with a sheet or light blanket. Electric light bulbs or heat lamps are not as comfortable as blowing heated air underneath the tent. This is easily accomplished with a portable hair dryer.

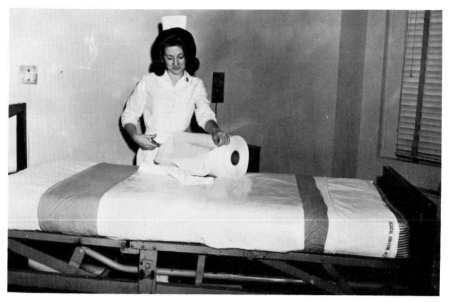

Figure 89. A new type of nonadherent sheeting developed by the 3M Company for use with burned patients. This dressing will not stick to an open wound. Should exudate from the wound dry and cause the dressing to adhere, a small amount of water on the back of the dressing will free it immediately. This type of dressing has been of tremendous value in burns because it removes the pain associated with the wound sticking to the sheet or dressing.

One of the most important facets in the conducting of the exposure method is the constant daily observations under a good light of the integrity of the crust or eschar. Frequently, small cracks develop in the crust, and fluid or pus collects beneath. The success of exposure depends upon the integrity of the crust. When there is a crack, the edges of the crust should be cut away and the area covered with a small piece of fine-mesh gauze.

The patient should be given a detailed explanation of the method. Patient cooperation contributes immeasurably to the success of exposure. The wound becomes very comfortable as the crust or eschar forms. A clear description of the aims and the method of exposure treatment must be given to the family before they are taken to the bedside to visit the patient. Relatives who are apprehensive and near exhaustion may suffer severe psychologic trauma at the sight of the exposed burn unless a complete explanation precedes the visit. This facet of care is necessary if faith is to be maintained in the physician and complete cooperation obtained.

Constricting Eschars

One of the problems in the exposure of full-thickness circumferential burns is the tight or constricting eschar. As the burned skin dries, it contracts, and the coagulated protein forms a stiff, inelastic eschar. A tight, constricting eschar after a circumferential burn of the chest will greatly limit respiratory exchange and can result in fatal hypoxia. Similarly, a circumferential full-thickness burn of the extremity that does not yield to the pressure of edema fluid within it forces pressure occlusion of the arterial supply to distal tissues. Both problems can be solved by escharotomy of the burned skin down to the deep fascia. No anesthesia is necessary. In the chest area, these are best made transversely at the rib margins and vertically at the anterior axillary line (Fig. 90). On extremities, the entire length of the third-degree burn is incised, with particular emphasis on the area of the major joints. Both sides of the extremity are incised if necessary, but only to the muscle.

Indications for Exposure

Most hospitalized burned patients do well when treated by exposure. Certainly the face and perineum are best treated by this method. Most burns of one side of the body surface should be exposed. Some deep dermal burns may do well under exposure, but they are probably best treated with Sulfamylon cream. Because deep dermal burns may become converted to full-thickness injury by infection, every effort should be made to minimize infection in such injuries. Extensive burns, because of

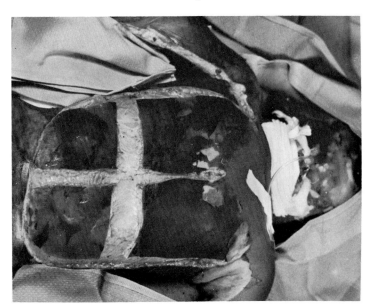

Figure 90. Not infrequently in deep, full-thickness circumferential burns, escharotomies are necessary. These are most commonly required in the lower extremities. Sometimes a circumferential third-degree burn of the chest constricts movement so much that respiration is embarrassed. Cutting through the eschar and into the subcutaneous tissue is not painful and releases the constriction.

the distinct possibility of life-threatening sepsis, do best when treated by either Sulfamylon cream or silver nitrate soaks.

SULFAMYLON CREAM

Studies in recent years have conclusively demonstrated that bacterial infection of the burn wound plays a dominant role in the genesis of mortality in the early postburn period and in the conversion of partial-thickness to full-thickness injury. In all full-thickness burns, there is progressive bacterial invasion of the wound that results in massive tissue involvement when the burn is extensive. Progressive bacterial invasion originating in the burn wound itself and spreading to adjacent normal tissue is termed *burn wound sepsis.*

The aim in local care is to prevent burn wound sepsis. In small burns this is minimal with almost any method of treatment. In extensively burned patients, burn wound sepsis is the most frequent cause of death unless the method of local care is such that it minimizes this complication. It has always been the hope, irrespective of whether treatment was accomplished by dressings or by exposure, that some type of chemotherapeutic agent could be used to prevent rapid and uncontrolled bacterial proliferation in and around the wound. The chief problem was that no agent would effectively penetrate the thick, heavy eschar.

In recent years, abundant laboratory and clinical experience has attested to the fact that Sulfamylon cream applied locally is an effective method of minimizing infection in burn wounds. Originally, Sulfamylon hydrochloride (para-aminomethylbenzene sulfonamide hydrochloride) was used. This hydrochloride salt led to acidosis in some burned patients unless its use was carefully managed. More recently, the acetate salt has become available, and with this, hypochloremic acidosis does not occur. A rapid respiratory rate may occur after application of the acetate, and this important facet is discussed in detail in the section on the use of the drug.

Sulfamylon cream is prepared as a 10 per cent concentration of Sulfamylon acetate in a water-soluble base. The drug is not strongly bactericidal in ordinary concentrations, but in the 10 per cent concentration, it is quite effective against the major pathogen isolated from burn wounds, namely, *Pseudomonas aeruginosa.* It is effective against a wide range of organisms, both gram-positive and gram-negative, and is particularly effective against anaerobes. Sulfamylon is soluble in water, actively diffuses into avascular tissue, is locally nontoxic and is broken down in the blood to produce p-carboxybenzene sulfonamide, an acid salt. The solubility of this acid salt breakdown product is such that crystalluria does not occur as has been so characteristic of other sulfonamides used in this same manner. Unique among the sulfonamides, this drug is not inhibited by blood or purulent discharge, nor is it antagonized by p-aminobenzoic acid.

Application of sulfonamide in a water-soluble base, which itself is 63 per cent water, has resulted in a significant decrease in the evaporative water loss from the burned surface. This reduction has been in the magnitude of 50 per cent, with the concomitant decrease in the metabolic drain on the patient. This has resulted not so much in a decreased requirement for electrolyte-free water, as the Diamox-like effect of this sulfonamide results in some diuresis, but more significantly it has resulted in a marked reduction in the magnitude of weight loss in the postburn period. This is the result of three factors: the first is the decrease in evaporative water loss from the burn wound itself; the second is the control of local sepsis with the concomitant decrease in metabolic demands of both; and the third is the increased caloric intake made possible by decreased trips to the operating room.

Technique of Use

After the burn wound has been cleansed, Sulfamylon cream is applied with the gloved hand much as one would apply soft butter. The entire wound is covered to a thickness of 5 mm. (Fig. 91). The medication is applied twice a day. It may be necessary during the day as the patient shifts position or the bed linens are changed to reapply the cream to certain areas. During the first 48 hours, when the burn wound itself is exuding copious quantities of protein-rich fluid, the topical medication may slip

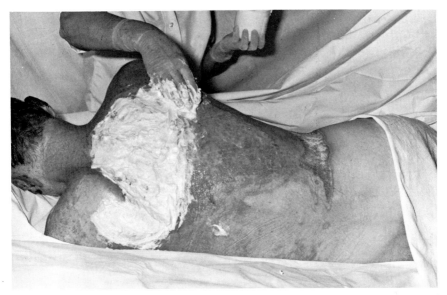

Figure 91. Photograph of back of patient with deep second-degree burn being treated with Sulfamylon. The Sulfamylon cream is put on in a thick layer with the gloved hand.

from the rounded surface of the trunk or extremities, and reapplication may be necessary rather frequently.

During the first few days, while the burn is fresh, a patient may complain of a local burning sensation for 15 to 30 minutes. This is usually not severe. Mostly it is marked discomfort rather than actual pain. But on occasions it requires analgesia. A maculopapular rash characteristic of sensitivity to sulfonamides has been seen in a few patients.

Application of the topical antibacterial agent is not an excuse for surgical neglect of the local burn wound itself. Each day the drug should be washed from the wound surface and an entirely new covering of the cream applied. In most patients, the best way to accomplish this is to put the patient in a Hubbard tank each morning (Fig. 92). This washes off the cream and any excess debris. It also encourages movement and makes the patient feel better. When it is not convenient to use the Hubbard tank, the cream is removed by gentle washing. No dressings are placed over the cream. In circumferential burns, it may be necessary to turn the patient from side to side. As the eschar begins to soften, it should be gently cut away. This progressive debridement of the burn wound, associated with

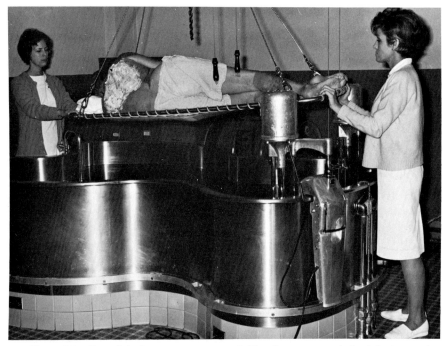

Figure 92.   One of the best ways to remove Sulfamylon cream each day is by immersing the patient in the Hubbard tank. Here a patient with Sulfamylon on his back is shown being placed in the tank to remove the cream. This permits the patient active movement.

hydrotherapy and removal of the topical medication, obviates the usual frequent surgical debridements accomplished in an operating room.

Sulfamylon is a strong carbonic anhydrase inhibitor and thus impairs the effectiveness of the renal tubular buffering mechanism in maintaining normal body pH. In extensively burned patients, the continuous use of Sulfamylon acetate, with its Diamox-like effect, may lead to pulmonary compensation. This results in the characteristic increase in the rate of respiration, with respiratory rates of 40 to 50 per minute. Usually this rapid respiratory rate will maintain the blood pH within normal limits. The effect of this rate over a prolonged period of time in a seriously ill patient is believed to be deleterious. Therefore, when the respiratory rate increases, irrespective of whether or not the patient's blood studies show an acidosis, Sulfamylon acetate should be discontinued for 2 or 3 days and then reapplied.

Control of bacterial proliferation within the burn wound itself has resulted in changes in management. Without topical therapy, separation of eschar is accomplished primarily by means of bacterial autolysis. With bacterial activity suppressed, such autolysis is impeded to the point that eschar separation is quite slow. It is not unusual to see densely adherent, dry, grossly uninfected eschar present 8 to 10 weeks after injury. Previous estimates of depth of dermal injury characteristically included the waxy, white, dry but still elastic burn as full-thickness dermal injury. Whereas previously these wounds required ultimate coverage by skin grafts, the successful control of the bacterial population has resulted in spontaneous healing of these wounds from the epithelial islands that remain.

Indications

The chief advantage of this topical method of therapy is the control of burn wound sepsis. It is one of the few means by which the almost universally fatal sepsis by *Pseudomonas* can be minimized. It is indicated in all extensive burns where it is expected that fatal sepsis might develop. It is very valuable in deep dermal burns because it minimizes infection and thereby prevents conversion to full-thickness injury.

Sulfamylon cream does not sterilize the burn wound. Bacterial proliferation is merely controlled and confined within the limits of the devitalized area. The total bacterial population of the burn wound is reduced from a magnitude of 10 million organisms to 10,000 organisms per gm. of tissue. Sulfamylon cream, although most effective when applied shortly after injury, may be of value as a method of local care in infected burns.

SILVER NITRATE SOAKS

In recent years, Moyer has introduced the use of 0.5 per cent silver nitrate soaks. There is evidence that this method of treatment, like Sulfamylon cream, diminishes infection in and around the burn wound. Its indications for use seem to be similar to those outlined for Sulfamylon cream.

Moyer states that an aqueous solution of silver nitrate (0.5 per cent, or 29.4 mEq. per liter) is an effective bacteriostatic agent *in vitro* and on burn wounds *in vivo* when used to wet thick dressings containing no impediment to diffusion and capillarity. It is nontoxic to man and argyria does not occur during or after its continuous application to burn wounds for as long as 120 days. It prevents the growth of such bacteria as *Staphylococcus aureus, Pseudomonas aeruginosa,* beta hemolytic streptococci and *Escherichia coli* on the burn wound, and it does not measurably interfere with epidermal proliferation. The range of concentration in which silver nitrate operates is narrow. A 1 per cent aqueous solution of silver nitrate kills newly grown epidermis, and a 0.1 per cent solution is not bacteriostatic *in vivo* on burn wounds. A 0.5 per cent solution of silver nitrate is not bacteriostatic for paracolon species, *Klebsiella* and a number of cutaneous saprophytes *in vitro* and *in vivo*.

Technique of Application

All loose epidermis from the burn surface is removed. This requires excision of all blisters and loose epidermis and the wiping off of the non-blistered epidermis that overlies deep burns. All greases or ointments that have been applied to the wounds are removed. This is important. For silver nitrate soaks to be effective, certain conditions must be met. The dressing that is the vehicle of delivery of the silver salt to the wound must contain no impediment to capillarity or diffusion, must be so thick that it holds a large volume of solution and must be in contact with the entire wound. Moyer suggests six to eight layers of four-ply, 9-inch dressing gauze that is thoroughly wet with solution before its application and closely coapted to the wound surface by spiraled elastic wrappings of two thicknesses of bias-cut stockinette 6 to 12 inches wide. This dressing complex is kept dripping wet by the addition of 0.5 per cent silver nitrate every 3 to 4 hours between daily changes of dressing. Kerlix gauze has been found to be unsatisfactory as the material constituting the body of the dressing; it coapts poorly to the wound surface and therefore does not serve as a proper transfer vehicle. The thick gauze dressing must not contain any cotton batting or paper filling. Such dressings will not permit the free flow of silver nitrate solution to the wound. A patient treated by wet dressings must be covered with a layer or two of dry cotton sheeting or a blanket to minimize evaporation and the loss of heat through the dressing.

The removal of eschar as soon as possible is also an important maneuver for securing bacteriostasis. Every day during the change of dressings, the edges of the entire wound are gently probed with a grooved dissector or the blade of flat forceps held horizontally with the smooth surface against the wound at the juncture of the visible pink margin of the wound and the eschar. The instrument is pushed toward the eschar center, and if a plane of cleavage is effected, the instrument is pushed until it meets high resistance or produces pain. The roof of the tunnel so made is cut with scissors, and the maneuver is repeated. Strips and pieces of eschar are then stripped off. Immersion of the patient in a warm water bath one to three times a week assists separation and removal of the eschar.

One of the disadvantages of the method is that on exposure to light silver nitrate stains black everything that it touches. The bed clothing, lounge wear and nurses' and physicians' clothing need to be segregated for laundry because they are unsightly for use except with the burned patient.

Precaution: Although silver nitrate dressings benefit the burned patient, they are dangerous. Depletion of body salts has occurred with the use of this dressing. Biologically dangerous sodium and chloride deficits with osmolar dilution occur in children who have large burns within a matter of a few hours after applying the hypotonic silver nitrate dressings to the fresh burn. It also occurs, but less rapidly, in adults. Potassium deficiency has been seen in cases involving full-thickness burns covering more than 30 per cent of the body surface within 3 to 10 weeks after the burn when inadequate potassium supplements were given. Calcium deficits have also been seen. The danger of sodium chloride depletion with the use of silver nitrate dressing is so immediate that the dressing should not be used without very frequent monitoring of serum sodium, chloride and bicarbonate. During the acute phase, these analyses must be done every 4 hours in infants and children with burns involving more than 10 per cent of the body surface and every 6 to 12 hours in adults with burns involving more than 20 per cent. This frequency must be kept up until adequate oral supplementation is possible, and then it may be reduced to once daily. It is absolutely essential that supplementary sodium chloride, potassium and calcium be given. These supplements may be administered intravenously at first and later orally. Calcium lactate, 4 to 8 gm., should be given each day. If the serum calcium level falls below 9 mg. per 100 ml. supplementary calcium gluconate, 2 to 4 gm. daily, is added. After the fourth postburn day, potassium, 40 to 80 mEq., is given. Daily, 10 gm. of sodium chloride and 30 to 50 ml. of molar sodium lactate are orally administered for burns covering up to 50 per cent of the body surface. This dosage is increased to 15 to 30 gm. of sodium chloride and 50 to 80 ml. of sodium lactate daily if the burns cover more than 50 per cent of the body surface. The above dosage schedules are for adults, correspondingly smaller doses are indicated for infants and children.

Indications

There are two distinct advantages to the use of silver nitrate dressings: improved control of infection and minimization of vaporization or water loss through the burn wound.

Certainly in Moyer's hands silver nitrate dressings have proved extremely beneficial. Their greatest use would seem to be in the very extensively burned patient, where life-threatening sepsis is prone to occur. Unfortunately, silver nitrate soaks are dangerous because of electrolyte depletion unless the patient is carefully monitored and replacement therapy maintained. Additional nursing care is required. The use of silver nitrate soaks is unpleasant because everything turns black. It is undoubtedly a good method of local care if appropriately applied, but it requires much hard work and extremely careful as well as time-consuming attention to detail.

REFERENCES

Bull, J. P., and Lennard-Jones, J. E.: The impairment of sensation in burns and its clinical application as a test of the depth of skin loss. *Clin. Sc.* **8**:155, 1949.

Davis, J. H., Jr., Artz, C. P., Reiss, E., and Amspacher, W. H.: Practical technics in the care of the burn patient. *Am. J. Surg.* **86**:713, 1953.

Monafo, W. W., and Moyer, C. A.: Effectiveness of dilute aqueous silver nitrate in the treatment of major burns. *A.M.A. Arch. Surg.* **91**:200, 1965.

Moncrief, J. A., Lindberg, R. B., Switzer, W. E., and Pruitt, B. A., Jr.: Use of topical antibacterial therapy in the treatment of the burn wound. *A.M.A. Arch. Surg.* **92**:558, 1966.

Moyer, C. A.: Burns. *In* Allen, J. G., Harkins, H. N., Moyer, C. A., and Rhoads, J. E.: *Surgery—Principles and Practice*. Philadelphia, J. B. Lippincott Company, 1957, p. 275.

Moyer, C. A., Brentano, L., Gravens, D. L., Margraf, H. W., and Monafo, W. W., Jr.: Treatment of large human burns with 0.5% silver nitrate solution. *A.M.A. Arch. Surg.* **90**:812, 1965.

Order, S. E., and Moncrief, J. A.: *The Burn Wound.* Springfield, Illinois, Charles C Thomas, 1965.

Chapter
Seven

ANESTHESIA FOR THE SEVERELY BURNED PATIENT

by Burton S. Epstein, M.D.

GENERAL ASPECTS OF THE BURN INJURY

For convenience, the course of the burn may be divided into three phases: initial resuscitative, definitive treatment and rehabilitative and reconstructive. These stages are more characteristic of the course followed by a patient with a large burn. A burn of 30 per cent total body surface in an adult, especially if this includes a sizable area of third-degree burn, may be classified as a large burn. Mortality is considerably increased in burns of this magnitude. With children and the aged, an increase in mortality is noted with less total body surface burn. A patient with a small burn may not pass through all of these phases. Location of the burn is also important. A more marked systemic response may follow deep burns of the face and neck than follows a burn of comparable magnitude in another area.

THE ROLE OF THE ANESTHESIOLOGIST IN THE TOTAL SURGICAL MANAGEMENT

Preoperative Evaluation of the Patient

An accurate appraisal of the physical and mental state of the patient must be made prior to each anesthetic, since the condition of the patient may change abruptly between operations. An adequate evaluation cannot be obtained unless the anesthesiologist is thoroughly familiar with the phases of burn injury and the associated complications. Only in this manner can future problems in the anesthetic management of the particular patient be fully anticipated.

169

Airway. The presence or absence of a face burn, oral and pharyngeal soft tissue swelling, trismus, laryngeal stridor or a tracheostomy will alter anesthetic management, particularly induction. The airway is not only a consideration in the acute burn phase, but must be reappraised prior to each anesthetic, since a face burn may heal, the tracheostomy may be allowed to close and contracture of the neck with limitation in head motion may develop.

Lower respiratory tract. Bronchospasm is a common sign of pulmonary irritation. It may occur during either the acute or treatment phase. It is probably most closely associated with irritation from copious purulent secretions originating in the upper airways, inhalation of smoke or combustion products and pulmonary edema. Atelectasis and pneumonia may be present as in any ill patient confined to bed for a prolonged period.

Circulation. Throughout the phases of initial resuscitation and definitive treatment, the volume and composition of the body fluids change. Protein loss with hypoalbuminemia and reversal of the A/G ratio are common. Electrolyte imbalance occurs. Red blood cells are lost initially, and blood destruction may occur later with septicemia, massive transfusion or increased red blood cell fragility. In addition, blood and plasma loss follow surgical excision, debridement and grafting. Hypovolemia and anemia are always a possibility during the initial resuscitative and definitive treatment stages. Frequent determinations of hemoglobin and hematocrit or blood volume measurements are valuable.

Bloodstream infection. Septicemia may be suspected even before the diagnosis is confirmed by a positive blood culture. Hyperthermia or hypothermia, paralytic ileus, tachycardia and a change in the mental state are highly suggestive. If septicemia has been diagnosed or is suspected any or all of these signs may occur and should be looked for at once.

General state. A patient subjected to multiple operations and anesthetics or even the burn injury alone is commonly in a state of physical and mental deterioration. At a time when food intake is essential, he may not eat. Weight loss and negative nitrogen balance occur almost inevitably regardless of oral intake. Even the patient without septicemia or specific pulmonary or circulatory problems may be exhausted or "washed out." This observation must be made prior to anesthesia, since a patient in this state must be managed with the least anesthesia and physiologic insult possible.

Establishment of Rapport with the Patient

The burned patient is subjected to the mental anguish and psychic trauma of multiple operative procedures and anesthetics. Unless the patient is disoriented, the anesthesiologist must attempt to become a friend—one who will supply comfort, gentleness and encouragement throughout the hospital course. Words of comfort and a soothing tone may also eliminate the necessity for depressant premedication. This takes time but is time well spent. This is best accomplished if one anesthesiologist is assigned to the patient for an extended period.

Maintenance of Nutrition in the Patient

Multiple operations and anesthetics are required to reduce mortality and morbidity and to provide as good a cosmetic and functional result as possible. In order to combat infection and withstand the massive assault produced by the burn injury, the patient must be in the best nutritional state possible. This can be insured only through oral intake of fluids and food. If the best state of nutrition is maintained at all times, it may mean the difference between survival and death. This is partly the responsibility of the anesthesiologist.

ANESTHETIC MANAGEMENT

INITIAL RESUSCITATIVE PHASE

During the early burn period, the surgeon is primarily interested in fluid replacement and insuring the patency of the airway. If the anesthesiologist is experienced in the management of the burned patient, he should assist in the evaluation of the airway and the adequacy of respiration. Signs of restlessness, hyperactivity and apprehension may be secondary to cerebral hypoxia. These signs may also be produced by pain or hysteria, and it is essential to differentiate between these three factors, since therapy will differ considerably in each case.

The only surgical procedure customarily performed in this period is the initial cleansing and superficial debridement. This can usually be accomplished on the ward, thereby minimizing unnecessary and potentially hazardous movement onto carts and through corridors. Debridement can be painful, but sufficient analgesia is usually afforded by the intravenous injection of a narcotic provided there are no signs of airway obstruction, respiratory depression or shock. The intravenous route should be used, since drugs administered subcutaneously or intramuscularly may be absorbed inefficiently by a slowed peripheral circulation. Later, as the circulation returns to normal, an agent previously deposited may be absorbed at once with undesirable consequences. In addition, if the drugs are given intravenously, the duration of action is shortened.

Narcotics should be given in small, divided doses, for example, morphine, 10 mg., or meperidine, 25 to 50 mg., for a previously healthy young male. If this proves insufficient, more can be added. The object is to make the patient comfortable, not to relieve all suffering. If the latter is attempted, too much narcotic may be needed, and this is hazardous in a patient liable to hypotension and respiratory obstruction. If a large dose of narcotic is administered, the patient may claim discomfort during the procedure; however, as the debridement is completed and the painful stimulus removed, he may become markedly depressed. Intravenous injection of a narcotic antagonist is recommended in this case although reversal of hypotension is not assured.

Occasionally, children or adults with very painful areas must be anesthetized by general anesthesia. If this is necessary, it can be accomplished with analgesic concentrations of nitrous oxide; that is, 20 to 40 per cent in the inspired mixture. Trichloroethylene would probably suffice in this situation although the author has no experience with this agent in the burned patient. Again, no attempt should be made to alleviate pain completely, because of the possible consequences of further depressing an already depressed patient.

DEFINITIVE TREATMENT PHASE

The anesthesiologist's responsibility in the initial resuscitative phase is not as extensive as in the definitive treatment phase. Indeed, the bulk of the problems of anesthetic management are confined to the treatment period. This will, therefore, be discussed in detail.

Preanesthetic Management

If sedation or relief of pain is desired, a minimum dose of depressant administered parenterally should be given preoperatively. An average or large dose of a narcotic for a healthy patient may precipitate hypotension, cause prolonged sleep postoperatively or initiate vomiting in a burned patient. If the patient's general condition is poor, the use of any depressant is best avoided.

Atropine or scopolamine in the usual therapeutic doses should be given to minimize secretions and to decrease vagal tone. These drugs are well tolerated even if hyperthermia or tachycardia is present. Hyperthermia is short lived, since body temperature decreases rapidly during operation. Heart rate is not significantly altered in the dosage used for the drying effect. Scopolamine may provide amnesia and sedation and is superior to atropine for decreasing secretions. If disorientation is present, atropine is preferred.

The patient should be encouraged to drink clear fluids up to within 6 hours of the procedure for an adult or 4 hours for a child. This is especially true if the patient depends solely upon oral fluids for hydration. If an ileus is suspected, or if it is impossible to judge the time of the operation, intravenous fluids should be given.

No standard preanesthetic regimen should be followed for all procedures in a given patient. Medication and fluid orders depend on an analysis of the state of the patient at the time of operation.

Initiation of Anesthesia

Establishing an intravenous route. The upper extremities are frequently burned and an intravenous infusion must be started in the foot or leg. Early in the course of the burn a cutdown may have been performed and a catheter inserted. This is an excellent means of access to the circulation either for induction of anesthesia or for administration of blood and fluids. One should determine in advance that the tubing is of sufficient size to accept large volumes of blood rapidly, that it is not leaking or kinked and that phlebitis is not present.

If a cannula is not in place, a foot vein may be sought. These are frequently small, and if an intravenous route is desired prior to induction of anesthesia, a 21- or 23-gauge scalp vein needle is often useful. It is frequently less traumatic to the patient to induce anesthesia by an inhalation agent and to start the infusion after the patient is asleep and veins become more prominent. This implies that the anesthesiologist has sufficient assistance and that there is no contraindication to this method of induction.

Monitoring. Monitoring may also be difficult. If the arms are burned, popliteal artery blood pressures may be taken by means of a cuff wrapped around the thigh. A leg cuff should be used if this is available because of the difference in size between the thigh and the arm. If a leg cuff is not available, any size cuff that can be wrapped around the extremity may be used. Blood pressure readings will usually be 20 to 30 mm. higher in the lower extremity than in the upper. It is important to establish a base line blood pressure so that any change during the procedure may be noted. The absolute value is of secondary importance. Occasionally, all extremities may be burned, or the surgeon may decide to use the unburned extremity as a donor site. In this case, no monitoring of pressure is done. Occasionally, it may be possible to auscultate a blood pressure through a burn eschar. If the surgeon is not operating in this area, this should be attempted.

The pulse or heart sounds should be monitored continuously for rate, rhythm and intensity. In the presence of a head and neck burn, a pulse is difficult to feel in this area. Here, a chest or esophageal stethoscope may prove valuable. Venous pressure should also be monitored, if possible.

Continuous observation of rectal or esophageal temperature may be helpful. A temperature decrease is almost invariably noted, especially in children, and is associated with prolonged exposure of a large segment of the body, use of cold solutions for cleansing, administration of cold blood and the use of an air-conditioned operating room. A reduction of body temperature to 92° F. is not uncommon.

Special considerations in choice of technique. The choice of a method for induction of anesthesia is affected by many factors. If the availability of a vein for starting an intravenous infusion can be disregarded for the moment, the prime factors to be considered are the presence of tracheostomy, edema of the oropharynx or larynx, trismus, face burn (its extent and depth and presence of edema) and vomiting or ileus.

TRACHEOSTOMY. If a tracheostomy is present, the cannula may be removed and a cuffed endotracheal or armored tube inserted after the trachea has been sprayed directly with a topical anesthetic. Unfortunately, all physicians performing a tracheotomy do not remove a segment of trachea; many merely incise it. The latter may give rise to many problems: (1) The incision may be small. In this case, a suction or oxygen catheter may be inserted initially as a guide and the tube then passed over the catheter. (2) The opening may be so small that only a tube of inadequate diameter can be inserted. The opening must then be enlarged. (3) It may take 4 or 5 days for a fistulous tract to develop. If the tracheal cannula is removed before a tract has formed and the patient is dependent upon the tracheostomy for breathing, respiratory obstruction may result unless the tube can quickly be inserted. This is not always possible. It is important for the patient to practice breathing through his mouth before the cannula is removed. If he cannot rely on unobstructed breathing through his upper airway, an orotracheal tube may be inserted while the tracheostomy cannula remains in place. The latter may be removed as the orotracheal tube passes through the larynx. A segment of trachea may then be excised for future use.

Surgeons vary in the choice of the tracheal ring selected for tracheotomy. The tracheal incision is frequently low. After the endotracheal tube is inserted through the tracheostomy stoma it may lie in a bronchus or upon the carina. Occasionally, it is impossible to insert the tube safely more than a few centimeters into the trachea before contacting the carina. In this case, it is better to recommend closure of the tracheostomy or incision at a higher level.

EDEMA OF THE OROPHARYNX AND LARYNX. A patient with swelling in either of these two regions will frequently show signs of soft tissue or laryngeal obstruction. Here a tracheotomy has usually been performed. If not, obstruction to breathing may be a threat to life during induction, and a tracheotomy or intubation of the patient while awake is the safest course to pursue.

TRISMUS. This is associated with a burn around the mouth. It is usually secondary to pain and is relieved after anesthesia is induced.

FACE BURN. It has frequently been advocated that a patient with a face burn requiring general anesthesia have a tracheostomy. This is not true unless there is concomitant airway obstruction. As mentioned previously, a tracheostomy not only solves problems but also creates them. The presence of a chronic foreign body in the trachea, the cannula, may be another source of infection and irritation, and this is often tolerated poorly. Ulcerative tracheitis secondary to tracheostomy is not uncommon in burned patients. The anesthesiologist should not routinely request that a tracheotomy be performed for use in anesthesia unless there is a firm basis for this position.

It has been stated that prolonged, firm pressure of a mask on the face is contraindicated if a burn is present. This is because of the danger of converting a burn of second degree into a third-degree injury. This point requires clarification. If a third-degree burn is already present, no harm can be done. This also applies to a superficial second-degree burn, unless excessive pressure is applied over a prolonged period of time. Firm pressure should not be applied over a deep second-degree face burn unless absolutely essential and then only momentarily, since it is most likely to be converted to a third-degree injury. In any situation, gentle application of a mask is well tolerated for a short time. Thus, it may be used for oxygenation prior to tracheal intubation. A mask should never be used during maintenance in the presence of an unhealed face burn. Edema of the face should cause concern only if associated with edema of the upper airway. If the patient has no edema of the oropharynx or larynx, the morbidity associated with repeated orotracheal intubation of the trachea is negligible compared to the prolonged use of a tracheostomy, where infection is so common and often so severe that it has been the primary or a contributory cause of death.

VOMITING OR ILEUS.   A patient actively vomiting or with an ileus should have a nasogastric tube inserted and stomach contents removed prior to induction. If vomiting occurs early in the initial resuscitative phase, a tracheostomy with insertion of a cuffed cannula may prevent aspiration. If a tracheostomy is not present, the patient should be managed as any other with a full stomach. Intubation of the patient while awake or intubation after induction with an inhalation agent is preferred. No relaxants should be administered, because of the increased danger of regurgitation.

METHOD OF INDUCTION.   It should be apparent that the choice of a method of induction is frequently a difficult one. In general, if a tracheostomy is present and a tube has been inserted into the trachea, anesthesia may be induced with an inhalation agent or with the intravenous injection of a small dose of a barbiturate.

If a patient has an extensive burn of the face and does not have a tracheostomy and any problems are anticipated, intubation is recommended while the patient is awake. If no problems are anticipated or the larynx has been visualized without difficulty during a previous intubation, a barbiturate and relaxant may be administered provided there is no other contraindication to their use such as shock or hypotension, hypovolemia or full stomach. Minimal doses of barbiturate necessary to produce sleep should be used. This should be preceded by a period of administration of 100 per cent oxygen with a mask gently applied to the face. If the intubation proves difficult, the patient may be ventilated by mask for a short time.

If a tracheotomy has been performed early in the burn course and is no longer necessary, it can be allowed to close and succeeding procedures done by mask or orotracheal intubation. Before allowing the tracheostomy to close, it is wise to visualize the larynx directly while the patient is anesthetized so that any problems in exposing the larynx can be noted while the cannula is still in the trachea. If it is extremely difficult or impossible to visualize the larynx and future intubation is anticipated, it may be wise to retain the tracheostomy solely for future anesthesia.

If no face burn is present, endotracheal intubation is advocated if the operation will be performed on the head or neck or the patient is to be turned to the prone position. This is no different from any other anesthetic situation.

A burned patient is frequently apprehensive, delirious or toxic. A violent excitement stage may be noted following induction with an inhalation agent. Small doses of a thiobarbiturate injected intravenously may minimize this reaction.

Maintenance of Anesthesia

Aims.   Although the administration of anesthesia can hardly be expected to improve the preoperative state of the patient, it should do little to alter it. This is true operatively and postoperatively. The patient's ability to maintain circulatory homeostasis and an adequate nutritional state cannot be accomplished if emergence from anesthesia is delayed or protracted vomiting occurs.

Depth of anesthesia.   The depth of anesthesia for maintenance depends upon the surgical procedure and the physical status of the patient. If the patient is a poor risk, anesthesia should be maintained at as light a level as necessary for the procedure. The only valid sign of light anesthesia with many agents is movement of the patient. If amnesia and analgesia are provided, there should be no attempt to inhibit these movements unless it is impossible for the surgery to be performed.

Anesthesia for dressing change and debridement should be conducted in the above manner. The only instances in which there should be no movement are the application or taking of a graft, the application of a dressing to prevent motion of an applied graft and the excision of an eschar in the area where meticulous surgical dissection is essential for a good functional or cosmetic result.

Even in these three categories, these specific procedures will only occupy a portion of the time of the entire operation. During the remainder of this time, anesthesia should be lightened.

Choice of agents and technique.   Nonvolatile drugs such as barbiturates should be avoided for maintenance of anesthesia. In a patient susceptible to hypotension and with possible hepatic and renal malfunction, these drugs may be poorly tolerated. They may not be easily detoxified or rapidly eliminated, and this is hazardous if an undesired effect has been produced. There have, however, been excellent reports with the use of the phencyclidine derivatives, CI-581, particularly in burned children. Investigators have been impressed with the use of maintenance of the airway, stability of the cardiovascular and respiratory systems, absence of nausea and vomiting, and immediate awakening.

There is no indication for use of muscle relaxants for maintenance. Short acting relaxants are well tolerated to assist in intubation of the trachea. In the world literature there are approximately 20 cases of cardiac arrest in burned patients ascribed to succinylcholine. In most instances it is impossible to separate the possible role of this agent from other factors, such as hypovolemia, electrolyte imbalance, positive pressure ventilation, autonomic discharge or general anesthesia. The report by Tolmie et al. illustrates clearly that succinylcholine can cause a large rise in serum potassium, which may lead to ventricular fibrillation. In the experience at the Surgical Research Unit, no cardiac arrest has been attributed to the use of this agent. Another muscle relaxant should be substituted for succinylcholine only if, following its administration, the effects of hyperkalemia are noted on the electrocardiograph.

The anesthesiologist should select an inhalation agent with which he is thoroughly familiar. As long as light anesthesia is provided, most agents are acceptable. There are, however, certain considerations that should be mentioned.

Nitrous oxide is well tolerated, especially if used as an analgesic. The technique of nitrous oxide analgesia requires a close, constant rapport between a motivated anesthesiologist and a cooperative, rational patient. Unfortunately, this combination is not always present. In many instances nitrous oxide does not provide sufficient analgesia for the procedure unless supplemented by agents injected intravenously or unless the oxygen concentration is compromised. These two techniques should be avoided. This agent may be satisfactorily supplemented by the addition of low concentrations of other inhalation agents, such as halothane, ether or trichloroethylene.

Cyclopropane is an excellent agent for anesthesia in the burned patient. It can be used for analgesia or anesthesia, a high oxygen concentration is provided, induction and emergence are rapid, it is well tolerated if hypotension is present and emesis is infrequent. Surprisingly, in the author's experience, cyclopropane has rarely produced retching or emesis in the burned patient. This is probably related to the following: (1) A minimum amount of the agent is used to provide, at most, first-plane, third-stage anesthesia. (2) Most operations are performed on extremities or the skin, and almost no operating is done inside the abdomen. (3) Postoperative pain is infrequent. Cyclopropane may be poorly tolerated if bronchospasm is noted. In this case, an increase in the depth of the agent or the addition of diethyl ether may eliminate the problem. Frequently, bronchospasm may persist in spite of these changes, and it may be advisable to change to another agent.

Halothane is useful provided there is an adequate means available for monitoring the blood pressure. Its use is usually not associated with prolonged sleep or emesis postoperatively. It is particularly useful in patients with bronchospasm. It should be administered with caution if hypovolemia is suspected or hypotension is present. Many authors have noted that the administration of multiple halothane anesthetics to the burned patient has not resulted in an increased evidence of hepatic necrosis.

Diethyl ether in anesthetic concentrations for a prolonged period of time is not recommended. Ether used in this manner is poorly tolerated if hypotension or hypovolemia is present. It may also produce emesis and prolonged depression postoperatively.

Spinal or epidural anesthesia is not usually administered for anesthesia in the burned patient. This is partly because of the likelihood of producing hypotension but largely due to the presence of skin contamination or a contaminated atmosphere in the operating room. The latter is of more than academic interest, especially if many burned patients are operated upon in the same operating room.

Regional infiltration of a local anesthetic may be all that is required for the taking of a small graft. Peripheral nerve blocks are occasionally useful in the latter situation and may also be considered for minor procedures such as incision and drainage of an abcess.

Hypnosis has been advocated to produce an analgesic state and to increase food intake on the ward. This technique is certainly desirable if repeated procedures are necessary, especially dressing changes and debridement. Unfortunately, it is not in widespread use primarily because only a few physicians are trained in this technique. Talking the patient to sleep while an inhalation anesthetic is being administered (a form of hypnosis) should be learned by all anesthesiologists. This is a particularly useful technique for inducing anesthesia in children for repeated procedures.

Controlled hypotension has been recommended by some to minimize blood loss during radical excisions. Again, many anesthesiologists are not familiar with this technique, and even if they are, the problem of monitoring the blood pressure on a burned patient should limit its acceptability.

Specific problems and their management. A patient who is burned may have a low blood volume or anemia at various times during the course of the burn. This should be diagnosed preoperatively and the volume or red cell deficit replaced at this time. Blood loss during extensive debridement or grafting procedures may be significant. Great quantities of blood may be lost rapidly during excision of an eschar. If acute blood loss is anticipated, and it will be after experience is gained, blood should be infused as anesthesia is begun. If the operation is well under way and blood pressure has already started to fall, it may be too late. Since it is often difficult to administer blood to a child rapidly, it has been helpful to infuse children with 10 ml. of blood per kg. body weight prior to surgery. This amount is well tolerated.

Measurement of blood loss is helpful if a method is available. Weighing of sponges may be difficult because of the frequent use of wet sponges. With experience, some degree of accuracy can be acquired in visually estimating blood loss for a given type of procedure. Initially, however, the estimate is invariably lower than the actual loss. Isotope dilution blood volume determinations, frequent observation of serial hematocrits and measurement of central venous pressure are useful if a base line has been obtained prior to surgery.

The use of tourniquets on the arms or legs for surgery of the extremity, particularly for excision of an eschar, is helpful in decreasing blood loss. This technique presents a few problems, however. Blood loss may be minimal while the tourniquets are inflated. There is frequently considerable loss of blood as the tourniquets are deflated. If this is not anticipated, the effect of release of the tourniquets with reactive hyperemia combined with acute loss of blood may result in shock. Even if the volume of blood loss is anticipated, it is easy to infuse too much blood when the tourniquets are inflated, since the effective circulation is diminished and a relative overtransfusion may occur. It is probably safest to infuse blood slowly while the tourniquets are inflated and increase the infusion rate rapidly if necessary as one tourniquet is released at a time. If the blood pressure falls precipitously, the tourniquet should be reinflated and more blood infused.

In heat regulation, the skin is the most important organ. A burn of the skin and the use of skin as a donor site will remove a considerable portion of the body's temperature-regulating mechanism. Septicemia and the use of bulky dressings may produce hyperthermia up to 105 or 106° F. Usually no extraordinary measures to lower body temperature are necessary preoperatively, since this temperature invariably falls rapidly once the patient has been in the operating room. Factors producing this fall have been mentioned previously. Hypothermia should be minimized, especially in children. This can be accomplished in part by turning off the air-conditioning unit, using warm rinse solutions, warming the blood before or during infusion and by use of anesthesia in low concentrations to minimize hypotension. Temperature drop is also directly proportional to the length of the procedure and results in constantly decreasing pulse rate. This is seen more often in children than in adults.

Patients who have been bedridden for months, who may be hypovolemic or who suffer acute blood loss during surgery tolerate changes in body position poorly. During the operation, turning the patient is frequently necessary, since the burn may involve multiple areas of the body. In addition, various portions of the body may serve as donor areas necessitating a change in position to take the graft. If a change in position is essential, it should be done slowly. Vital signs should be carefully noted before and after a turn. If a patient is critically ill, it may be best not to turn him at all. Anesthesia should be lightened prior to turning to allow the patient full use of his compensatory reflexes. Blood replacement must be adequate before turning.

Tachycardia of 140 to 200 beats per minute is not uncommon if septicemia or hyperthermia is present. It may be difficult to decrease this rate during anesthesia, but usually it is fairly well tolerated. A change in pulse volume, rate or rhythm is usually more significant than the rate itself. It is especially important to use as light a level of anesthesia as possible in any of these conditions to avoid myocardial depression. This is also true if myocarditis or endocarditis is suspected with septicemia.

Bronchospasm occurs repeatedly in certain patients. As has been reported in bronchial asthma, halothane is particularly effective in reversing or preventing bronchospasm in the burned patient. Cyanosis has been reported during emergence, particularly in a patient with pre-existing pulmonary problems. Although the specific cause of this is somewhat obscure, 100 per cent oxygen should be administered and the patient retained in the operating room until the cause has been determined or the situation reversed.

Emergence from Anesthesia

Many operative procedures for burns are not painful. Even when they are, however, the routine injection of narcotics before the end of the operation is not recommended. In many patients, the pain is well tolerated even without the use of narcotics. Analgesics can be administered once undue reaction to pain has been demonstrated. If they are used routinely, the patient will be depressed postoperatively, or vomiting may extend the time before which he may resume oral feedings.

Before leaving the operating room, the anesthesiologist should be convinced that the patient can tolerate a move onto a litter, through the corridors, possibly in an elevator and back to his bed. It is easier to treat any problems in the operating room, where equipment and personnel are available. This may be impossible if the patient is in transit.

REHABILITATIVE AND RECONSTRUCTIVE PHASE

Usually, further grafting and cosmetic and functional reconstructive procedures are performed in this stage. The patient is generally in better health and can be handled like any other patient coming to surgery. There is, however, one problem that requires elaboration. This is a neck contracture.

A third-degree burn of the neck may be associated with considerable scarring and contraction of this area in the late treatment or rehabilitative and reconstructive phase. The chin frequently is pulled down to rest on the chest. Extension of the head is frequently impossible. If further operations are required, and they most certainly will be at least to release this contracture, tracheal intubation may be difficult or impossible. It is probably best to attempt intubation through the nose or mouth while the patient is awake. In children, it may be necessary to attempt intubation during administration of an inhalation agent. If these efforts are unsuccessful and a tracheal tube is needed, the surgeon may incise the contracture while the patient is under light anesthesia. Once the tension of the contracture is relieved, extension of the head and intubation may prove easier. CI-581 may also be useful in the patient with a contracture of the neck, since airway destruction may not occur, even when adequate analgesia is provided.

Some surgeons prefer to perform a tracheotomy using local anesthesia. Since contractures frequently occur months after the burn injury, a tracheotomy should not be performed early in the burn course even if a contracture is anticipated. The tracheostomy may be poorly tolerated for this length of time and may be a source of chronic irritation and infection. If this operation is performed late in the course of the burn, when the patient is well and requires little or no suctioning, it produces little or no complications. A tracheostomy at this time will not only serve as a route for induction of anesthesia but also will insure the patency of the airway postoperatively if a bulky dressing is placed around the neck to minimize motion of the graft.

STERILIZATION OF EQUIPMENT

A burned patient is usually heavily contaminated with bacteria. If a deep burn is present in or around the head and neck area, the anesthetic equipment may be contaminated. Following the anesthetic, all equipment should be rinsed and scrubbed with water and then sterilized. Autoclaving is injurious to much of the equipment, particularly rubber. Antiseptic solutions may be effective in eliminating bacteria from sources that they can reach and diminish the degree of contamination in other areas; however, it is frequently impossible to eradicate completely bacteria from the rebreathing bag and tubing. This is probably because the solution cannot enter every crevice in these areas. The only way to sterilize completely all the equipment without excessive injury is by the use of ethylene oxide. If available, this method is recommended.

REFERENCES

Allen, C. R., and Slocum, H. C.: The function of the anesthesiologist in the management of the patient with extensive burns. *Anesthesiology* 13:65, 1952.

Artz, C. P., and Reiss, E.: *The Treatment of Burns*, 1st ed. Philadelphia, W. B. Saunders Company, 1957.

Beecher, H. W.: Resuscitation and sedation of patients with burns which include the airway. *Ann. Surg.* 117:825, 1942.

Belin, R. P., and Karleen, C. I.: Cardiac arrest in the burned patient following succinyldicholine administration. *Anesthesiology* 27:516, 1966.

Benway, R. E., Maier, E. S., and Jenicek, J. A.: Anesthetic management of the severely burned patient. *Am. J. Surg.* 103:677, 1962.

Bernstein, N. R.: Observations on the use of hypnosis with burned children on a pediatric ward. *Internat. J. Clin. Exper. Hypnosis* 13:1, 1965.

Burns and the airway, a challenge in anesthesia. *New York J. Med.* **62**:2023, 1962.

Bush, G. H., Graham, H. A. P., Littlewood, A. H. M., and Scott, L. B.: Dangers of suxamethonium and endotracheal intubation in anesthesia for burns. *Brit. M. J.* **2**:1081, 1962.

Crasilneck, H. B., Stirman, J. A., Wilson, B. J., McCranie, E. J., and Fogelman, M. J.: Use of hypnosis in the management of patients with burns. *J.A.M.A.* **158**:103, 1955.

Epstein, B. S., Hardy, D. L., Harrison, H. N., Teplitz, C., Villarreal, Y., and Mason, A. D.: Hypoxemia in the burned patient: a clinical pathologic study. *Ann. Surg.* **158**:924, 1963.

Epstein, B. S., Rose, L. R., Teplitz, C., and Moncrief, J. A.: Experiences with low tracheostomy in the burn patient. *J.A.M.A.* **183**:966, 1963.

Epstein, B. S., Rudman H., Hardy, D. L., and Downes, H.: Comparison of orotracheal intubation with tracheostomy for anesthesia in patients with face and neck burns. *Anesth. & Analg.* **43**:352, 1966.

Lowenstein, E.: Succinylcholine administration in the burned patient. *Anesthesiology* **27**:494, 1966.

McCaughey, T. J.: Burn mortality and the anaesthetist. *Canad. Anaesth. Soc. J.* **10**:501, 1963.

Middleton, H. G.: Anesthesia for burned children. *Proc. Roy. Soc. Med.* **50**:888, 1957.

Middleton, H. G., and Wolfson, L. J.: Anaesthesia in burns. *Brit. M. Bull.* **14**:42, 1958.

Paton, W. D. M.: Mode of action of neuromuscular blocking agents. *Brit. J. Anaesth.* **28**:470, 1956.

Pickrell, K. L., Stephen, C. R., Broadbent, T. R., Masters, F. W., and Georgiade, N. G.: Self-induced "trilene" analgesia in plastic surgery, with special reference to the burned patient. *Plast. & Reconstruct. Surg.* **9**:345, 1952.

Roe, C. F., Kinney, J. M., and Blair, C. S.: The effect of anesthesia on energy exchange in third degree burns. *Surg. Gynec. & Obst.* **120**:1207, 1965.

Shannon, D. W.: An anaesthetist looks at a burnt child. *Lancet* **1**:111, 1955.

Snow, J. C., Mangiaracine, A. B., and Anderson, M. L.: Sterilization of anesthesia equipment with ethylene oxide. *New England J. Med.* **266**:443, 1962.

Teplitz, C., Epstein, B. S., Rose, L. R., and Moncrief, J. A.: Necrotizing tracheitis induced by tracheostomy tube. *A.M.A. Arch. Path.* **77**:6, 1964.

Teplitz, C., Epstein, B. S., Rose, L. R., and Moncrief, J. A.: Pathology of low tracheostomy in children. *Am. J. Clin. Path.* **42**:58, 1964.

Tolmie, J. D., Joyce, T. H., and Mitchell, G. D.: Succinylcholine danger in the burned patient. *Anesthesiology* **28**:467, 1967.

Visser, E. R., and Tarrow, A. B.: Fluothane for multiple burn dressing anesthetics. *Anesth. & Analg.* **38**:301, 1959.

Wilson, R. D., Nichols, R. J., and McCoy, N. R.: Dissociative anesthesia with CI-581 in burned children. *Anesth. & Analg.* **46**:719, 1966.

Chapter
Eight

REPAIR OF
FULL-THICKNESS BURNS

The closure of the full-thickness burn wound may be accomplished in many ways. Much depends upon the type of local care, the configuration of the burn and the general physical condition of the patient. Since the ultimate aim in the care of a burned patient is the closure of the burn wound, its repair is extremely important. It should be approached with a definite degree of aggressiveness. The sooner the eschar is removed and a skin graft applied, the quicker the recovery. The burn wound is a continuing insult to the body, and it should be closed as early as possible to avoid general debilitation of the patient.

In some small burns, the eschar can be excised early and the skin graft applied. In patients with larger injuries, bold excision of massive amounts of tissue is more than the patient can withstand; therefore, it is wise to wait until the eschar has separated and then apply a graft. The general attitude should be to make an attempt to remove the eschar and accomplish the grafting as early and as rapidly as the patient's general condition will permit. In large wounds, separation of the third-degree area can usually be accomplished by the fourth postburn week, by which time the accompanying second-degree burn has healed. Irrespective of the size of the injury, the general condition of the patient or the type of local care, the first grafting procedure should be accomplished at least by the thirtieth postburn day. When the newer local antibacterial treatments are used, the eschar remains firmly attached and free of infection for a much longer period than when dressings or simple exposure methods are used. Local antibacterial treatment, however, has a tendency to delay grafting somewhat. If by the thirtieth day the eschar has not started to loosen, surgical removal of this eschar should be accomplished and the underlying tissue prepared for skin grafting while the patient is under anesthesia.

INITIAL EXCISION OF
FULL-THICKNESS BURNS

Initial or immediate excision is a very desirable method of management for some small full-thickness burn wounds. The indications and a description of management for this technique are given in Chapter Six.

REMOVAL OF ESCHAR

One of the most difficult aspects of the repair of full-thickness burns is the removal of the eschar. As long as the eschar remains in place, it provides dead tissue for the rapid proliferation of underlying bacteria. In spite of intensive investigation with various enzymes and chemicals, no solution or agent has been found that will dissolve the eschar.

There are several acceptable techniques for removal of the eschar, and their desirability depends upon the type of local care, location and extent of burn, general condition of the patient and the facilities available. These methods include repeated changes of dry dressings, daily soaking in a Hubbard tank, wet soaks and surgical excision under anesthesia. The surgeon usually selects the method best suited to his patient and his institution. Sometimes two or three methods are used for the same patient.

Repeated change of dry dressings is an acceptable technique, especially in burns of limited extent treated initially by the occlusive dressing method. The dressing is usually changed every 4 or 5 days. This helps to keep the area clean and provides for adequate drainage. When dressings are used, the dead skin softens, and bacterial activity beneath the eschar causes it to loosen. Third-degree burn wounds treated by dressings usually have a much greater degree of infection than those treated by other methods. This large growth of bacteria beneath the eschar causes it to loosen and sequestrate. This means that an area treated by dressings is usually ready for grafting earlier than one treated by other methods of local care, but there is always an increased amount of infection. If repeated changes of dry dressings are used as a method of removal of eschar, particular attention must be paid to the degree of infection on the burn wound. If infection gets out of control, then another method of local care, such as daily baths in the Hubbard tank or wet soaks, should be used.

With repeated changes of dry dressings, it may be necessary to accomplish the change in an operating room under light general anesthesia. When this is done, all loose tissue should be removed. A good rule of thumb is to use a pair of scissors to cut the collagen strands that hold the eschar but not to cut deeply enough to cause bleeding. Invasive infection is a constant danger during the sloughing stage; therefore, removal of the eschar must be accomplished as gently and expeditiously as possible. The surgeon should remove the dead tissue in such a way that a good granulating barrier develops as the eschar is removed.

A daily bath in the Hubbard tank is an excellent method of removing eschar. It provides excellent drainage for the wound, keeps the area clean and softens the eschar, thus hastening its removal. This method requires a Hubbard tank and a team of people devoted to the care of burned patients. It is an especially good method when local care is accomplished by the use of Sulfamylon cream.

The patient is bathed each day in a Hubbard tank; this provides gentle cleansing of the burn wound and an excellent opportunity for movement of all joints. Since water is hypotonic, the patient should remain in the tank only 15 or 20 minutes. The most comfortable water temperature is 100°F. Loose dead tissue is pulled or gently cut away while the patient is in the tank or immediately thereafter. Usually the patient is very cold after he is removed from the tank and considerable nursing care is required to keep him warm. After the bath the burn surface may be covered with Sulfamylon cream or with one layer of fine-mesh gauze. Most patients like this technique because they feel good when they are in the water, and they are able to maintain motion in the extremities. When this technique is used, it is advantageous to ask the physical therapist to work with the patient for continued exercise between baths. Since this technique is so desirable, every burn unit or ward should have a Hubbard tank in the area.

Wet soaks are a good method of removing eschar and preparing the recipient site for grafting. The wet dressings keep the eschar soft, and when they are changed, any loose areas of dead tissue are removed. When the wound is severely infected, the wet soak method is particularly desirable. It provides good drainage, accomplishes some debridement and permits frequent inspection of the area. The best technique is the application of comfortable wet saline soaks with coarse-mesh gauze every 4 hours. Frequent removal of the wet gauze pads pulls away dead tissue. The dressings are more comfortable when kept warm. Although this is difficult, an Aqua-K pad over the wet dressings will provide heat and comfort. At least once a day, forceps should be used to clean the wound as thoroughly as possible. As soon as the eschar loosens, scissors may be used to cut the collagenous bands that hold the eschar. The wound should be inspected each day, and a concentrated effort should be made to remove any dead loose tissue. Although wet soaks are an excellent method of removing eschar, this method is a time-consuming one. A tremendous amount of nursing care is required to apply dressings properly and on schedule. Soaks must be kept moist, and gentleness is essential in making the change of dressing. The wet soak method is good for many areas of the body but is of especial value in removing eschars from the face.

When silver nitrate soaks are used, the eschar softens during the course of therapy. As the eschar begins to loosen, great care should be taken to remove gently the dead skin as it begins to sequestrate. Blunt scissors may be pushed gently beneath the eschar and used to cut the collagen bands. Active bleeding should be avoided.

Surgical debridement is the quickest method for removing an eschar, but it has some serious disadvantages. If the patient has suffered extensive burns, cutting away the eschar is a formidable procedure that entails general anesthesia and considerable blood loss. It may predispose to a breakdown of the body's defense mechanisms against infection. It may open avenues for invasive infection. If the wound is not too large and the patient is in good condition, it is a desirable method for removal of eschar. In some burns that are not too extensive, it can be accomplished on the tenth to the twelfth day. In more extensive burns where the difference between partial- and full-thickness injury is not so obvious in the first 2 weeks, surgical excision can be performed on approximately the twenty-first day. In treatment with Sulfamylon, it may be necessary to remove the eschar on approximately the twenty-eighth day. Surgical debridement is usually accompanied by considerable blood loss; it is imperative that the patient's blood volume be at a normal level before this is undertaken. There is always more blood loss than the surgeon anticipates; an adequate quantity of blood should be ready for use during the operative procedure. The eschar is cut away as gently and as rapidly as possible. If it has started to loosen, it may be pulled away with a limited amount of sharp dissection. The surgical debridement should include only the dead burned area, not the entire subcutaneous tissue. After the dead tissue is excised, great care must be taken to obtain good hemostasis. The area may then be covered by a large bulky dry dressing, wet soaks or homografts. Sometimes it is advantageous to remove the dry dressing in 3 or 4 days and apply wet soaks to prepare the recipient site for grafting.

PREPARATION OF RECIPIENT SITE FOR GRAFTING

In most instances continuation of the method used for removal of eschar yields a surface upon which an optimal graft take may be expected. As soon as all the dead tissue is off the wound, the graft should be applied. One should not wait for thick, abundant granulations. The sooner the graft is applied, the better will be the take.

It is almost impossible and certainly unnecessary to sterilize the granulating surface. If the amount of purulent material and bacterial proliferation is minimal, a graft will usually take unless the surface is contaminated by certain organisms, such as group A beta hemolytic streptococci. When a large amount of purulent material caused by any bacteria is present, the graft may not adhere to the underlying surface. In such instances wet soaks usually provide good drainage and are an excellent technique for clearing the wound of pus. If group A beta hemolytic streptococci are present, an antibiotic should be given systemically and local chemotherapeutic agents applied to the wound.

One of the best ways to prepare the recipient site is frequent changes of homografts. Placing homograft skin over the area, permitting it to stay for 4 days, removing it and putting on another homograft is an excellent way to keep the wound clean. This usually produces a flat granulating surface with a minimal number of bacteria.

When grafting has been delayed for some reason, soft, pale, edematous granulation tissue is often present. A skin graft does not take well on such granulations. They must be shaved or scraped down to the base, and a dressing must be applied for 2 days. If grafts are applied immediately after removing the granulations, hematomas will form beneath the grafts and cause a poor take. In old wounds, if for some reason it was impossible to apply a graft, there may be a considerable amount of fibrous tissue beneath the granulations. In such instances it is advisable to excise the entire area down to the fascia and apply a dressing, then graft 2 or 3 days later.

PLANNING THE GRAFTING

As the eschar is being removed and the recipient site prepared, the patient must be kept in the best possible nutritional state; blood transfusions are given in an effort to maintain the hematocrit at 40 or above. One should plan the grafting procedure, keeping in mind the priority of certain areas for skin coverage and the availability of donor sites. Since skin grafts take best in the early postburn period, plans should be made to cover as much of the burn wound as possible at the first grafting procedure. If a patient is extensively burned, it is advantageous to have three or four surgeons assist in the transfer of skin. When it is not possible to autograft all of the wound and the patient's general condition is endangered by serious infection, available autografts may be used to cover as much of the wound as possible and homografts used for the remainder. Plastic foams and other types of artificial skin have been tried as temporary cover of the wound, but at present none is of any value.

If more than one grafting procedure appears to be necessary, it is wise to set up a tentative time schedule with plans to cover one surface at one time and another surface at a specific time several days later. Subsequent grafting procedures should be performed as soon as reasonable. The grafting should be planned with the patient's ultimate rehabilitation in mind. If, for instance, by the application of a small graft to one arm the patient would be able to feed himself, high priority should be given to grafting that area. At an early stage, the initial application of a few skin grafts to the lower extremity may permit the patient to be out of bed. This hastens his convalescence.

Priority of Areas for Skin Coverage

Certain areas of the body should be given consideration for coverage before others (Fig. 93). Areas around joints should be grafted before the large, flat surfaces. Priority for skin coverage is as follows: hands and face

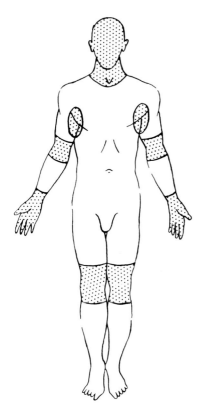

Figure 93. Priority areas for skin coverage. The hands and face must be given the highest priority for skin coverage. Areas of motion, such as the axilla, elbows, and knees, should be covered early to prevent contracture and to allow for early return of function.

first, with special priority to the hands; then areas of motion, especially those about the elbow. It is wise to obtain skin coverage of the arms and hands as early as possible; this permits the patient to do things for himself and improves his morale. When a leg is burned, the area around the knee should be covered first. Next in order of preference is the anterior aspect of the lower leg and then the posterior aspect of the lower leg. The thighs may wait until later. An attempt should be made to cover the areas of motion to lessen fibrosis and scarring. Large, flat surfaces may be covered last unless the patient has a very extensive burn and it is believed that covering of large areas might be a life-saving measure; in this case, all available skin should be used to cover as much of the wound as possible.

It is usually difficult to obtain a good take around the perineum; hence, this area should be given lowest priority.

Selection of Donor Sites

Donor areas should be selected on the basis of availability, accessibility, rehabilitation and cosmetic results. The easiest and most accessible area from which to take skin is the anterior aspect of the thigh. A large quantity of skin may be obtained rapidly from this area with the Brown dermatome. It is an easy area to expose. If only a small amount of skin is needed and it is desirable to get the patient out of bed early, the lower abdomen is a good donor site. The drum-type dermatomes work on this area better than the Brown dermatome.

Selection of a donor area is usually determined by the distribution of the surfaces to be grafted. For example, if the entire recipient site is on the posterior aspect of the body, it is wise to take the donor skin from posterior areas if they are available. This permits the patient to be placed on his abdomen, and both graft and donor sites can be exposed. When there are circumferential burns, it is advantageous to cover the anterior wound with skin taken from donor areas on the anterior surfaces of the body at the first grafting. Then the patient may be turned on the abdomen, and skin may be taken from the posterior aspect of the body to cover recipient sites on the back at a later procedure.

The skin over the tibia should be avoided whenever possible. If there is a choice between using the chest and the abdomen, the selection will probably depend upon the type of dermatome used. With a Brown dermatome it is much easier to take skin from the chest than from the abdomen. The abdomen and the buttocks, on the other hand, are excellent areas from which to take skin, especially in girls, because scars will not show. It is best to select donor areas on the anterior surface of the body rather than the posterior when there is a choice because the patient is more comfortable on his back during the convalescent period.

Skin may be obtained easily from the arms if necessary, but it is best not to incapacitate the arms if skin is available on other surfaces, because the patient uses his arms for eating and moving about in bed. It is inadvisable to take skin from areas of motion or flexion creases if these areas can be avoided. The popliteal area, the groin and the antecubital area should be spared whenever possible. Sometimes it is necessary to take skin from any place that it is available. In such instances, the dorsum of the foot or the scalp may be used. Small strips of skin may be taken with the Brown dermatome from almost any area. In extensive burns, every donor area available must be used in an attempt to achieve skin coverage as rapidly as possible.

Several crops of skin may be taken from the same area if a patient has extensive burns. Depending on the thickness of the skin, a second crop can be taken approximately 4 weeks after the first graft has been removed. The thinner the donor site is cut, the more rapid the healing of the area and the earlier a second crop of skin may be removed.

OBTAINING THE SKIN GRAFT

Skin used to cover burn wounds is generally between 0.008 and 0.012 of an inch in thickness. The thinner the graft, the better the take; the thicker the graft, the better the cosmetic result. When certain areas of function are to be covered, such as the knee joint, a somewhat thicker graft should be applied. Hands and the soles of the feet require a split-thickness graft of about 0.018 of an inch. In infants and children, the graft must be very thin. The important aspect in taking the skin is that a quantity be obtained that is sufficient to cover the wound completely. Too often an insufficient amount of skin is taken, and when it does not quite cover the wound, large spaces are left between strips of skin, and these require a long time for healing. The dermatome should never be taken from the operating table until all the skin has been applied. The surgeon never knows when he may have to use the dermatome to take one or two additional strips of skin to complete the coverage. Some surgeons favor taking a little extra skin and placing it in the refrigerator, so that if some skin is lost, an extra supply is available for regrafting on the third or fourth postoperative day. Although general anesthesia is usually used for grafting, skin may be cut under local anesthesia if the patient is seriously ill or if he needs coverage of only a small area.

The donor area selected should be shaved and washed with soap and water. Some surgeons prefer to shave this area on the night before operation. It is easier and much more comfortable to shave the area while the patient is under anesthesia immediately before the graft is taken. There are many ways to prepare the skin, but washing with some type of hexachlorophene detergent or soap appears to be as good as any method.

Skin may be cut for grafting with a variety of instruments. The type of instrument to be used varies according to the experience of the operator. One important fact must be kept in mind, however, and that is the sharpness of the blade. Regardless of the skill of the surgeon or the construction of the instrument, a good skin graft cannot be removed with a dull or nicked blade. The surgeon must become familiar with the instrument to be used and must be responsible for the sharpness of the blade. Even new blades sometimes are nicked or dull.

Brown Dermatome

The Brown dermatome is one of the most useful instruments for cutting skin for grafting because many sheets of thin skin can be removed rapidly. In addition, the use of certain areas for donor sites, such as the dorsum of the foot, scalp and wrist, is possible with the Brown instrument and not with other dermatomes. Initially the instrument was driven by electricity. The Brown electric dermatome was a very satisfactory instrument and was used for many years. More recently the dermatome has been powered by an air-driven motor, and this seems to be advantageous (Fig. 94). This dermatome takes a strip of skin 3 inches in width. Its construction is simple, and little experience is required for the successful removal of a large amount of skin. The only real disadvantage to using the dermatome is that a flat firm surface must be available. It will take a thin sheet

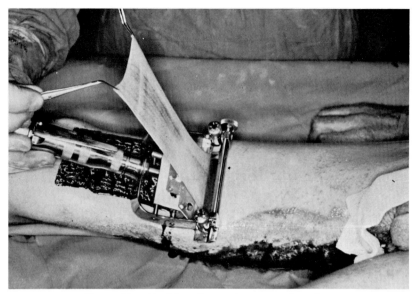

Figure 94.   Air-driven Brown dermatome in action.

of skin better than it will take a thick one. Usually the skin thins out at the edges.

Before any skin is removed, the area must be lubricated lightly with mineral oil or water. The dermatome is held in one hand by the handle. The air-driven instrument is activated by a lever on the handle. The thumb and forefinger of the other hand are placed over the forward part of the instrument (Fig. 95). This permits the application of increased pressure from one side to the other. Usually an assistant picks up the skin with forceps to enable the surgeon to visualize the depth of the cut. One of the most important aspects in the use of this dermatome is the trial cut. The instrument should be set for the desired depth and placed on the skin, and a cut should be made about 1 inch long. Then the instrument should be stopped but left in place. The surgeon should look at the skin to make sure it is of the appropriate depth and that the instrument is cutting well. If the instrument does not cut well in the trial, another blade should be inserted. There is no excuse for a poor piece of skin when the Brown dermatome is used. If it is properly adjusted and properly used and a good sharp blade has been inserted, a good strip of skin will be obtained. If the instrument is not working when the trial piece of skin is taken, then other adjustments should be made before it is used further.

During extensive grafting procedures, the period of anesthesia is shortened considerably by the use of the Brown dermatome. The instrument is also valuable in removing skin from children because of the easy manner in which a very thin strip of skin may be cut. Sometimes it is

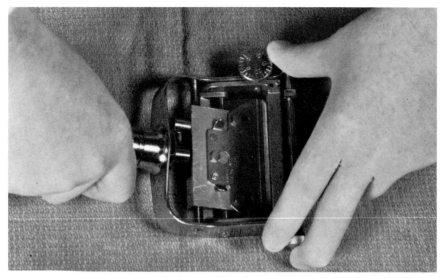

Figure 95. The best method of controlling the Brown dermatome is with the thumb and forefinger placed on front of the instrument.

necessary to take small postage stamp grafts from a limited area. The Brown dermatome works very well in such instances. It has throw-away blades; they are good for only a short time and are difficult to resharpen. In extensive grafting procedures, it may require two new blades to get an adequate amount of skin.

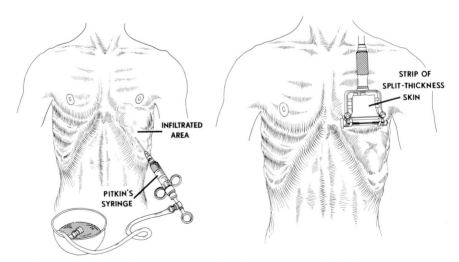

Figure 96. When skin must be taken from irregular areas with the Brown dermatome, infiltration of the areas with saline provides a smooth surface for cutting the graft. The saline is rapidly infiltrated by means of a Pitkin's syringe.

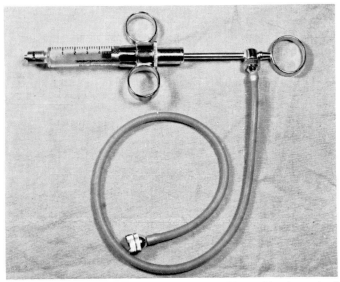

Figure 97. Pitkin's syringe. The free end of the rubber tubing is put in the solution to be injected. The syringe refills as the plunger is withdrawn. This apparatus permits rapid injections of local anesthetics or saline into the subcutaneous tissue.

Infiltration of donor area with saline. A flat, smooth surface is hard to obtain in certain areas, particularly over the abdomen, the chest and on the extremities of children. When the area is irregular, a much better graft can be obtained if saline is injected into the subcutaneous tissue to make the area smooth (Fig. 96). This procedure is very time consuming if an ordinary 10-ml. syringe is used, but large areas can be infiltrated rapidly by using a Pitkin's syringe (Fig. 97). The availability of a Pitkin's syringe and a pan of saline when grafts are being taken is very advantageous. Ballooning the skin over a bony chest or a scaphoid abdomen helps immeasurably in obtaining a good skin graft. The technique is also of considerable value around the ankle, over the dorsum of the foot and on small, thin extremities.

Drum-type Dermatomes

There are two drum-type dermatomes in common use—the Padgett and the Reese.

Padgett dermatome. The Padgett dermatome is particularly useful in obtaining grafts from uneven surfaces (Fig. 98). This instrument furnishes the best method of cutting skin when a thicker piece of skin is desired. A wider piece of skin can be removed than with the Brown dermatome, but the piece will not be as long, since the standard Padgett instrument cuts an area only 10 by 20 cm. Smaller and larger instruments are available. The Padgett dermatome is particularly useful in removing skin for coverage of hands or areas about joints.

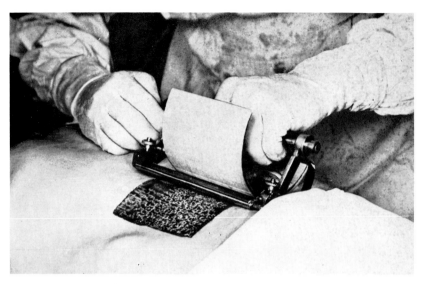

Figure 98. The Padgett dermatome in action. A full drum of skin measures 10 by 20 cm. This dermatome is particularly useful in removing skin for coverage of areas of motion.

A considerable amount of practice is required before this dermatome can be used with agility. Certain factors must be considered if a full size piece of skin is to be obtained. All skin oils and any water remaining after the preliminary preparation of the skin must be removed. This procedure is best accomplished by washing the area with ether and then permitting it to dry.

The area to be used as the donor site must be covered evenly by a thin layer of dermatome glue. Since the successful use of this dermatome depends upon the adherence of the skin to the drum, great care must be taken in preparing a donor site. If powder from the surgeon's glove falls on the donor site, or if a small amount of blood, water or skin oil remains on the region, the glue will not stick in that area, and a full drum of skin cannot be obtained. Glue that has remained in a container for a long time may be too thick. It may be thinned by adding a small amount of ether. It is best to pour the glue from its sealed container just before it is used. When glue is allowed to stand open on the table, it becomes quite thick; hence, it cannot be spread evenly on the dermatome.

The drum is prepared by first cleansing it with ether to remove any oil. Then a thin layer of glue is applied over the entire drum. The glue must be spread evenly and completely to the edges of the drum. This is accomplished by using a small brush or, better still, a piece of gauze folded and grasped with sponge forceps. It is a common mistake to apply too little glue rather than too much. Care must be taken to place an adequate amount of glue on the leading edge of the dermatome because it is particularly important to have proper adhesiveness in this area. If the drum does not stick at the leading edge when the graft is started, it is very difficult to obtain a good drum of skin. The glue on the drum and the skin is permitted to dry or set for several minutes; a period of 3 to 5 minutes is usually adequate. If ether has been used to thin the glue, a longer drying period is indicated.

A considerable advance has been made in the use of this dermatome because of the availability of a special type of cellophane tape with adhesive surfaces on both sides (Fig. 99). This tape adheres tightly to the dermatome, and on the other side, the adhesive material sticks well to the skin. A small amount of petrolatum ointment or mineral oil placed on the back of the blade holder causes it to slip over the skin smoothly.

The depth of the cut is determined by a lever on the side of the handle. The distance between the blade and the surface of the drum may be altered by rotating this lever, thus varying the depth of the cut. It is always advisable to look at the alignment between the blade and the surface of the drum before starting to cut the graft. Occasionally the drum is warped or the blade is out of alignment, and unless the instrument is checked before use, an uneven cut may be obtained.

To achieve a good initial sealing between skin and drum, pressure must be used in applying the leading edge of the drum to the donor site. As soon as a satisfactory seal is made, the cut is started. The area from

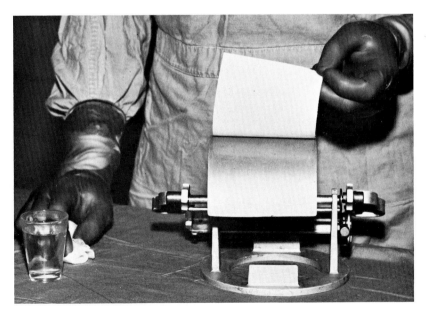

Figure 99. A double adhesive cellophane tape (3M Company) for use on drum-type dermatomes. The tape sticks to the drum, and when the protective paper sheet is removed, there is an adhesive surface that adheres tightly to the skin as the graft is being cut.

which the skin is to be removed is measured carefully by eye before the drum is applied. The drum is placed on the skin in such a way that there is ample space for the cutting hand to move the blade. For example, if skin is to be taken from the left side of the patient's chest by a right-handed surgeon, the leading edge is placed on the lower part of the chest, and the cut starts at the bottom and is directed upward toward the axilla. This permits freedom of the cutting hand.

The hand holding the dermatome must remain steady at all times. Because the hand that operates the blade is moving back and forth constantly, it is not uncommon for the opposite hand, which controls the drum, to be in rhythm with the hand on the blade. As a result, the drum moves back and forth over the donor surface. This can be corrected only by practice. It is important to move the drum along a straight line over the skin rather than to twist it at an angle. The blade cuts the skin much more smoothly if it is worked back and forth in a sawing motion while the drum is being advanced slowly. The drum should not be rotated too rapidly. Constant pressure should be exerted on the drum in an upward and forward direction to feed the skin into the blade. If excessive pressure is exerted, however, a wider piece of skin will be fed into the blade. This results in deep overcuts (Fig. 100). On the other hand, if the drum is pulled away too fast, the full width desired will not be obtained (Fig. 101).

The operator must focus his attention at all times on the point at which he is cutting to make sure that the blade does not overcut and that a full drum of skin is removed. It is advantageous for the operator to watch the right side of the drum and let his assistant observe the left side. If a full drum of skin is not being removed, a little more pressure must be exerted by the drum hand, and the cutting stroke must be shortened. If there is a tendency to overcut, the drum is pulled away a little more rapidly and the stroke is lengthened slightly.

There are several methods of removing the skin from the dermatome. The most common method is simply to cut the skin free of the site with a sharp knife, place the dermatome in its rack and peel the skin away with several hemostats. The disadvantage in using this method is that the glue on the back of the skin is still present and causes the skin to wrinkle and stick together. This makes it difficult to handle.

A better method for removing skin from the dermatome is to loosen the skin while it is still attached to the donor site. Upon reaching the end of the graft, slight tension may be exerted on the drum to pull the skin away from the drum as far as the leading edge (Fig. 102). The glued surface and the base of the skin are then covered with blood from the donor site. This procedure eliminates the stickiness and also avoids tearing the skin as it is being removed from the drum. The skin remains suspended between the donor site and the leading edge of the dermatome; it can easily be cut free from the donor site by a pair of scissors or a knife. Care must be taken when a knife is used or the blade may cut into the subcutaneous tissue.

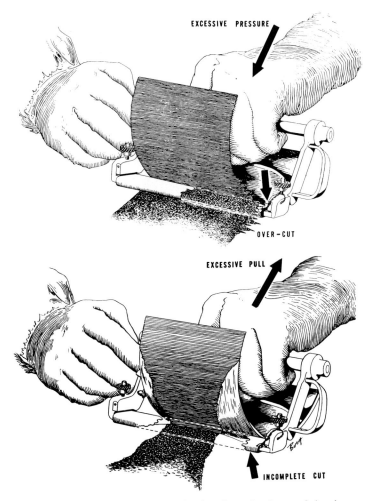

Figure 100. When excessive pressure is placed on the drum of the dermatome, the skin will be fed into the blade too rapidly and a deep overcut will result.

Figure 101. If the drum of the dermatome is pulled away too rapidly, an incomplete cut results. Unless the skin is fed into the blade by even pressure, a narrow strip of skin will be obtained rather than a strip of skin the entire width of the drum.

After the skin is removed from the drum, the dermatome is placed on its stand. The drum is then cleaned and reglued to be ready to take the next sheet of skin. The simplest method of cleaning a dermatome is to rub the drum surface vigorously with a dry sponge. Since the glue is a plastic-like material, it will roll up and separate readily from the instrument. The drum should be further cleansed with ether before a new application of glue is made.

Several sheets of skin may be removed from the front and back of the trunk if the donor areas are properly placed (Fig. 103).

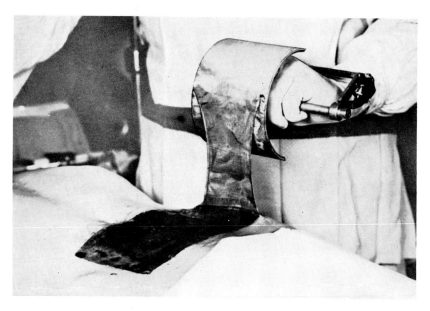

Figure 102. Method for removing skin from the dermatome drum. The glued surface and the base of the skin are covered with blood from the donor site. This procedure eliminates the stickiness and avoids tearing the skin as it is removed from the drum.

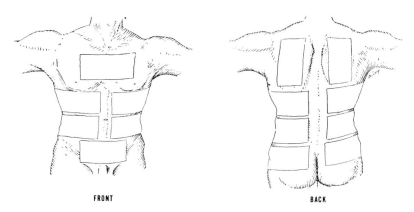

FRONT   BACK

Figure 103. The number of sheets of skin that can be removed from any surface depends upon the size of the patient. Outlines in the diagrams above provide a maximum amount of skin without interfering with critical areas. The area over the anterior superior iliac spine should be avoided. The area near the anterior axillary fold must not be used, because motion of the arms prevents optimum healing in that area. It is easier to take skin transversely over the lower chest and center of the back than longitudinally. It is difficult to remove a strip of skin in a longitudinal direction from the side of the chest by means of the drum-type dermatome.

Reese dermatome. The Reese dermatome is essentially a modification of the Padgett dermatome. The instruments are identical in basic design. The Reese dermatome is a much heavier instrument, and it is more solidly built (Fig. 104). This is advantageous in that it helps the surgeon to hold the instrument steady while he is cutting the skin.

The method of regulating the depth of cut has been modified on the Reese dermatome. A series of shims are supplied with the instrument; these are fitted between the blade and blade holder to regulate the thickness of the skin to be cut. This modification produces an absolutely uniform thickness of skin which does not change during the process of cutting. For a beginner, the Reese dermatome is nearly foolproof, and as a result, a full drum of skin can usually be taken by an inexperienced operator. The Reese instrument is heavier and more cumbersome than the Padgett dermatome and cannot be used with the same agility.

The one outstanding advantage of the Reese dermatome is the addition of dermatape as a backing for the skin. This green, rubberized material fits over the back of the drum. It is attached at one end and then is placed over the drum and tightened by means of a worm gear spool at the other end. Once the dermatape is applied tightly, the dermatome is ready for use. Dermatome cement is painted on the skin. The green dermatape is covered with a white, glazed linen backing which is peeled off before the dermatome is used (Fig. 105). The adhesive layer of the green rubber backing is thereby protected from becoming soiled before

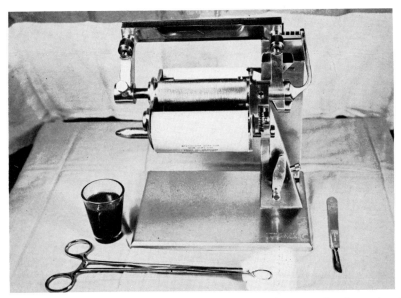

Figure 104. The Reese dermatome on its stand. The dermatape has been placed on the dermatome, but the white linen backing has not been removed. The medicine glass holds liquid cement to be painted on the skin. Gauze is folded and grasped with sponge forceps to be used for painting the skin.

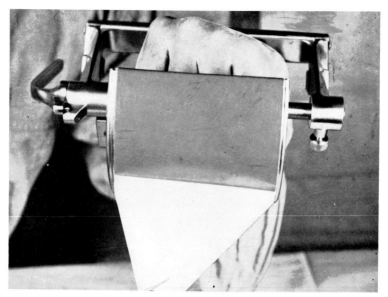

Figure 105.   Immediately prior to placing the dermatome on the skin, the linen backing is removed from the dermatape. This linen backing protects the adhesiveness of the dermatape.

being used. The dermatapes are sterilized by soaking in a cold sterilization solution.

This instrument can be used more rapidly than the Padgett dermatome because the drum does not have to be cleansed between grafting
procedures. The surgeon simply removes the dermatape backing with
the skin attached and then places another dermatape on the drum. The
skin is always removed from the dermatape before application.

Freehand Knife

The earliest method of obtaining split-thickness grafts was by means
of the freehand knife. A straight edge razor may be used, but the width
of the graft will be limited. A double edge razor blade grasped between
the jaws of a straight hemostat is sometimes used to obtain small pieces
of skin. The preferred instrument for freehand cutting, however, is either
the Blair-Brown knife or the Ferris-Smith knife. These instruments have
a blade that is approximately 5 or 6 inches in length.

A freehand knife has the advantage that it is inexpensive and requires
no power. It has three distinct disadvantages, however: (1) To use the knife
properly, a great amount of skill is required. (2) Regardless of the skill
in cutting with a freehand knife, it is almost impossible to remove a sheet
with uniform depth throughout the entire width of the cut. (3) It takes
much more time to obtain skin with a freehand knife than with other instruments.

If a knife is used, it is advantageous to apply a small amount of mineral oil to the back of the blade to make it slide easily over the surface. Before an attempt is made to cut a graft, the skin should be stretched tight either with a suction cup or with two skin boards. The graft is cut with long, even strokes of the knife, and the surgeon must work about 1 or 2 inches behind the lead board (Fig. 106). As the skin is cut, the loose end may be held by an assistant. It must be held in such a manner that the surgeon is able to observe the thickness of the graft.

With the many instruments available today, very few grafts are cut with the knife except in certain instances where a few small pieces of skin are needed for the application of postage stamp grafts. If only one piece of skin is required, a razor blade or freehand knife may be used rather than taking the time to set up a Brown dermatome.

Mesh Dermatome

In 1963, Tanner introduced the mesh skin graft. A strip of skin is taken by any type dermatome and then put through the mesh instrument. With this instrument, which consists of two 4-inch rollers with cutting blades, a piece of skin can be meshed so that it can be stretched to cover an area twice its initial size (Fig. 107). Mesh grafts seem to take as well if not better than sheet grafts because there is no fluid accumulation beneath

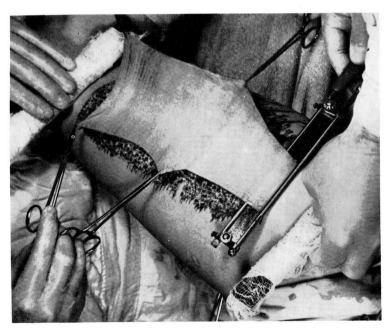

Figure 106. Cutting skin with a freehand Blair-Brown knife. Considerable practice is required to obtain large sheets of split-thickness skin by this method.

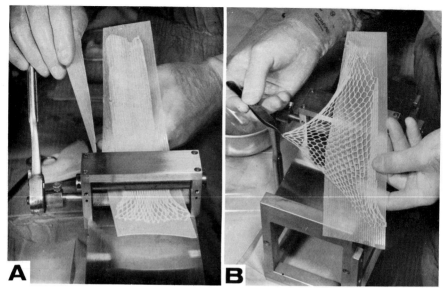

Figure 107. Latest model of the Tanner mesh dermatome. (Courtesy of Bruce Mac-Millan, M.D., Cincinnati, Ohio.)

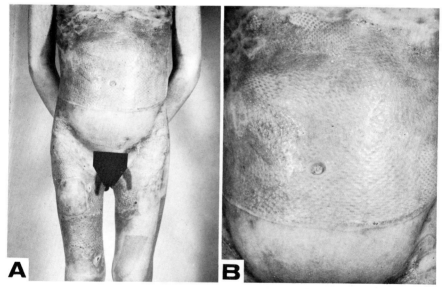

Figure 108. Healed areas after mesh graft. *A*, Skin has been stretched to cover larger area of trunk. *B*, Closeup photograph shows excellent healing between the interstices of the mesh. (Courtesy of Bruce MacMillan, M.D., Cincinnati, Ohio.)

them. The mesh is very strong and can be sewn over a defect with moderate tension. The grafts must be covered with a bulky dressing for 48 hours. The openings in the mesh seem to fill in with epithelial cells in about 10 days. Some surgeons feel that the mesh graft does not contract as much as a sheet graft. Its particular advantage, however, is that a larger recipient area is covered by a smaller piece of skin. Mesh grafts are particularly suitable for use on the trunk, especially in children (Fig. 108). They should not be used below the knee or over joints.

EXPOSURE OF DONOR SITES

The best method of treating donor sites in burns is the exposure method. Immediatcly after the skin graft has been removed, the donor area is covered with dry fine-mesh gauze. A thick wet gauze pad is then applied to achieve hemostasis. Sometimes weak epinephrine solution is used on the pads. At the end of the operation, the gauze pad is removed. The blood-soaked, fine-mesh gauze is allowed to remain as the only covering of the wound. All free edges of the gauze are trimmed away. The area of the donor site is permitted to remain exposed to the air. A firm coagu-

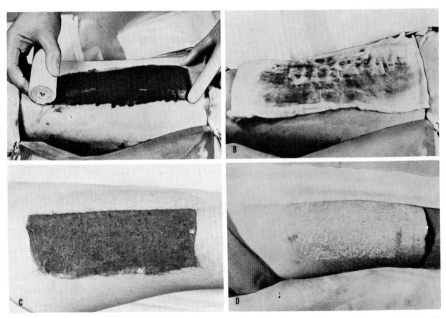

Figure 109. *A*, After the graft has been removed, a layer of fine-mesh gauze is placed over the donor area. *B*, A warm, moist laparotomy pad is placed over the donor site for hemostasis. This is removed at the end of the operative procedure. *C*, Blood has coagulated in the interstices of the fine-mesh gauze. This forms a hard coagulum that serves as a protective cover for the wound. *D*, The twelfth postoperative day. Epithelial growth has occurred beneath the fine-mesh gauze coagulum.

lum is soon formed by the blood that is caught in the interlacing fibers of the gauze. This coagulum dries within 24 hours and when hardened serves as a protective covering for the wound (Fig. 109). Sometimes, if the patient is moving around a great deal, it may be wise to fix a pad or bandage over the fine-mesh gauze for 10 to 12 hours until the coagulum has formed. This prevents the patient from tearing away the layer of gauze.

There may be a moderate amount of pain until the coagulum dries, but this is not severe. After a good coagulum is formed there is no further discomfort from the donor area. Epithelization proceeds beneath the coagulum. As healing progresses, the protective covering loosens at the edges and must be trimmed. When healing is complete, the covering falls off, leaving a well epithelized surface. Exposed donor sites are more comfortable, less frequently complicated by infection and easily observed.

A time-honored method for a small donor site is the application of a large, bulky petrolatum gauze dressing. The dressing is usually allowed to remain in place for about 8 days, changed and replaced until the area is healed 14 days later. Although this is an excellent technique for a small, isolated area, in extensive burns where the donor sites must be interspersed between infected granulating areas, infection occurs because it is difficult to isolate the donor area with an adequate occlusive dressing. Occasionally the grafted area and the donor site are in the same region, and it is essential to dress the grafted areas. In such instances the donor site must be dressed. When the site is dressed, the dressing must be changed about every 5 days or the donor area will become severely infected and might be converted to a full-thickness granulating surface.

APPLICATION OF SKIN TO THE WOUND

In the operating room, preparation of the recipient site should be simple and nontraumatic. It is unwise to attempt to scrub granulation tissue or use any type of antiseptic soap or detergent on it. The area around the granulating bed should be shaved and prepared with hexachlorophene soap and water. The granulations should be irrigated with saline. Further attempts at cleansing are unnecessary and may cause troublesome bleeding.

As soon as the skin has been removed from the donor site, it is put into a pan of saline solution. The scrub nurse can then place strips of skin on petrolatum-impregnated gauze to make handling easier.

The simplest way to impregnate fine-mesh gauze with petrolatum or Carbowax is to place a 3-inch roller bandage in a pint jar and add 2 ml. of water along with the ointment until the jar is about one-third full, cover the jar and place it in the autoclave. The pressure and heat of the autoclave cause the petrolatum to penetrate the meshes of the roller bandage. The roll is easy to handle, and an excessive amount of petrolatum does not adhere to the gauze.

This impregnated gauze is put on a sterile skin board; as each strip of skin is cut, it is placed on the gauze with the external surface next to the gauze (Fig. 110). Strips of skin usually curl, but if they are kept moist in saline and pressed firmly against the petrolatum-impregnated gauze, they remain flat and are easy to handle. Each strip of skin placed on petrolatum gauze may be folded over and kept between moist gauze pads until the surgeon is ready to apply the skin.

There are several acceptable methods for the application of skin to the wound. Usually a combination of techniques is used. In most instances for large, flat surfaces the best method of application is to take a large strip of skin and lay it on the surface. This lay-on method is very effective. The sheet of skin is placed over the recipient area; then the petrolatum-impregnated gauze is removed. The sheets are placed in close apposition. This is extremely important; areas of granulation tissue should not be left between grafts. After this, the grafts may be exposed or a bulky dressing used to hold the grafts in place.

Sometimes grafts must be sutured. This is especially true over irregular surfaces and points of motion, such as the chin, neck, feet and hands and around the knee and elbow. Very fine 4-0 silk sutures may be used on a sharp cutting needle. Deep bites into the underlying tissue must be taken to prevent excess bleeding. Little time is required to suture grafts in place if the areas to be grafted are small. When extensive areas are to be grafted, however, suturing of all the sheets of skin prolongs the

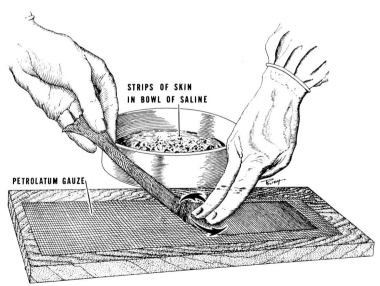

Figure 110. Strips of skin are placed in a bowl of saline as soon as they are removed. The nurse places the strips of skin with the epithelial side next to the petrolatum gauze. This makes the sheets of skin easy to handle.

operative procedure unduly. When a mesh graft is applied, it is essential that it be sutured in place to maintain the stretch.

It is usually unnecessary to perforate the grafts except in rare instances. If the surface is uneven and a dependent area might be a focal point for the collection of serum, the graft should be perforated at that point.

Occasionally if the mesh dermatome is not available and the recipient site is so extensive that only limited amounts of skin are available for grafting, the postage stamp method may be used. This is not a good method for general use, because it takes a long time for the areas between the grafts to heal, and the ultimate result is an uneven surface. Postage stamp grafts may be used on certain flat surfaces, such as the thigh and the back, when there is truly a serious shortage of skin. Sometimes when large surfaces are to be grafted and the recipient site is not in good condition, postage stamp grafts permit drainage between the grafts; hence, the take is better than if large sheets are applied. If there is a good recipient site, sheet grafts by the lay-on method result in less scarring and more rapid closure of the wound.

It is extremely important that all of the recipient areas be well covered with skin if it is available. In fact, it is judicious to take a little extra skin to make sure that an adequate amount is available for coverage. If there is a little skin left over after the grafts have been applied, it can be stored in a refrigerator. After the first dressing change, this excess skin may be used for patching areas in which grafts have not taken.

Exposure of Grafts

Most grafts take better if they are exposed rather than put under a dressing. Unfortunately not all grafted surfaces lend themselves to exposure. If the grafting can be planned in such a way that the area can be exposed, there is usually a better take. Certainly, when there is a poor recipient site, a better take can be expected with exposure than when a graft is placed under a dressing. Flat surfaces are easily exposed (Fig. 115). It is difficult to expose a circumferential area unless it is on an extremity and the extremity can be suspended by some means. It is simple to suspend an arm by wrapping the hand and attaching it to a standard. It is a little more difficult to suspend a lower extremity, especially in an adult, and usually a circumferential graft is dressed. Sometimes, however, it may be wise to suspend the extremity by skeletal traction.

If exposure is used, great care should be taken to place the grafts in close approximation. There should be little or no space between the grafts. The graft must be given daily care. This includes using an applicator to roll out the serum and blood that may collect beneath the graft. One of the advantages of exposure is that the graft can be observed, and if fluid is collecting beneath it, it can be evacuated. The patient should be kept as quiet as possible during the first 24 hours after grafting to prevent dislodgment of the grafts. After 24 hours, the grafts are moderately well fixed in place.

Application of Dressing over Graft

When dressings are placed over a graft, the procedure must be performed with great care. The dressing must be firm, bulky and capable of producing even compression. As soon as the grafts are applied, a layer of fine-mesh gauze is placed over them to hold them in place. Moist 4- by 4-inch gauze pads may be placed over this area to fix the grafts, and on top of this, a large amount of fluffed gauze may be placed to make a bulky dressing. Some type of elastic bandage is then applied to provide splinting and even, firm compression.

Although the grafting procedure is almost complete at the time a bandage is to be applied, the anesthesiologist must be cautioned that this is an important time to keep the patient asleep and free from motion. Too frequently, an anesthesiologist thinks that the patient should be awakening as the operative procedure draws to a close, and as a result, the patient will move at the time when the dressing is being applied. Motion disturbs the position of the grafts and prevents a good take.

A poor dressing is often applied because the surgeon is fatigued after a 3- or 4-hour operation. If extensive burns are being grafted, it is usually advisable for one member of the team to withdraw for a few minutes to rest prior to the conclusion of the operation. After the grafts are in place, he may rescrub and apply a good dressing. If a leg has been grafted it is advisable to include the foot in the dressing to keep it in a position of function and to exert even compression over the entire leg and foot. By placing the dressing over the joints both above and below the graft, better immobilization is obtained.

On-lay Gauze (Stent) Dressings

On-lay gauze dressings, commonly known as stent dressings, are extremely valuable for holding grafts in place over irregular surfaces. They are most advantageous over grafts on the head, the neck, around the shoulders and on the buttocks. Heavy silk sutures are placed in the normal tissue surrounding the area and tied over a large amount of fluffed gauze (Fig. 111). This not only immobilizes the graft, but also maintains even compression. Stent dressings are used when it is felt that firm compression is necessary and cannot be maintained by the usual type of dressing. They are usually removed after 4 days.

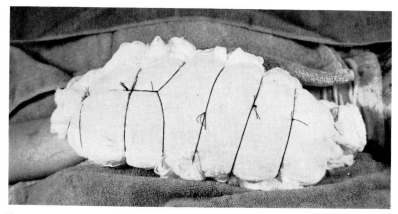

Figure 111. On-lay gauze dressing, or stent dressing. Heavy black silk sutures are placed in the normal skin surrounding the grafts. These are then tied over the large bulky gauze dressing. Such a dressing holds the grafts firmly in place and serves as a splint to the area. Stent dressings are particularly indicated over rough, irregular surfaces.

AFTERCARE OF GRAFTS

One of the common causes of failure of take is slippage of the graft from either direct trauma or movement under the dressing. Inadequate fixation or undue voluntary motion of the grafted area may displace grafts in the early postoperative period. For this reason, the grafted part needs to be observed carefully during the postoperative period to make sure that the patient does not move the area excessively. In extensive grafting procedures, especially when exposure is used, it is sometimes necessary to place the patient under sedation for 24 hours to insure immobilization.

If dressings have been applied, they should be changed between the second and fifth day. If the surface on which the graft was applied was in poor condition, the grafts should be inspected on the second day. When the recipient site appears to be free from infection, it is safe to allow the dressing to remain in place for 5 days. At the first dressing change, great care must be exercised to prevent pulling away grafts that are not firmly fixed. When graft and gauze are adherent, irrigation with a bulb syringe can be used to loosen the gauze and thus prevent grafts from being torn from their base. It is not always necessary to perform dressing changes under anesthesia, but it is advisable to use anesthesia at least at the first dressing change.

It is often difficult to estimate the percentage of take of a graft after it has been in place for only 3 to 5 days. Some areas may not appear to have taken, although a good take is observable at subsequent dressing changes.

After the initial dressing change, other changes should be done at 2- to 5-day intervals. Dressings must be removed as soon as there is a good graft take and coverage of all areas. If small areas do not seem to have a good take and excess skin has been stored in the refrigerator, it may be applied.

The Hubbard tank is an excellent method for stimulating motion and keeping the grafted areas clean (Fig. 112). As soon as the dressings have been removed on an extensively burned patient, it is advantageous that he be placed in a Hubbard tank at least once a day. If the areas have been treated by exposure, the patient can usually go in the Hubbard tank on the third or fourth postoperative day. When muscular tone returns to the lower extremities, the patient may become ambulatory. Early motion and early ambulation are desirable.

When a patient with burns of the lower legs becomes ambulatory, he should wear an elastic rubberized bandage. Such a bandage is worn over the grafts or the donor sites on the lower extremities for a period of 2 or 3 months. This support for freshly grafted areas and donor sites is necessary to prevent breakdown of the epithelium and subsequent small ulcerations. The patient usually has a burning or stinging sensation when he stands if the circulation in the lower extremities is unsupported.

Occupational therapy stimulates the patient's desire to rehabilitate himself and also improves his morale. As soon as the granulating wounds are covered, a complete change occurs in the general condition of the patient. He suffers less pain, feels much better, his appetite improves and he begins to gain weight. A patient may lose as much as 1 pound per day

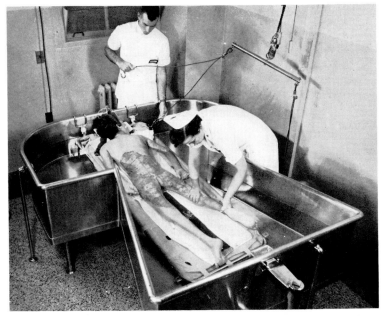

Figure 112. Patient in a Hubbard tank. As soon as grafts have taken, a patient may be placed in a Hubbard tank. This stimulates motion and keeps the grafted areas clean.

during the early period following a burn, but he is able to gain back from 1/2 to 1 pound per day after the wounds have been closed.

USE OF HOMOGRAFTS

Undoubtedly the best dressing for a burn wound is a homograft. When it is impossible or injudicious to apply an autograft, a homograft makes an excellent biological skin dressing. It temporarily closes the wound, eliminates infection and prevents fluid and protein losses. Homografts may be very advantageous in a variety of ways in the treatment of burns. Their chief indications are as follows:

1. They are extremely valuable in the critically burned patient who has a large open wound but who is too ill to withstand an autografting procedure. Viable skin homografts may be placed over the wound in lay-on fashion without anesthesia. This temporarily closes the wound and permits the patient's general condition to improve. Autografts can then be applied to close the wound permanently. Such a technique is very useful in patients who have developed a severe complication, such as septicemia, or who are seriously debilitated and have wounds with large, open granulating areas.

2. In some very extensively burned patients with large, open granulating wounds, there may be only enough autograft skin available to close a portion of the wound. In such instances, homografts may be used on the remaining areas as temporary cover. When more autograft skin becomes available, the homografts may be removed and replaced by autografts.

3. One of the best methods of preparing the recipient site for grafting is by the temporary use of homografts. By placing homograft skin strips on the recipient site and replacing them every 4 days, the recipient site can be cleansed and prepared for a good autograft take (Fig. 113). The use of a homograft in this fashion provides a good test of the recipient site prior to autografting. If the recipient bed is questionable and a large area must be grafted, or if the donor sites are limited, testing with a homograft is very advantageous. The homograft is applied and then pulled off about 4 days later. If it does not start to take in these 4 days, the surface is probably not ready for grafting and another homograft should be applied. With each application, the underlying bed usually improves.

4. Acceleration of the healing process of partial-thickness burns occurs beneath a homograft. The mechanism of this phenomenon is not clear, but in some way the homografts provide a more favorable environment for proliferation of persisting epithelial remnants present in partial-thickness burn wounds. In the early stages of healing, it may be difficult to differentiate a deep second-degree burn from a superficial third-degree burn, or both may be present. In such instances the application of homografts will allow a differentiation to be made, since the areas of partial-

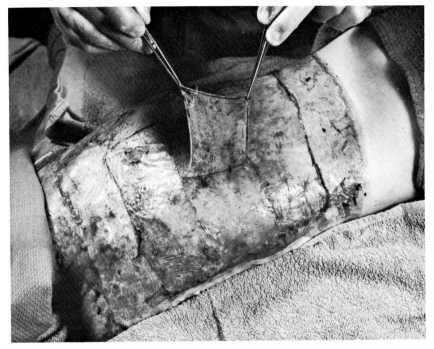

Figure 113. Homograft skin is in place over a recipient site being prepared for grafting. After 3 days the homograft is pulled off and replaced by another homograft. If the homograft is left in place longer, it cannot be pulled away without producing bleeding.

thickness burn will re-epithelize rapidly under the homografts, and the homografts will take on the areas in which there is full-thickness injury.

Homografts may survive for 4 or 5 weeks before being rejected. Usually they are only needed for about 10 days if applied for cover of a large granulating wound. After this period, however, the homograft may be well attached to the underlying surface and difficult to remove except by sharp dissection. If allowed to remain in place less than 4 days, it may be peeled away easily. After this time the homograft must be cut away or allowed to remain until rejection.

There are many benefits to be achieved by homografting but probably the greatest is the limitation of infection and the diminution in loss of water, electrolytes and protein. In a large, open wound a homograft diminishes the energy requirement because it minimizes the large obligatory water loss through the wound. One of the most rewarding effects of a homograft is its reduction of pain. As soon as a wound is closed by a homograft, the area is more comfortable, the patient's psychological outlook improves and his appetite increases.

The chief problem with the use of homografts is their availability. In large burn centers, it is possible to maintain a good supply of viable postmortem homografts. It is much more difficult to have homografts available in the hospital that cares for only an occasional severely burned patient. Every burn ward or burn unit should keep on hand an adequate supply of postmortem homografts. If such a bank is not available, arrangements should be made for homografts when an extensively burned patient is under care, since there are so many uses for homografts. A crop of skin should be taken from a recently deceased body and stored in the refrigerator. If an emergency need develops for homografts and postmortem skin is not available, then skin should be taken from a relative or friend. The latter procedure is not justified unless the homografts seem to be needed as a life-saving measure.

There are many ways of storing homografts. Lyophilized skin is almost as good as viable skin that is kept for a short period of time. Prolonged storage can be made possible by quick freezing. The best method of storage is short term storage in a refrigerator.

Postmortem homografts function as well as those procured from living donors. Specific permission for postmortem skin donation must be obtained from the deceased donor's next of kin. Most deceased bodies are acceptable as donors except those that are of patients who have died from communicable diseases, sepsis, blood dyscrasias or malignancies with cutaneous metastasis or those with cutaneous lesions in the potential donor areas. As soon after death as possible but not more than 12 hours post mortem, the cadaver should be taken to the operating room and the donor sites shaved, prepared and draped as for any sterile surgical procedure. With the Brown dermatome, split-thickness grafts, 0.010 to 0.015 of an inch, are removed from all available surfaces except the head, neck and distal portion of extremities. The skin is spread on fine-mesh gauze that is lightly impregnated with petrolatum. The raw surface is away from the gauze. The graft strips are placed in large sterile Petri dishes, sealed with tape and stored in a refrigerator at 4°C. immediately beneath the freezing compartment. One million units of penicillin and 1 gm. of streptomycin in 30 ml. of saline are added to each Petri dish as antibacterial agents.

Although homografts are useful 2 or 3 weeks after removal, a better take is obtained with early application.

REFERENCES

Artz, C. P.: Understanding thermal burns and principles of management. *In* Davis, J. H. (ed.): *Current Concepts in Surgery.* New York, McGraw-Hill Book Company, 1965, p. 247.

Artz, C. P., Becker, J. M., Sako, Y., and Bronwell, A. W.: Postmortem skin homografts in the treatment of extensive burns. *A. M. A. Arch. Surg.* **71**:682, 1955.

Artz, C. P., Bronwell, A. W., and Sako, Y.: The exposure treatment of donor sites. *Ann. Surg.* **142**:248, 1955.

Davis, J. H.: Evaluation of dermatomes. *Surgery* **36**:92, 1954.

Haynes, B. W.: Skin homografts—a life-saving measure in severely burned children. *J. Trauma* **3**:217, 1963.

Larson, D. L.: Closure of the burn wound. *J. Trauma* **5**:254, 1965.

Moyer, C. A., Brentano, L., Gravens, D. L., Margraf, H. W., and Monafo, W. W., Jr.: Treatment of large human burns with 0.5 per cent silver nitrate solution. *A. M. A. Arch. Surg.* **90**:812, 1965.

Switzer, W. E., Jones, J. W., and Moncrief, J. A.: Evaluation of early excision of burns in children. *J. Trauma* **5**:540, 1965.

Tanner, J. C., Jr., Vandeput, J., and Olley, J. F.: The mesh skin graft. *Plast. & Reconstruct. Surg.* **34**:287, 1964.

Zaroff, L. I., Mills, W., Jr., Puckett, J. W., Jr., Switzer, W. E., and Moncrief, J. A.: Multiple uses of viable cutaneous homografts in the burned patient. *Surgery* **59**:368, 1966.

Chapter
Nine

SPECIAL
TYPES OF BURNS

ELECTRICAL INJURIES

In electrical injuries there is a far greater variety of lesions than ordinarily realized. The capacity of an electrical current to cause injury when some part of the body is interposed between two conductors having different electrical potentials varies enormously. At one extreme is the fracture dislocation caused by the disruptive stress of violent unopposed muscular contraction; at the other there is deep burning caused by the current.

The first man-made electric shock of which we have any record occurred in Holland in 1746, when two Dutch physicists unintentionally discharged a Leyden jar and the current went through their bodies. After the introduction of the dynamo, a stagehand was killed at Lyons, France, in 1879. In the United States and Canada, the number of fatalities due to electricity each year is estimated at seven per million of population. The hazards from the use of electricity are electric shock, electric tissue damage, fire and explosion and eye flash.

Factors Determining Effect of the Current

Our knowledge of the effects of electricity on the human body stems from the early research of Prevost and Batelli, Jellinek, and Jaffe in the 1920's. Kouwenhoven has more recently provided information about pathologic changes from the effects of electricity. He has pointed out that there are six factors that must be taken into consideration when the effects of the passage of an electric current through the body are determined. These are type of circuit, voltage of circuit, resistance offered by the body, value of the current that flows through the tissues, pathway of the current through the body and duration of the contact.

The type of circuit and the voltage with which contact is made have a

214

profound effect upon the resulting injury. Direct current does not produce the same contraction of the muscles that is found with alternating current. Low voltage direct current is not as dangerous as the corresponding alternating current. On the other hand, contact with high voltage direct current is more apt to be fatal than contact with alternating current of the same voltage. The response of the human body is practically uniform for frequency ranging from 10 to 300 cycles per second. At 1000 cycles, a somewhat greater value current is required to produce a given reaction, while very high frequencies, such as are used in diathermy, have only a heating effect. High voltages are dangerous. There are a number of cases on record in which contact with 60- or 65-volt circuits of commercial frequency have resulted in fatal accidents. It is probable that circuits of 24 volts or less may be considered safe under practically all conditions.

The resistance of the body consists of two parts—that offered by the skin at the point of contact and the internal resistance. The epidermis is nonvascular, and when dry it has a very high resistance, which may reach 100,000 ohms per sq. cm. The resistance offered by the dermis is low because this layer contains blood vessels, and body fluids are good conductors. The only poor conductors inside the body are the bones. The internal resistance of the body, therefore, is relatively small. The soles of the feet and the palms of the hands are considerably more resistant than other areas because of the thick layer of epidermis. The resistance of the skin is not constant. It varies with the amount of moisture that it contains, the temperature and the applied voltage. Under thoroughly wet conditions, the resistance of the epidermis may fall to as low as 1/100 of its dry value. If contact with a circuit continues for any length of time, the skin loses its protection because of the formation of blisters. At 50 volts, blisters form in 6 or 7 seconds. Kragh and Erich point out that, if the resistance is less than 1200 ohms, current of 110 volts may be fatal. With favorable contact between the skin and external conductors, the resistance of the human body may be reduced to less than 1000 ohms. Accidental electrocution in bathtubs and fatal electrocutions of sweating workmen who contact conductors of 110 volts fall into this category. Sweating may decrease the resistance from 30,000 to 25,000 ohms in the skin. Small superficial injuries such as scratches, small cuts and abrasions lower the skin's resistance.

The value of the alternating current that flows through the body when contact is made with an electric circuit is of extreme importance, as it determines the resulting injury. The current that will produce only a tingling sensation at the point of contact is of the order of 1 or 2 milliamperes. Contact with an electric circuit produces a contraction of the muscles. This contraction may be so severe as to prevent the victim from freeing himself from the circuit. The let-go current is that value which an individual can withstand without harmful effects for at least the time required for him to release his hold on the circuit. The value of the let-go current varies with the individual but it is believed for men to be between 8 and 22 milliamperes. In certain accidents, the current holds the individual frozen to the circuit. Contact on the palmar aspect of the hand is therefore more dangerous than on the dorsal surface because the former causes flexion of the fingers and consequent grasping of the contact, while the latter causes such an extension of the fingers that the contact is usually knocked away. A current of 100 milliamperes flowing from the hands to the feet is sufficient to throw the ventricles of the heart into fibrillation. The current that will produce a block or partial paralysis in the nervous system is somewhat less. When such a block occurs, there is respiratory arrest, and the patient is usually unconscious. If the victim of an electric shock retains consciousness during and following the contact, there is often a ringing in the ears and partial deafness for a time. In addition, there may be visual disorders such as flashes and brilliant luminous spots.

The pathway that the current traverses in its passage through the body is of extreme importance. Obviously, if the current passes through vital organs such as the heart and the brain, the resulting injury is greater. It is always difficult, however, to tell from the cutaneous injury the exact pathway that the electrical current has taken. The difference in the susceptibility of the heart to electrical injury at different times in its contraction cycle also seems important. The longer the duration of contact, the greater the amount of damage.

Conduction of the Current Through Various Tissues

The resistance to electric current in tissue varies in order from the greatest to least as follows: bone, fat, tendon, skin, muscle, blood, nerve.

The resistance of the skin varies from person to person and from one area of the body to another. Thin skin is less resistant, of course, than thick skin. After an electric current has penetrated the skin, it passes rapidly through the body along lines of least resistance, that is, through the tissue fluids and along blood vessels, leading to degeneration of vessel walls and formation of thrombi. This vascular injury often occurs at some distance from the site of injury and accounts for the apparent progressive nature of the lesion.

If the resistance of the skin is low at the time it interrupts the electric current, the current passes readily into the body, causing proportionately more severe systemic disturbances. If the skin maintains its resistance during contact, however, the current may be retarded and the systemic damage may be somewhat less. Other things being equal, the greater the skin resistance, the more severe the local burn; similarly, the less the resistance, the greater the systemic effect of the current.

Death from electric shock may be the result of a number of causes or a combination of two or more. In general, low voltage kills through the mechanism of ventricular fibrillation and high voltage causes respiratory failure, either because of direct depression of respiratory center or hemorrhages in the region of the fourth ventricle.

Pathologic Effects

Because of the different types of burns associated with electrical accidents, there is a wide variation in electrical injury. Most skin burns occur at the entrance and exit of the current. Damage at the current entry is generally more severe than at the exit. The burns may vary from small, circular spots to large areas of charred destruction. The depth and the extent of burning are often grossly underestimated when first seen. Usually, the lesion appears as an ischemic, whitish yellow, coagulated area, or it may be charred. It is dry and painless. The edges are usually well defined initially, but necrosis is the dominant feature of the lesion, and therefore, it is always more extensive than originally anticipated. This later extension of necrosis is at least partly due to ischemia from arterial thrombi. Necrosis deep to the lesion in the subcutaneous tissues and muscles is common. A limb may appear viable soon after an electric accident, but in a few days it becomes ischemic and, finally, gangrenous. Extreme spasm and thrombosis of arteries and necrosis of the walls may extend the area of necrosis. Parts of the media of vessels may be weakened by cellular disintegration, and if thrombosis does not occur, the lesions may lead to serious hemorrhage.

The histologic appearance of the dead muscle varies. Immediate heat coagulative changes cause a pale appearance in the muscle; some muscle becomes soft. The death of muscle bundles usually is very uneven. As time progresses, it can easily be seen that some muscle fibers are viable and adjacent ones are not. It is not infrequent, after the first 5 or 6 days, to find nonviable muscle present where there is a good size nutrient artery in normal condition supplying the muscle bundle. This unevenness of destruction is particularly typical of electrical muscle damage.

Burns associated with electricity may be divided into the following three categories:

1. True electrical injury is caused by an electric current passing through the skin after contact with a conductor. There is some disagreement as to the immediate cause of the damage. On one hand, it is held that the damage is due to heat generated by the passage of current; on the other, it held that it is due to a specific action of the current on the tissues. It is true that hot temperatures may be produced by the passage of electric currents through tissues, but the natural history of electrical burns differs so clearly from that of thermal burns that it is impossible to avoid the conclusion that some specific effect of the electric current is at least partially responsible for the damage. It is well known that the current follows blood vessels and that thrombosis, even at some distance from the original injury, is common. This thrombosis is partly responsible for the fact that more tissue is always destroyed in electrical injury than is apparent at first inspection.

2. Electrothermal burns are the result of electrical generation of heat outside the skin, such as flash or arc burns. The burns which follow the

leaping of an electric arc from the conductor to the skin are mainly associated with high tension current. They are severe and deep because an electric arc has a temperature of approximately 2500°C.

The arcing problem is of particular medicolegal interest. It is generally believed that under ordinary atmospheric conditions arcing occurs on a high tension line approximately 1 inch for each 20,000 volts. Once an arc is established, it can be drawn away by the person in contact to a distance of about 10 feet with the highest line voltages. The mineral content and other conditions of the soil at the site of an arcing accident play some part in the intensity of current which the individual receives when he is grounded.

3. Flame burns result from the ignition of clothing by electrical sparks and arcing. Many times the extensive area of flame burn is much greater than the other lesions.

It is little wonder that burns associated with an electrical injury are so different. The lesion varies according to the type of accident. Many times, all three types—electric contact, electrothermal and flame burns—may be evident.

One of the immediate effects of an electric injury is tetanic contraction of the muscle. This may be so severe that fractures and dislocations occur. A delayed effect of an electrical injury, especially about the head, is the development of cataracts; such changes may be unilateral or bilateral and may be stationary or progressive. In electric cataracts, the point of contact is usually, although not always, near the involved eye and becomes evident 4 to 6 months after the accident.

Cardiorespiratory manifestations. The severe cardiorespiratory manifestations usually occur at the time of the initial injury. Respiratory paralysis and ventricular fibrillation are the principal causes of immediate death. Taylor reported electrocardiographic changes in a few patients who showed either right bundle branch block, ectopic focus arrhythmias or supraventricular tachycardia. Probably the most extensive experience with cardiovascular disturbances after electrical injury is that of Andreuzzi of Italy, a report of which was given at the International Symposium on Electrical Accidents. He reported having observed several types of disturbance: disturbances of rhythm consisting essentially of extrasystoles, disturbances in atrioventricular and intraventricular conduction, clinically and electrocardiographically established manifestations of acute coronary insufficiency and subjective disturbances consisting of precordial pains of a constricting type, palpitations and tachycardial attacks.

Abdominal burns. A most distressing diagnostic problem occurs in electrical injuries to the abdomen. It is very difficult to determine whether or not intra-abdominal injury is present. Taylor described two cases of abdominal involvement. The first patient was struck by lightning, the discharge entering through the back and leaving through both feet. Abdominal symptoms were noted on the second day and death followed after 4 days. Autopsy revealed hemorrhagic necrosis of the descending and sigmoid colon. The other patient developed abdominal symptoms on the second day after a high tension injury and later succumbed. Autopsy disclosed subserous hemorrhagic necrosis of the gallbladder. Both of these cases received vasopressor drugs. Therefore, it is difficult to state that the abdominal findings at autopsy were totally due to electrical injury. Almgard reported three cases of electrical burns of the abdomen with intra-abdominal injury; all had intestinal damage.

Careful assessment of intra-abdominal signs and symptoms is important. One must beware making a diagnosis of paralytic ileus associated with the electrical injury and forgetting that intestinal damage may be present.

Renal manifestations. Electrical injuries have a higher incidence of renal failure than burns. Renal damage is most likely caused by one or a combination of the following: the initial severe shock, direct electric current damage to the kidney or renal vessels or abnormal protein breakdown from the damaged tissue. Since muscle is involved, it would appear that renal damage may be similar to that seen in the crush syndrome. Certainly, patients with electrical injury show a greater incidence of hemoglobinuria and hematuria than burned patients. Sachatello and Stephenson found that four of nine patients had marked hemoglobinuria and hematuria. Renal failure occurred in seven of 31 patients reported by Taylor et al.

The most likely cause of renal damage is the toxic products released by the damaged muscle. In some patients, it may be difficult to obtain a good urinary output, in spite of massive quantities of fluid, until after the dead and devitalized muscle is excised.

Platts and Rozner reported two cases of acute tubular necrosis following high tension electrical burns treated by hemodialysis. One patient had 30 days of oliguria and the other 40. Both patients survived but required hemodialysis eight times.

TREATMENT

First Aid

The victim of an electrical shock should be freed from the electric current as quickly as possible. The rescuer must make sure that the current is off before touching the victim to avoid being injured by the current. The current may be switched off or the wires may be cut with a wooden handled axe or properly insulated pliers. Artificial respiration must be started immediately if the victim is not breathing. Mouth-to-mouth resuscitation has saved many lives. If the heart is not beating, there is probably ventricular fibrillation; cardiac massage should be instituted until the patient is removed to a facility where defibrillation is possible.

Fluid Therapy

The amount and type of replacement therapy after electrical injury depends upon the type and extent of the injury. For minor low voltage burns, very little replacement therapy is necessary. When there is true electrical injury, with damage to muscle as well as skin and subcutaneous tissue, large volumes of fluid may be required. Such an injury is very similar to crush injury, and therefore the principles associated with replacement therapy after crush injury are applicable (Fig. 114). In true electrical injury of a major degree, a massive quantity of fluid must be used for replacement. Too often, the clinician looks at the area of electrical injury, finds that it covers only a small percentage of the body surface and therefore determines the amount of fluid to be given on the basis of per cent of skin involvement. When there is damage to the muscle, much larger volumes of tissue have been destroyed than is frequently anticipated; thus, replacement therapy is always greater than expected. There is no formula that can be used to determine the amount of replacement solution for true electrical injury. Resuscitative fluid administration is based primarily on the urinary output. The incidence of renal failure in electrical injury is out of proportion to the total extent of skin involvement, and in this area, electrical injury is similar to crush injury. Renal damage is most likely caused by the precipitation of myoglobin in the renal tubules following muscle death. Some clinicians feel that the administration of an alkaline solution immediately after electrical injury prevents

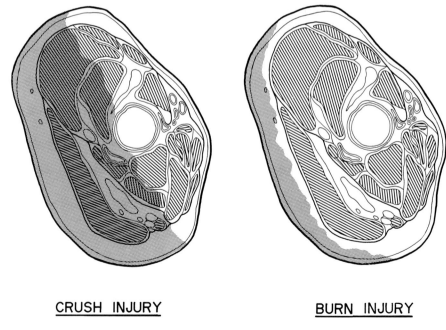

CRUSH INJURY   BURN INJURY

Figure 114.   Electrical injury simulates crush injury.

renal complications. The value of the administration of a sodium bicarbonate solution has not been established. The real aim in preventing renal damage should be the administration of an adequate amount of resuscitative fluids to provide good renal perfusion. Resuscitative fluids should include colloids, such as plasma, dextran and possibly whole blood, lactated Ringer's solution in large quantities and glucose in water. Such fluids should be given at a rate sufficient to maintain a urinary output of approximately 30 ml. per hour. When urine flow is not adequate, mannitol may be of considerable value. In extensive injuries it is always wise to put a catheter into a major venous channel so that central venous pressure can be measured. Monitoring the venous pressure will prevent overloading of the circulation and pulmonary edema. If there is a massive amount of dead tissue, emergency operation to amputate the part or remove the dead tissue may be necessary before an adequate urine volume can be obtained. In some instances it is impossible to combat shock until the dead tissue is removed.

When the injury is merely a thermal burn and there is no evidence of true electrical injury, fluid management should follow the usual principles for replacement in thermal burns, according to the extent and depth of the injury.

Local Wound Management

The principles of local wound management depend upon the type of injury. If there is no evidence of tissue damage beneath the skin and subcutaneous tissue, the area should be treated according to the principles for full-thickness thermal burns. The surgeon's first responsibility, however, is to make sure that there is no underlying muscle damage. This can usually be ascertained by incising one or two areas and looking at the muscle beneath.

If there is dead muscle, the patient should be taken to the operating room as soon as his general physical condition permits and all of the dead skin, subcutaneous tissue and muscle excised (Fig. 115). Again, such an injury is similar to crush injury, and dead muscle must be removed. Clostridial myositis is a common complication of electrical injury. It develops because of inadequate excision of dead muscle. When the electrical injury is adequately debrided in the first 24 hours, clostridial myositis does not occur. After all the dead muscle has been cut away, a dressing should be applied and the wound inspected 3 or 4 days later. Usually a second, and sometimes a third, debridement will be required. Thrombosis, common after electrical injury, deprives muscle fibers of their blood supply and their death follows. This makes the lesion of electrical injury seem somewhat progressive. Since the effect of electrical current on arterial walls weakens them, secondary hemorrhage is common. When an extremity has major damage, it is usually necessary to amputate (Fig. 116). The stump should be allowed to remain open because frequently it becomes necessary to amputate again a few inches higher.

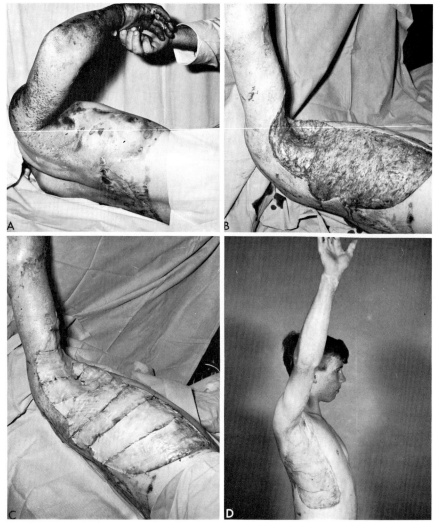

Figure 115. Electrical injury from 11,000 volts in 16-year-old boy. *A*, Full-thickness thermal burn of right chest and true electrical injury to shoulder and deltoid muscle. *B*, Entire area of dead muscle and full-thickness skin loss excised 24 hours after injury. *C*, On the sixth postinjury day, split-thickness autografts were applied in lay-on fashion and exposed. *D*, Follow-up photograph taken 3 months after injury.

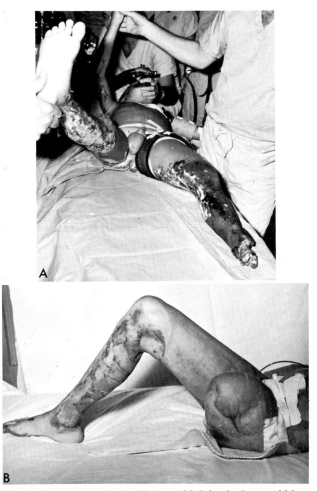

Figure 116. *A*, Severe true electrical injury of left leg in 8-year-old boy who came in contact with a high voltage line. Amputation with further amputation was required. *B*, Healed amputation stump after delayed primary closure.

After debridement, the wound should be inspected every 2 or 3 days. As soon as there is no further evidence of dead tissue, the wound should be closed by delayed primary closure after amputation or by a split-thickness skin graft after excision of a broad area.

When the burn is small and of low voltage, like that seen after injury from house current, it should be treated conservatively. Excision is usually not required. Certainly in lesions of the lips, initial conservative treatment allowing the wound to slough and heal, followed by plastic reconstruction at a later date, is the preferred method of management.

When there is only a thermal burn and there is no evidence of deeper electrical damage, the principles associated with local management of thermal burns should pertain. If the area is small and obviously full thickness, primary excision, with grafting 4 days later, is an excellent method of management. If the area is more extensive, a local chemotherapeutic regimen should be used.

CHEMICAL BURNS

Most lethal chemical burns are the result of industrial accidents or military conflict. However, domestic and laboratory mishaps and deliberate criminal assaults lead to the greatest frequency of these burns, which, though smaller in area, cause significant morbidity.

The mechanism of injury is a combination of chemical and thermal alteration of tissue. In Table 15 are listed the more common agents encountered, and it will be noted that only in burns by phosphorus is the thermal component the major factor. In such cases, the histologic picture is one of thermal destruction of a localized but frequently deeply penetrating nature. The thermal damage is intense in the limited area of involvement.

Tissue study of those burns in which chemical alteration, such as denaturation, precipitation and alkalization, is predominant reveals intra- and intercellular edema of skin and subcutaneous tissue, nuclear vacuolization of the skin, separation of dermis from epidermis, disorganization of the cellular architecture of the dermal appendages and widening and coalescence of collagen bundles (Table 16). Severity and depth of cellular damage is a function of duration of exposure and concentration and, with the longer periods thrombosis of deep capillary, venular and arteriolar networks, results in progressive tissue necrosis.

Acid Burns

The distribution of acid burns depends upon the nature of exposure as well as duration and concentration. Immersion in acid slurries, such as may occur in industrial plants, results in a predictable distribution covering the immersed body area. Wearing apparel may influence this to some extent but only if exposure is brief. The more frequent and more typical acid burn is due to spill or splatter, with contact being spotty or in the form of rivulets coursing down the body.

Characteristically, the wound is extremely painful, and the pain often persists for long periods because of the continued chemical reaction. Appearance varies, according to depth of burn, from erythema in the more superficial to gray, yellowish brown or black in the deeper lesions. Though leathery in texture in most instances, the superficial wounds are soft.

Systemic complications of acid burns are not of significance except in the case of hydrofluoric acid burns, in which immobilization of fluoride may cause alterations in clotting mechanisms. When this occurs, however, the burn is so extensive that it is an initially fatal wound.

Table 15. Pathophysiology of Chemical Injury

AGENT	MECHANISM OF ACTION	APPEARANCE	TEXTURE
Acid Burns			
Sulfuric Nitric Hydrochloric Trichloroacetic Phenol	Exothermic reaction, cellular dehydration and protein precipitation	Gray, yellow, brown or black, depending on duration of exposure	Soft to leathery eschar, depending on duration of exposure
Hydrofluoric	Same as other acids plus liquefaction and decalcification	Erythema with central necrosis	Painful, leathery eschar
Alkali Burns			
Potassium hydroxide Sodium hydroxide Lime	Exothermic reaction, hygroscopic cellular dehydration with saponification of fat and protein precipitation	Erythema with bullae	Painful, "soapy" or slick eschar
Ammonia	Same as other bases plus laryngeal and pulmonary edema	Gray, yellow, brown or black, often very deep	Soft to leathery, depending on duration
Phosphorus	Thermal effect, melts at body temperature, runs, ignites at 34°C., acid effect of H_2PO_4	Gray or blue green, glows in dark	Depressed, leathery eschar
Mustard gas	Vesicant, alkalization effect	Marked erythema with vesicles and bullae	Painful, soft vesicles and bullae
Tear gas	Weak acid effect	Similar to mild second-degree flame burn	Soft and wet

Table 16. Histology — Acid and Alkali Burns

Epidermis may appear intact but is not

Cytoplasmic edema

Epidermal perinuclear vacuolization with elongated pyknotic nuclei

Dermal — epidermal separation

Collagen banding and loss of collagen

Intercellular edema with separation and irregularity of cells of sebaceous and sweat glands

Endothelial thickening and thrombosis of deep dermal capillaries

Concomitant with exposure to acids in industrial accidents, there may be inhalation of acid fumes. In such instances, a chemical tracheobronchitis of varying severity may markedly limit respiratory exchange. Tracheostomy and pulmonary hygiene with ventilatory support is mandatory.

Treatment of acid burns is most effectively accomplished immediately after onset and thus becomes both a first aid and a definitive action. Except in industrial and some laboratory areas, where specific antidotes are often available, the most readily available substance for effective treatment is water. Copious rinsing with plain water as soon as possible is the most effective practical method of therapy. This simple dilution of the agent is quite effective.

Should specific antidotes be readily available, these are used, but

Table 17. MANAGEMENT OF CHEMICAL BURNS

AGENT	CLEANSING	NEUTRALIZATION	DEBRIDEMENT
Acid Burns			
Sulfuric Nitric Hydrochloric Trichloroacetic	Water	Sodium bicarbonate solution	Debride loose, nonviable tissue
Phenol	Ethyl alcohol	Sodium bicarbonate solution	Debride loose, nonviable tissue
Hydrofluoric	Water	Same as other acids plus magnesium oxide, glycerin paste, local injection, calcium gluconate	Debride loose, nonviable tissue
Alkali Burns			
Potassium hydroxide Sodium hydroxide Ammonia	Water	0.5–5.0% acetic acid or 5.0% ammonium chloride	Debride loose, nonviable tissue
Lime	Brush off powder	0.5–5.0% acetic acid or 5.0% ammonium chloride	Debride loose, nonviable tissue
Phosphorus	Water	Copper sulfate soaks	Debride and remove particles of phosphorus
Mustard gas	Water	M-5 ointment	Aspirate; then excise blebs during flushing with water
Tear gas	Water	Sodium bicarbonate solution	Debride loose tissue

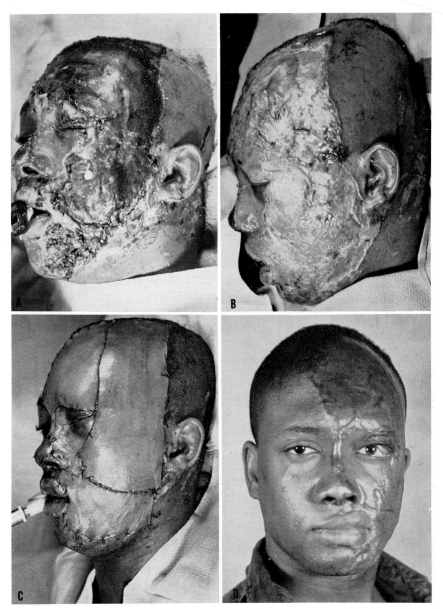

Figure 117. *A*, The fourteenth postburn day. Sulfuric acid burn of the face. Although excision of eschars on the face is rarely indicated, it was required in this instance because of the tight adherence of the tough eschar.

B, Appearance immediately after excision on the fourteenth postburn day. The area is clean and ready for application of a dressing.

C, The nineteenth postburn day. Thick split-thickness grafts taken with a Padgett dermatome are sutured in place.

D, The graft is completely healed, but further plastic procedures were necessary to correct the contractures around the eye and the lips.

therapy with water should never be delayed while these agents are being secured (see Table 17). After rinsing with water and treatment with specific antidotes, debridement of loose, nonviable tissue is accomplished.

General support and fluid resuscitation are the same as for a flame burn. Close observation of cardiopulmonary response is mandatory, however, as depth of burn and pulmonary damage are difficult to assess. After initial care, the local treatment of acid burns is the same as that for thermal injuries (Fig. 117).

Alkali Burns

Circumstances of burning, distribution of burn, appearance and treatment of alkali burns is essentially the same as that for acid burns. Some important differences do exist, however, and should be understood in regard to burns by phosphorus.

While of little import to the civilian surgeon, phosphorus burns are an extremely painful and common injury in modern warfare. This substance melts at body temperature and penetrates deeply into tissue. The wound can be seen to emit smoke if the phosphorus is exposed to air, and in the dark, the wounds glow with an eerie bluish green color.

For decades it has been advocated that copper sulfate is the optimum substance for the therapy of burns due to organic phosphorus. The use of copper sulfate is based on its reaction with the phosphorus to produce an inert shell of cupric phosphide over the surface of the organic phosphorus. This inactivates the phosphorus and stops the tissue destruction. The chemical must then be surgically removed from the tissue.

The reaction is quite effective in stopping the combustion of phosphorus, but it may result in copper toxicity, manifested primarily by massive hemolysis of red blood cells and subsequent acute renal tubular necrosis. To obviate this occurrence when copper sulfate is used, an active urine flow must be maintained either by means of a fluid load or mannitol.

Burns resulting from ammonia are often quite deep, and the persistent pain may divert attention from a much more lethal aspect of the exposure, the pulmonary component. Severe laryngeal and tracheobronchial edema is a common complication of inhalation of concentrated ammonia fumes. Tracheostomy, pulmonary hygiene and effective ventilatory support are the essentials to successful therapy.

A rare occurrence even in military casualties today is that due to mustard gas. Such burns result from training accidents and, fortunately, involve dilute concentrations of the agent. This vesicant gas causes the rapid appearance of progressively enlarging blisters, or bullae, at points of contact with the skin (Fig. 118). These painful lesions must be ruptured, but only during copious rinsing with water to prevent the chemical contacting adjacent skin in effective concentration. The wound is then left exposed.

General support and fluid resuscitation are the same as with a flame burn, but the same precautions are taken as with the acid burn.

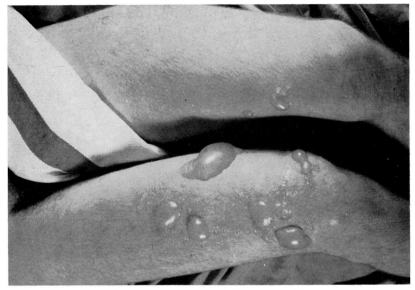

Figure 118. Mustard gas burn at 27 hours after injury. The large blebs surrounded by a wide zone of erythema are typical.

In any chemical burn of the eyes, extreme care must be exercised. Copious rinsing and specific antidotes as soon as possible are mandatory to prevent extensive and irreversible damage.

Subsequent to removal or neutralization of the chemical agent, the burn wound is handled in the same manner as a flame burn. Frequently the burn, although appearing deep and well circumscribed initially, will heal quite rapidly by peripheral contracture and proliferation. This is particularly true in the splash or spill burns and surprisingly so in many burns by phosphorus.

Magnesium Burns

Burns from ignited magnesium are relatively uncommon. Usually they occur among workers in munitions factories or among persons subjected to incendiary bombing. Magnesium burns produce ulcers which are small at first but gradually enlarge to form extensive lesions. Wilson and Egeberg have pointed out that the deeper part of the ulcer is usually quite irregular. They believe that at first the ignited magnesium is only on the skin and then penetrates irregularly into the deeper tissue. By scraping the outer layers of the skin under local anesthesia soon after injury, most of the magnesium may be removed. Magnesium may be a rapid or slow burning ember, depending upon the size of the particles involved. If the slow burning embers penetrate deeper than the outer layers of the skin, they must be excised completely, and the wound must be closed by means of delayed primary suture or by skin grafting.

REFERENCES

Almgard, L.-E., Liljedahl, S.-O., and Nylen, B.: Electric burns of the abdomen. *Acta chir. scandinav.* **130**:550, 1965.

Artz, C. P., Electrical injury simulates crush injury. *Surg. Gynec. & Obst.* **125**:1316, 1967.

Brown, K. L., and Moritz, A. R.: Electrical injuries. *J. Trauma* **4**:608, 1964.

Kouwenhoven, W. B.: Effects of electricity on the human body. *Electrical Engineering* **68**:199, 1949.

Kragh, L. V., and Erich, J. B.: Treatment of severe electric injuries. *Am. J. Surg.* **101**:419, 1961.

Mills, W., Jr., Switzer, W. E., and Moncrief, J. A.: Electrical injuries. *J.A.M.A.* **195**:852, 1966.

Muir, I. F. K.: The management of electrical burns. *Postgrad. M.J.* **33**:219, 1957.

Platts, M. M., and Rozner, L.: Survival after high tension electrical burns complicated by acute tubular necrosis. *Brit. M. J.* **1**:781, 1966.

Proceedings of the International Symposium on Electrical Accidents. Geneva, Switzerland, International Occupational Safety and Health Information Centre, International Labour Office, 1964.

Rabinowitch, I. M.: Treatment of phosphorus burns. *Canad. M.A.J.* **48**:291, 1943.

Sachatello, C. R., and Stephenson, S. E., Jr.: Management of high voltage electrical burns. *Am. Surgeon* **31**:807, 1965.

Sevitt, S.: *Burns — Pathology and Therapeutic Applications.* London, Butterworth & Co., Ltd., 1957.

Taylor, P. H., Pugsley, L. Q., and Vogel, E. H., Jr.: The intriguing electrical burn, *J. Trauma* **2**:309, 1962.

Terry, H.: Caustic soda burns, their prevention and treatment. *Brit. M.J.* **1**:756, 1943.

Wilson, J. A., and Egeberg, B.: Treatment of burns of the skin due to molten magnesium. *Indust. Med.* **11**:433, 1942.

Chapter
Ten

BURNS OF
SPECIFIC AREAS

Burns in certain regions of the body present some special difficulties. Recommendations for therapy of these specific areas may be helpful.

BURNS ABOUT THE HEAD

Management of burns about the head is particularly difficult because of the many important functional organs involved. For some unexplained reason, a more marked systemic response appears to be associated with deep burns about the face and neck than with burns of comparable extent in other areas. Extensive edema occurs because the loose areolar tissues around the face and neck offer little tissue pressure to oppose extravasation of edema fluid. Convulsions occurring in children with head burns are frequently reported in the British literature. Cerebral edema has been demonstrated by special autopsy techniques in these instances. Such episodes are rare in our experience. (See Chapter Eleven.)

Burns of the Face

Rapidly developing edema is characteristic of most burns of the face. If the burn is a deep third-degree one with a leathery, inelastic eschar, little swelling can occur outwardly and thus swelling is manifested mainly by edema of the posterior pharynx and other soft tissues of the neck. The eyelids become edematous and are usually closed tightly within 6 to 8 hours after injury. Most of the edema occurs in the first 24 hours, although it does not reach its maximum formation until about 48 hours (see Fig. 88, Chapter Six). It is difficult to determine accurately the initial depth of a burn on the face. Occasionally the injury appears to be third degree initially, but with proper care epithelization occurs in many areas from the lining of the hair follicles. This is particularly true in the beard area in adult males.

The principal initial problem in burns about the face and neck is to determine the presence of respiratory tract irritation. When such involvement is seen, an early tracheostomy is indicated (see Respiratory Tract Damage, p. 241).

Initial cleansing and removal of all detached epithelium are indicated. Unless this is done, an accurate appraisal of depth and distribution cannot be made. If the burn involves the hair or is near the hairline, the hair should be removed by clippers when the initial cleansing is performed (Fig. 119). This allows a cleaner wound than would be possible otherwise. Inspissated crusts must be removed from the nose and an adequate nasal airway assured if possible. Edema of the face and lips often precludes mouth breathing. Both second- and third-degree burns of the face do well when treated by the exposure method, and the advent of effective topical therapy has greatly improved results. Dressings are difficult to apply, extremely uncomfortable, and should not be used. Both the patient and his family should be informed of the impending formation of edema. They should be forewarned particularly about the closure of the eyelids for the first 48 to 72 hours.

Superficial second-degree burns usually heal uneventfully without scarring in 14 to 21 days (Fig. 120). Thick crusts are particularly prone to occur in second-degree burns of the face, and infection is readily hid-

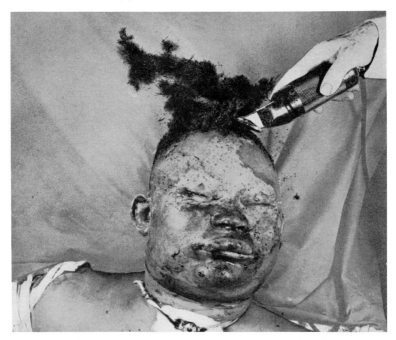

Figure 119. The hair should be clipped during initial cleansing of the face, especially if the burn involves the hairline. This patient had a partial- and full-thickness burn of the face that was cleansed gently with soap and water. An elective tracheotomy was performed 12 hours after the burn, before appreciable edema had occurred in the neck.

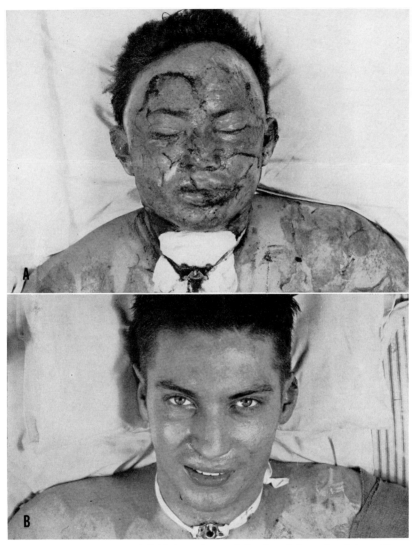

Figure 120. *A*, Deep partial-thickness burn of the face 2 days after injury. The area was cleansed with soap and water. All devitalized epithelium was removed, and hair adjacent to the burn was clipped. The face was treated by the exposure method. A tracheotomy was done prophylactically on this patient. Subsequent experience indicates that such a burn does not usually require this type of airway if close observation can be maintained. *B*, A month later, the face is completely healed, and there is little evidence of scarring. The tracheostomy should not remain in place only for administration of anesthesia, as was done in this case; it should be removed after 5 to 10 days.

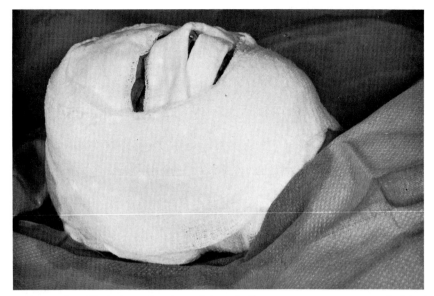

Figure 121. Typical wet dressings of face. Ordinary gauze sponges are applied to the face with apertures left for eyes, nares and mouth. Sponges are held in place by conforming gauze roll loosely wrapped. Dressing is soaked with saline every 4 hours and changed twice daily.

den beneath them. This is often precipitated by the moisture about the eyes and mouth and the bacteria ubiquitous in the deep follicles of the beard area. The crust may crack as the beard grows. When the crusts become wet or infection appears beneath them, wet dressings should be applied to hasten the removal of the crust and to prevent infection from destroying the underlying epithelium (Fig. 121). With few exceptions, dressing changes three times daily are required by the end of the first week. The vermilion portion of the lips and angles of the mouth crust and crack readily and healing may thus be retarded. Generous application of glycerin to the lips softens crusts and allows less traumatic removal.

Healing of second-degree burns tightens the skin of the face and removes wrinkles and skin creases. This gives a pleasing result in superficial injury, but the deeper second-degree burn heals with webbing of the mouth, loss of the nasolabial fold and often ectropion.

When full-thickness burns are exposed, the devitalized skin dries and serves as a temporary protective cover. About the end of the first week, when bacterial autolysis begins, wet saline dressings applied every

---

Illustration on opposite page.

Figure 122. *A*, Third-degree burn of the face at 24 hours following injury. Edema of the eyelids has resulted in their closure. The tight eschar of the full-thickness burn directs the edema inward, except for the typically everted lips. Compare this with Figure 119, a second-degree burn. The tracheostomy makes it possible to maintain an adequate airway

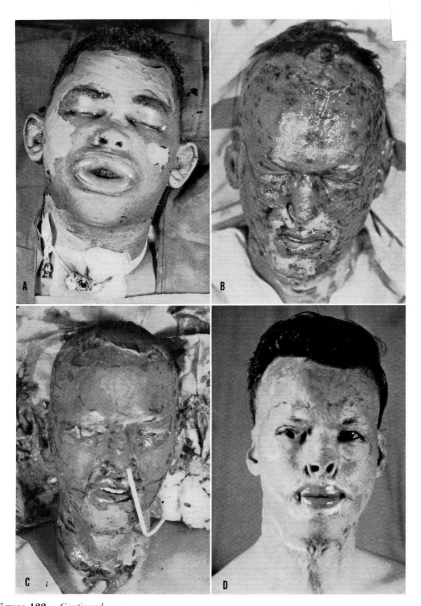

Figure 122. *Continued*

and prevents aspiration of vomitus. Regurgitation is common, and the inelastic eschar pro-
hibits opening of the mouth to permit egress of the fluid. The burn was treated by the exposure method. *B,* The twenty-sixth postburn day. Wet dressings were applied to the face,
beginning on the eighth postburn day. The entire eschar has been removed, and the area
is ready for grafting. *C,* The thirtieth postburn day. At the initial grafting procedure, a tarsorrhaphy was performed on each eye. Almost all of the face was covered by split-thickness
grafts. The plastic nasogastric tube was used for feeding purposes. Anesthesia is being administered through an endotracheal tube placed in the tracheostomy opening. *D,* Seven months
after injury. The tarsorrhaphy on the left eye has been opened, and a small skin graft has
been placed beneath the lower lid. The right tarsorrhapy is still intact. Considerable loss of
cartilage resulted from deep burns of both ears. A contracture about the mouth required
correction.

4 hours soften the eschar and hasten its sequestration and subsequent removal. Grafting can usually be performed by the eighteenth to twenty-first day (Fig. 122). Excision of eschars of the face is indicated only in rare instances.

Grafting of the scalp or beard area is fraught with difficulty, even in areas covered with confluent, healthy appearing granulations. Graft take is poor unless special techniques are used. Failure is due to the persistence, even in deep burns, of the hair follicles and the remaining perifollicular epithelium beneath the tissue destruction. When autografts are placed over these areas, proliferation of the epithelial buds is stimulated. This is often extremely rapid, occurring in 4 to 6 hours, associated with auto-lytic purulence, and resulting in graft loss.

To prevent such tragedy, close attention should be directed toward the wound, which should be left exposed after grafting to facilitate access. The simplest technique is to cover the areas with fresh homograft, as loss of this skin is of no consequence. The epithelial stimulation occurs as well as with autograft, and with equal swiftness the purulence appears beneath the grafts. Every 6 to 8 hours, the homografts are removed simply by peeling them off, and fresh ones are applied. As healing progresses, the intervals are longer. In 7 to 10 days, complete healing has usually occurred.

If autografts are used, the area must be inspected every 4 to 6 hours until final healing. Dressings are not used and grafts are laid on without sutures. During inspection, areas of purulence which identify hair follicles or epithelial islands are unroofed. This allows the autograft to fuse with the margins of the expanding epithelial islands.

Although free of deep follicles, burns of the forehead, temples and malar areas are best grafted without sutures. Adequate dressings are a rarity in these areas and are not needed.

Several weeks after complete coverage of the hairy areas, grafts may break down because of delayed hair follicle proliferation. Homografts and soap-and-water cleansing help.

Burns of the face and the hands should be given first priority for skin cover. Split-thickness sheets of skin must be applied. Additional plastic procedures for cosmetic and functional purposes are usually not indicated for at least 6 months and preferably 18 months. Occasionally, if there is significant functional impairment, it may be necessary to reconstruct eyelids or relieve contractures about the mouth prior to 6 months.

Burns of the Eyelids

All face burns demand close examination of the eyes and ophthalmologic consultation, particularly with deeper burns. Injury by blast or foreign body must be kept in mind.

Burns of the eyelids occur frequently when the face is burned. However, burns of the sclera and cornea are rare. Usually the eyelids close by reflex action and the cornea and sclera are not damaged. In addition, the constantly wet conjunctiva provides insulation. Occasionally a flash burn affects these areas, but the mild irritation produced usually heals within 2 days.

In partial-thickness burns of the eyelids, edema closes the eyes for a period of 48 to 72 hours. The important therapy during this period is routine eye care, such as irrigation with saline and the instillation of an antibiotic ophthalmic ointment to prevent infection. It is particularly important to realize that the eye itself need not be involved directly with thermal injury for serious damage and even blindness to occur. The infection present in the periocular skin can rapidly extend to the globe structures, particularly the cornea. Every effort must be made to avoid such an occurrence.

In full-thickness burns of the eyelids, the chief danger is rapid contracture and ectropion formation. The resulting incomplete closure of the lids causes drying of the cornea and ulcer formation. If infection then supervenes, a panophthalmitis may develop. The important aim in treating burns of the eyelids, therefore, is protection of the cornea. It is sometimes necessary in the early postburn period to suture the lids or tarsal plates together to protect the cornea while the wound is being prepared for grafting. As soon as the eschar is removed, the area is grafted in such a way as to prevent ectropion formation.

The procedure used to prevent contracture depends upon the amount of involvement of the surrounding skin (Figs. 123 and 124). If the skin adjacent to the lower lid is burned and the skin adjacent to the upper lid is normal, only the lower lid is likely to become contracted and vice versa. In such instances, the affected lid should be overcorrected in such a way as to make allowance for a certain amount of inevitable contracture. Contracture is delayed but inexorable, particularly in the malar area, with only flattening of the nasolabial fold in mild cases but extreme ectropion and elevation of the corner of the mouth in others. Unless allowance is made for further contracture with maturation, another correction will be necessary. Sutures are placed along the margin of the lid and tension is applied. An incision is made through the superficial tissue of the lid to release any contracture of scar tissue that may have occurred. If the lashes are greatly everted and a rim of conjunctiva is easily seen, there is evidence of rolling of the lid margin along with the ectropion. In such cases, the incision must be made very close to the lid margin to allow it to roll back to its normal position.

A split-thickness graft may be sutured into place and a stent dressing applied. If so, the stent should be removed in 48 hours to prevent necrosis of the margin of the wound. There is so little motion by this time that the graft is quite safe. Graft sutures are removed after 3 days.

A simpler and equally effective method is to suture the lid margins together (blepharorrhaphy) and merely lay the graft free on the defect

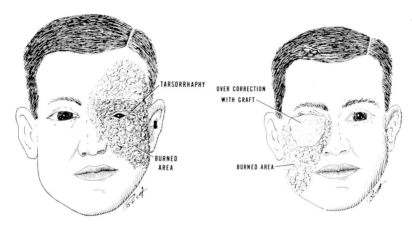

Figure 123   **Figure 124**

Figure 123. Diagram to illustrate the type of burn requiring a tarsorrhaphy. When the burned area involves an appreciable amount of skin adjacent to both the upper and lower eyelids, a tarsorrhaphy must be performed to prevent contracture of the lids and ectropion formation. The tarsorrhaphy is done at the time a skin graft is applied.

Figure 124. Diagrammatic outline to show the corrective procedure required when a third-degree burn is adjacent to only one eyelid. In this instance, there was a burn of the lower eyelid and the adjacent skin of the cheek. The upper eyelid was not involved. Such configuration of burn does not require a tarsorrhaphy, but an overcorrection of the lower eyelid is made when the initial skin graft is applied. Tarsorrhaphy is indicated if both eyelids are involved; but if only one eyelid is involved, overcorrection with a graft is the procedure of choice.

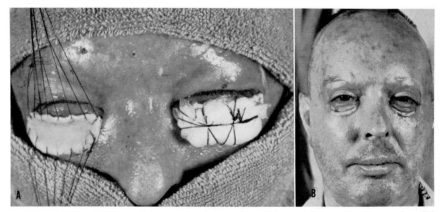

Figure 125. *A,* This patient sustained deep dermal burns of the entire face and eyelids 6 weeks prior to this photograph. There was contracture of both lower eyelids. After releasing these contractures, an overcorrection graft was applied. The graft on the right eye has been sutured in place and is ready to be dressed. A stent-type dressing has been completed over the graft on the left lower eyelid. *B,* Both eyelids have healed completely. The thick, split-thickness skin grafts are quite evident. The graft did not contract; hence a good functional and cosmetic result was obtained.

without sutures or dressings. This allows constant inspection and evacuation of any fluid which may collect beneath the graft. Results are as good as with any other method.

In deep dermal burns, contracture of the lids sometimes occurs after epithelization. Overcorrection with grafts is the acceptable corrective procedure (Fig. 125). In these instances, split grafts of intermediate thickness give the best results. The same techniques are used.

In more extensive, full-thickness burns about the eye involving both upper and lower eyelids, a tarsorrhaphy may be performed at the time the graft is applied. Tarsorrhaphy was once considered essential to minimizing ectropion of both lids because of contracture of the surrounding skin. However, it will not obviate the scar contracture, only distort it. Simple blepharorrhaphy will usually suffice even if the lids are pulled apart in a few days. If the tarsorrhaphy is to hold, it must be of the tongue-in-groove type (Fig. 126). This is done at the time the graft is applied.

A small peephole is left in the center of the lid with medial and lateral apertures for irrigation. Stents are removed at 48 hours to gain access to the eye for mandatory irrigations. As soon as the grafts are well attached (3 days), the tarsorrhaphy may be divided under local anesthesia. The slow but unrelenting contracture of adjacent scar cannot be resisted effectively by lid apposition, and free access to the eye is of much greater importance.

Burns of the Ears

Thermal injury to the skin of the external ear may result in direct destruction of the cartilage or necrosis subsequent to infection. The early inflammatory necrosis is not usually associated with demonstrable bacterial involvement. As the process progresses, more cartilage is liquefied and an abscess of the auricle is formed. This is characterized by a swollen, tender, extremely painful helix. Other areas are less often involved but are not immune. The purulent chondritis which occurs may be associated with either partial- or full-thickness burns of the ear but is completely unpredictable in occurrence.

Once chondritis has developed, the aim is to minimize infection and prevent further destruction of the cartilage. The best method of treatment is wet soaks and, if necessary, early and wide excision of the necrotic cartilage. A fishmouth-type incision is made extending along the entire area of involved helix. The devitalized cartilage may thus be exposed and removed (Fig. 127). Since chondritis cannot be predicted, prophylactic surgery is not indicated. Topical antibacterial therapy has shown no ability to diminish the incidence, reflecting the lack of evidence that infection is the primary cause.

Free drainage can be accomplished by separating the layers of the wound with loose gauze and by applying warm, wet compresses continuously. The wound must not be packed, as this obstructs the drainage. The warm compresses also alleviate pain. When the necrosis subsides, the

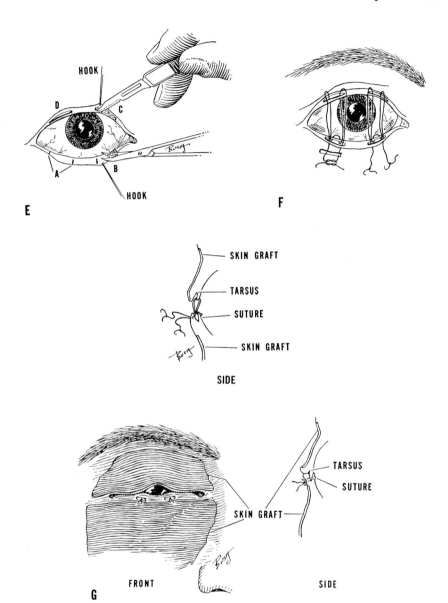

Figure 126. *E.* Initial steps in technique of tongue-in-groove type tarsorrhaphy. Areas are prepared at *A, B, C* and *D* to use the tarsal plate on the upper eyelid as the tongue to be placed in a groove prepared in the lower eyelid. This makes an attachment of the lids on either side of the iris, allowing a peephole in the center. After the sites are selected, the first step is to make small transverse incisions as shown in *A*. A pair of scissors is used to remove a thin strip of epithelium between these incisions as shown in *B*. A knife is used to separate the anterior and posterior layers of the lid as shown in *C*. This separation on the upper lid is done anterior to the tarsal plate. Area *D* is then ready for suturing as shown in *F*.

F, The lids are sutured together with 5-0 silk. A needle is placed on either end of the suture and the sutures are started from the posterior aspect of the lower lid. They are carried up through the posterior lip of the upper lid and out through the anterior portion of the

Legend continues on opposite page.

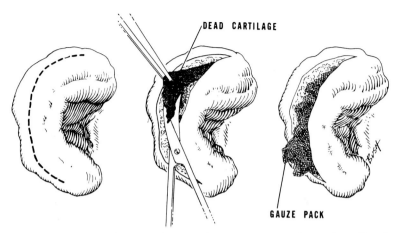

Figure 127. In partial- or full-thickness burns of the ear, the cartilage liquefies and becomes infected. Usually there is considerable edema of the auricle. The preferred method of treatment is a wide, fishmouth-type incision along the helix. The dead cartilage is removed and the two layers of the ear are held apart with a light gauze wick. Packing is to be avoided, since it obstructs drainage. Wet dressings are applied, and the gauze is changed each day. The ear heals by secondary intention.

ear heals by secondary intention. In such burns of the ear, subsequent plastic reconstruction may be desired but is not necessary for auditory acuity which suffers little with loss of auricle.

RESPIRATORY TRACT DAMAGE ASSOCIATED WITH BURNS

Respiratory tract damage is most frequently associated with burns about the face and neck, especially in individuals burned in a closed space. However, it is known to occur in any type of burn. Respiratory irritation results from inhalation of noxious fumes and gases and should be termed inhalation injury, not burn. For clinical purposes, respiratory tract injury may be divided into two parts: damage to the upper respiratory tract, and damage to the lower respiratory tract (Fig. 128).

Injury of the upper respiratory tract includes irritation of the pos-

Figure 126. *Continued.*
lower lid. This brings the posterior portion of the upper lid (the part containing the tarsus) into the groove of the lower lid. The sutures are tied over a small piece of rubber catheter. Excessive tension must be avoided.

G, Skin grafts are applied after the tarsorrhaphy has been completed. The split-thickness skin should be placed near the margins of the lid and anchored in place with fine interrupted sutures. The sutures in the tarsorrhaphy may be removed between the eighth and tenth postoperative day.

UPPER RESPIRATORY TRACT

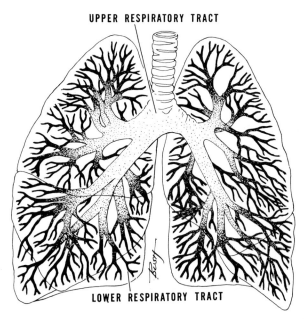

LOWER RESPIRATORY TRACT

Figure 128. Diagrammatic outline of the respiratory tract. The clear areas show the upper respiratory tract, particularly the trachea and larger bronchi. If these areas are injured by the inhalation of noxious gases and fumes, a marked amount of secretion will result; but these larger air passages can be kept free if a tracheotomy is performed. The heavily shaded areas represent the lower respiratory tract. Irritation of this area leads to damage in the alveoli. A tracheostomy is indicated in treatment; however, most patients who experience injury to the lower respiratory tract do not survive.

terior pharynx, trachea and larger bronchi. Injury of the lower respiratory tract involves the bronchioles and alveoli. Since air is such a poor conductor of heat (air:water = 1:4000), an actual burn of the respiratory passages does not occur except in certain experimental situations or with the inhalation of steam. Even those individuals burned while inhaling 100 per cent oxygen sustain actual thermal damage only as far down as the larynx. Carbon particles, while heaviest in the same area, may extend down further. The most common cause of respiratory tract damage in association with a burn is inhalation of combustion products. This occurs most often when the individual is burned in a closed space. However, marked alterations in pulmonary dynamics may occur in the absence of any direct involvement of the respiratory tree, suggesting a systemic response to thermal injury.

Inhalation injury is recognized clinically by redness and edema in the posterior pharynx, coughing and hoarseness. Singeing of the nasal hairs may be present but is not often seen. A delay of hours to 2 or 3 days in appearance of clinical signs is characteristic of this damage. Later signs, occurring a few hours to 2 days after injury, are rales, dyspnea and increased respiratory rate. Bronchospasm with prolonged wheezing may be a prominent finding, and increased bronchial markings may be apparent on roentgenographic examination (Fig. 129).

It is important to realize that clinical evidence of pulmonary involvement usually exists many hours before roentgenographic changes are noted. This is particularly true of rales, ronchi and the wheezing of bronchospasm. In damage to the upper respiratory tract, profuse secretions may be present, and a secretional type of obstruction may occur unless a tracheotomy is performed promptly.

Injury to the lower respiratory tract may produce (1) obstruction of the airway because of bronchial constriction, congestion, edema, or desquamation, (2) congestion of the alveolar walls, or (3) pulmonary edema. Any or all of these effects may markedly alter the resistance to breathing, the distribution of inspired air or diffusion of gases across the alveolar membrane and result in serious hypoventilation.

Appreciable injury to the lower respiratory tract is difficult to treat successfully. Usually the patient's condition deteriorates rapidly until death occurs within a few hours of injury. Characteristically this is associated with progressive severe pulmonary edema.

Studies of ventilatory efficiency in burned patients, as manifested by pCO_2, pO_2 and oxyhemoglobin saturation, show that depth and extent

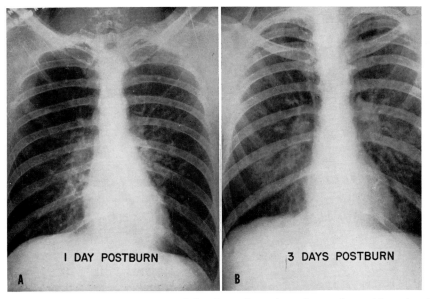

Figure 129. *A*, Roentgenogram of the chest of a patient who was burned in a closed space when a mattress caught fire. He received appreciable damage through inhalation. On the first day after the burn, there is only a slight increase in bronchial markings in the lung fields. *B*, The third postburn day. Roentgenogram shows a marked infiltration and increase of hilar markings in both lung fields. A tracheotomy was performed on this patient as soon as he was admitted and he experienced an uneventful recovery. It was believed that he had irritation of only the upper respiratory tract.

of burn rather than location are the significant factors. Early postburn difficulty is almost exclusively irritational, while pulmonary complications secondary to fluid overloading, atelectasis and secretional obstruction occur later. Trauma to the upper tract from mechanical efforts at cleansing is often a significant factor in morbidity and mortality.

While extensive atelectasis or hyaline membrane formation is frequently seen in such patients at autopsy, ventilatory studies do not differentiate distributional problems from those of diffusion. Hyaline membranes are seen as often in those without respirator support as in those with it.

Irrespective of the areas involved, the treatment of respiratory tract damage associated with burns is the same. Treatment consists of the maintenance of adequate ventilation by any means available. This often includes tracheostomy followed by diligent gentle aspiration of tracheobronchial secretions and the administration of wet oxygen. Ventilatory support must be provided as soon as respiratory insufficiency is suspected. The patient may suffer serious hypoxia if such support is delayed until respiratory difficulty and cyanosis are obvious.

The primary object is to provide sufficient oxygenation of the blood to meet body demands. The simplest method is to assure a patent airway from mouth to alveolar membrane. This may be accomplished by (1) removing obstruction secretions and sloughing mucosa by frequent gentle aspiration with the assistance of mucolytic agents, (2) expanding atelectatic segments by coughing and intermittent positive pressure breathing (IPPB), (3) relieving bronchospasm with bronchodilator agents (including intravenous steroids), and (4) diminishing functional dead space by means of tracheostomy.

All of these simpler means may be of no avail, however, and the use of respirator support is often mandatory. While the pressure cycle type (Bird) is simple to use, it is usually ineffectual in such cases. Although not the final answer by any means and requiring much more immediate attention, the piston-type, volume-controlled respirator (Morsch) provides more effective and dependable ventilation. Until he learns to cooperate with the ventilator, the patient may require rather heavy sedation to overcome his conscious resistance.

In using respirators, it is important to be familiar with the characteristics and dangers of each type, to provide humidified air for inspiration and to "sigh" the patient frequently to prevent atelectasis and wash out alveolar CO_2.

THE USE OF TRACHEOSTOMY IN BURNED PATIENTS

For a number of years, tracheostomy was used only to treat established respiratory obstruction. In recent years, tracheostomy has been advocated as a prophylactic measure. It is not advisable to perform a tracheotomy on a strictly prophylactic basis, as many will be done unnecessarily; nor should one wait for established obstruction. Rather, the patient must be observed closely and the requirement anticipated. The three basic reasons for performing tracheotomy are to prevent or treat mechanical airway obstruction, to accomplish adequate tracheobronchial toilet by removing secretions and stimulating coughing and to prevent aspiration of swallowed substances.

Tracheostomy is indicated in patients who have clinical evidence of respiratory tract damage. These patients are in danger of asphyxia both from swelling of the air passages and from accumulated excessive secretions. The danger is lessened if early tracheotomy is performed and efficient tracheobronchial toilet is maintained. It is important to realize that the primary function of endotracheal suction is to stimulate coughing which effectively expands alveoli and moves the secretions up to a point from which they can be readily aspirated. Vigorous suctioning with insertion of the catheter deep into the tracheobronchial tree is never indicated, as it only worsens the mucosal damage already present. Bronchoscopy through the tracheostomy stoma (or the mouth if a stoma is not present) should be utilized without hesitation if good clearing of the respiratory tree and alveolar expansion cannot be assured by other means. It is often a life-saving procedure.

Respiratory embarrassment may follow a severe burn of the neck in which there is edema of the pharyngeal mucosa and epiglottis, as well as the soft tissues of the neck. Some patients are unwilling to cough because of discomfort; others are unable to clear their respiratory passages spontaneously because of age, extent of injury or debility. A tracheostomy may be indicated in all of these patients to maintain an adequate airway.

It is advisable to consider an elective tracheotomy on all patients sustaining deep burns of the face (Fig. 130). Since a tracheostomy can be potentially dangerous, selection of patients for application is made with care. The deep face burn results in inelastic eschar which will not stretch with the edema. The tight compartment of the facial skin thus forces edema to be manifested primarily in the yielding soft tissues of the neck and posterior pharynx. Respiratory obstruction may be quite sudden. These patients can be recognized by the tight eschar limiting jaw movement and prominent edematous eversion of the lips. External facial edema is not so prominent as in the more yielding second-degree burn which usually will not need tracheostomy. However, the patient must be observed closely. Tracheotomy is usually performed within the first 24 to 48 hours following thermal injury, but may be indicated at later periods. It is much easier to perform a tracheotomy in burns about the head and neck as an elective procedure before extensive edema occurs. Tracheostomy lessens the danger of respiratory difficulty from mechanical or secretional obstruction.

A tracheotomy should not be done merely for anesthesia purposes,

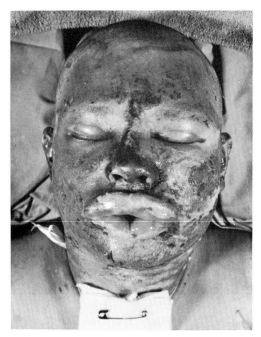

Figure 130. Typical distortion of the face with a deep burn. Eyes are tightly closed, face is rounded, lips are everted and the burn wound is tightly binding the jaws so the mouth cannot be opened adequately. This patient had nausea and vomiting, as well as thick, copious secretions. A tracheotomy was done to prevent aspiration.

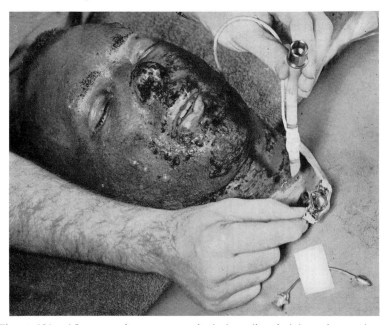

Figure 131. After a tracheotomy, anesthesia is easily administered to patients with deep burns of the face if the tracheostomy tube is replaced with a short endotracheal tube. The tube is inserted after the trachea has been sprayed with a local anesthetic agent.

but when present it offers several advantages in administering anesthesia to patients who must have repeated operative procedures.

1. The surgical field is free from anesthetic equipment.

2. The danger of increasing damage to the burned surface from pressure or irritation is avoided. Sometimes when an anesthesia mask is applied over face grafts or a recently healed partial-thickness burn, the area is converted to a deeper injury.

3. Intubation is simpler by way of the tracheostomy opening. It can be accomplished in most instances after topical anesthesia of the trachea; the use of deep anesthesia or muscle relaxants for intubation is thus avoided (Fig. 131). It may be difficult to insert an endotracheal tube through the mouth because of contracture. Intubation through the nose is troublesome and may carry infection to the lungs.

4. There is less difficulty from aspiration following anesthesia.

Technique of Tracheotomy

Better technique and more accurate placing of the cannula are possible if a tracheotomy is performed as an elective rather than an emergency procedure. Either a vertical or transverse incision may be used. The vertical incision offers better exposure if the tracheotomy must be done hurriedly. A transverse incision is preferred if the operation is an elective one. The optimal level for the tracheostomy opening is at the third to fifth tracheal ring. Above this level erosion by the tracheostomy tube may cause late laryngeal stenosis. Of more immediate consideration is the danger of serious complications of low lying tracheostomy. Particularly if the patient has a forceful, grunting expiratory phase, the apical pleura is apt to be opened under such circumstances. Especially in children, impingement by the standard tracheostomy tube on the carina causes coughing, bronchospasm and obstruction. At this level, the standard tube can readily slip down one mainstem bronchus and obstruct the other.

Positioning with the shoulders elevated and head extended gives better access to the trachea, but this also pulls the trachea up, which predisposes to opening the trachea at too low a level. This is best avoided by identifying the lower border of the thyroid cartilage and then moving inferiorly to the opening between the second and third rings. At this level, the thyroid isthmus rarely causes difficulty. If it does, it can be retracted or transected.

Tracheotomy must never be performed without auscultation of the chest afterward to ascertain the presence of pneumothorax or obstruction of a bronchus. This is particularly important in children.

A most important feature in technique is the excision of a segment of one of the tracheal cartilages (Fig. 132). Such an opening permits easier insertion of the tracheostomy tube; it prevents the edges of the trachea from approximating if the tube slips out; and it provides a patent opening for easier entry of the endotracheal tube during anesthesia. Oc-

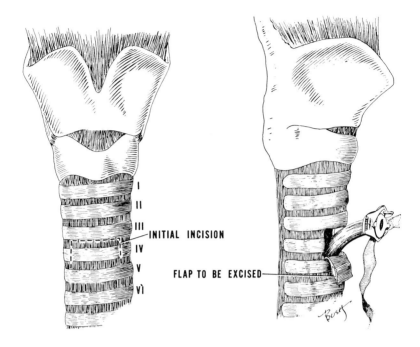

Figure 132. An acceptable technique for tracheotomy. A segment of the anterior tracheal wall is removed. As soon as the trachea is located, an inverted U-shaped incision is made
beginning at the upper border of the fifth tracheal cartilage and extending across the fourth.
The flap of the anterior tracheal wall is pulled out and a tracheostomy tube is inserted. The
flap is then cut away with a scalpel and the tracheostomy tube is left in place. Removal of a
small segment of the anterior tracheal wall gives assurance that the airway will be patent,
even though the tracheostomy tube slips out. It is easier to introduce an endotracheal tube
for anesthesia if a small segment of the trachea has been removed. Removal of a block of
tissue does not result in any problems of healing later. Avoid the low tracheostomy.

casionally, it may be necessary to perform bronchoscopy through the
tracheostomy opening. Such a procedure is much easier if a segment of
the anterior tracheal wall has been excised. The excision technique causes
no complications or delay in healing of the tracheostomy wound.

The standard Jackson tracheostomy tube, with its 90-degree curve,
abuts forcefully on the anterior tracheal wall. Erosion and, in extreme
cases, acute perforation may occur. Metal tubes with a 60-degree curve
lessen the danger. The softer, flexible plastic tubes, though theoretically
better, have resulted in no lessening of the complications.

A tracheostomy may do more harm than good unless careful attention is paid to proper aftercare. The trachea and major bronchi should be
aspirated frequently but gently. Unnecessary trauma to the tracheal epithelium must be avoided. Moist air must be provided for inhalation to
prevent disastrous drying of tracheobronchial mucosa (Fig. 133). This
moisture cannot be provided by oxygen delivered through a water trap
from a compressor gas outlet, as the cooling resulting from rapid gas ex-

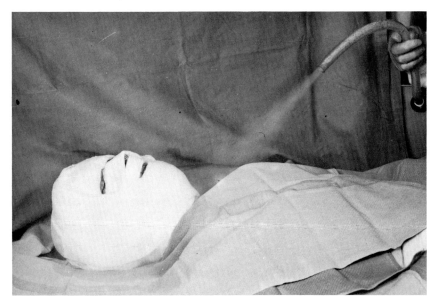

Figure 133. In proper tracheostomy care, moist air must be provided for inhalation. The ultrasonic nebulizer is quite an effective means of securing this. The heated vaporizers are also effective but more difficult to maintain.

pansion precludes water vapor pickup. Some superheated systems deliver adequate quantities but the ultrasonic nebulizers are more effective and simpler to operate.

BURNS OF THE HANDS

Burns of the hands are common because of their exposed position and because the hands are used to combat the fire. In wartime, especially in airplane accidents, hands are often burned severely. Individuals in the vicinity of explosions place their hands over their faces; thus flash burns of the dorsum of the hands are common.

The most common type of burn of the hand involves the dorsum of the fingers, hands and wrist. Burns of the palm frequently occur but are rarely full thickness unless due to electricity, chemicals or contact with a hot object.

High priority should be given to early treatment of burns· of the hands. It is most important to obtain early skin coverage in this area to achieve a good functional result. The principles of initial local care applicable to all burns are also applicable to burns of the hands. Superficial and deep second-degree burns of the hands do well when treated by exposure.

When not being actively exercised, it is mandatory that the hands be elevated. This hastens resolution of edema or prevents its recurrence. Organization of protein-rich edema fluid is a major cause of fibrosis of intrinsic muscles of the hand.

Active motion in a whirlpool is begun as soon as the patient's general condition will tolerate it, usually by 48 to 72 hours post burn (Fig. 134). Motion must be vigorously pursued, both in the water and out. When not moving, the hand should be kept in a position of function by light splinting. Dressings are rarely indicated.

The patient must be encouraged to use his hands, although it may be awkward and painful at first. This is by far the best and simplest physical therapy. Assistance can be provided by altering eating utensils (Fig. 135) in a manner which allows the patient to feed himself. This accomplishes two purposes. It initiates and maintains active physical therapy, and it demonstrates to the patient that he still has useful hands, a very important factor.

The simple, superficial second-degree burn will heal uneventfully regardless of the type of therapy instituted, providing infection is not allowed to occur beneath the crust which forms and joint motion is maintained by active movement and use of the hand. The whirlpool serves both objectives adequately; it allows thorough and repeated cleansing and provides a comfortable medium for exercise.

The deep dermal burn of the dorsum poses a more difficult problem because of slower healing during which pain and discomfort persist and

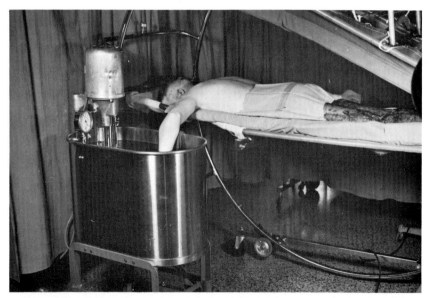

Figure 134. Early active motion of the hands is mandatory and is best accomplished in a whirlpool or hydrotherapy tank. If the patient cannot go to the hydrotherapy area, the tank should be brought to the bedside.

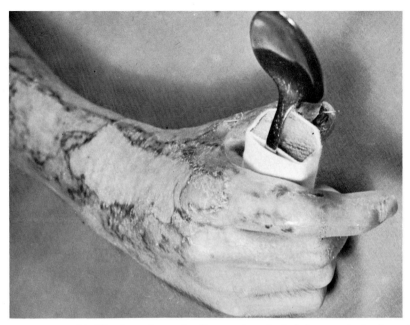

Figure 135. Modification of utensils allows active physical therapy. A simple taping of eating utensils to a balsa block allows encouraging self-help activity. Such activities on the part of the patient are great encouragement and boost his morale.

the ease with which the wound is converted by infection to full-thickness loss with attendant loss of tendon structures. Whirlpool hydrotherapy to maintain motion and simultaneous debridement are essential for success in these cases. The wound must be kept clean and the joints moving.

Homografts are particularly useful in both third-degree and second-degree burns, particularly the latter. As soon as the wound is essentially clear of nonviable elements, homografts are applied without sutures or dressings as lay-on grafts. This biologic dressing eliminates pain, thus allowing comfortable active motion, and stimulates epithelial regrowth. The homografts are changed every 3 to 4 days or sooner if necessary and when in place 24 hours will withstand gentle hydrotherapy associated with active motion (Fig. 136).

Optimal therapy of burns of the dorsum of the hand must include topical antibacterial therapy directed at control of bacterial proliferation and prevention of conversion of second-degree burns and destruction of the delicate tendon mechanisms which may remain viable following deep dermal or full-thickness burns. At present, either 0.5 per cent silver nitrate or 10 per cent Sulfamylon cream is the method of choice.

Upon admission, the topical therapy is instituted along with hydrotherapy and active motion. The latter is more readily accomplished with Sulfamylon than the silver nitrate because of the motion-limiting effects

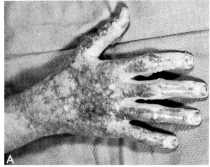
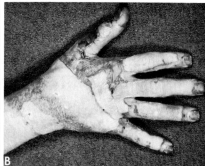
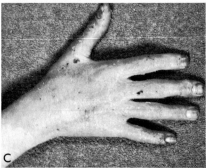

Figure 136. Homograft can be of great value in healing deep dermal wounds by its power to stimulate epithelial proliferation. In hand burns, the immediate relief of pain attendant upon its application allows full and active motion of the hand. In *A* the deep dermal burn of the dorsum is seen 12 days post burn after daily hydrotherapy and debridement. In *B* homograft is applied in strips with no dressings, as dressings would restrict motion. The original homograft was stripped away gently after 48 hours and another crop applied. This latter separated readily after another 48 hours, revealing a healed wound *(C)*. From Moncrief, J. A.: Management of burns. *Monogr. Surg. Sci.* **3**:175, 1966.

of 'the dressings in silver nitrate therapy. Active motion must be maintained. Wound debridement is accomplished at least daily between applications of the cream or dressing changes and vigorous physical therapy and hand motion pursued until autografting is initiated. Homografting may precede autografting and is of unequaled value in second-degree burns as previously emphasized.

Effective topical therapy should be used even in deep burns of the hand, since preservation of whatever function remains following the thermal insult is of irreplaceable value to the patient. This is particularly true of the thumb and index finger.

If effective topical therapy is not possible, the eschar should be removed as soon as practical. If the area of full-thickness burn can be well delineated and tendon destruction by deep burn is not obvious, it should be excised as soon as the general condition of the patient permits. If the deep structures are destroyed, excision offers nothing.

Excision of the palm is not technically feasible unless the burn is a well localized area such as electrical injury or contact burn. The optimum time for definitive excision is between the second and fifth postburn day. Surgical excision removes all dead tissue, and grafting provides skin cover, thereby avoiding the whole phase of natural slough separation, granulation and especially fibrosis. The healing time is shortened, and the hands can be actively exercised as soon as the grafts are stable, usually about 6 or

7 days after grafting. The limitation attendant upon prior immobilization prevents excessive motion, which would disturb the graft. If conditions
prevent early excision and topical therapy is not available, separation of
the eschar should be hastened by wet saline soaks.

To provide a bloodless field for operation, surgical excision is best
done under tourniquet constriction. Before a tourniquet is applied, the
hand should be elevated and the blood forced proximally by the use of an
Esmarch rubber bandage. If excision is performed early, a plane of edema
usually underlies the eschar and makes dissection easy. The webbed spaces
between the fingers and between the index finger and the thumb are seldom burned. However, a better functional result is achieved if they are
excised (Fig. 137). The tourniquet is released after excision and all bleeding points are ligated. A bandage is applied and the area is grafted 2 days
later.

Split-thickness skin (0.018 of an inch) is applied. Strips of skin are
first placed transversely over the metacarpophalangeal joints; then small
strips may be added longitudinally over the fingers. Other strips are placed
transversely across the dorsum of the hand. When grafts are placed longitudinally on the back of the hand, the suture lines contract and interfere
with function. Grafts on the back of the hand must be carefully sutured in
place and covered with a bulky, well splinted dressing (Fig. 138).

The best functional results are obtained when early excision is accomplished in burns which are waxy white and insensitive but still relatively soft. This type of burn is usually termed third degree but actually

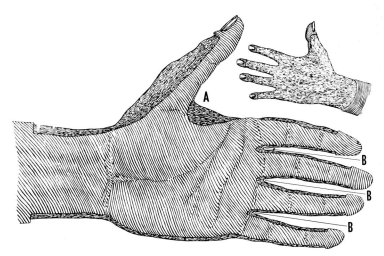

Figure 137. Diagram of areas of excision for full-thickness burns of the dorsum of the
hand. The small insert shows that dead skin of the dorsum of the hand has been removed.
The lines of incision are shown on the drawing of the palmar surface. It is extremely important to excise the skin of the entire webbed space at *A*. Likewise, at *B*, the webbed spaces
between the fingers should be excised, even though they are unburned. Less contracture
occurs in these areas if the webbed spaces are excised and covered with a graft.

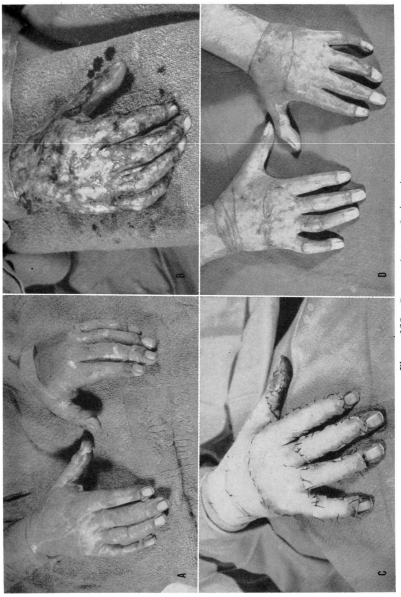

Figure 138. *See opposite page for legend.*

Figure 138. *A,* Full-thickness burns of the dorsum of both hands at 20 hours after injury.

B, The third postburn day. The dead skin of the dorsum of the hands was excised after the application of a tourniquet. The tourniquet was released and all bleeding points were ligated. An occlusive dressing was applied.

C, The fifth postburn day. A thick, split-thickness graft has been sutured in place. Note that the webbed spaces have been excised and a graft has been placed in these areas on the right hand.

D, Photograph at time of discharge. The function of both hands is excellent. A slightly better result was obtained on the right hand because the webbed spaces were excised. On the left hand, a slight contracture at the base of the fingers occurred because the unburned webbed spaces were not excised.

---

heals spontaneously when bacterial autolysis is suppressed by effective topical chemotherapy. If the latter can be accomplished, early excision is not indicated. If it cannot, excision will provide a good functioning hand. Nothing is gained by excision in deeper burns of the hand.

Deep burns of the hand are often very deforming in spite of active, vigorous therapy instituted early. Distortion and loss of function are due primarily to destruction or fibrosis of joint capsules and loss of continuity of the extensor tendons. The characteristic deformity is hyperextension of the metacarpophalangeal joints and extreme flexion of the interphalangeal joints. Distal interphalangeal hyperextension often occurs. If extensor tendons or joints are involved, several procedures to preserve maximum function are indicated. Nonviable tendons are excised. Proximal interphalangeal joints are fused in a position of function to prevent severe flexion contracture. This procedure may be done at the time of grafting. The articular cartilage is removed and flexion is maintained at approximately 30 degrees by the insertion of Kirschner wires (Fig. 139). Fusion becomes solid in approximately 4 to 6 weeks, and the wires are then removed if they have not spontaneously extruded. The extensor mechanism of the little finger is particularly weak. Therefore, after burns of the little finger, a special effort must be made to prevent flexion contracture. If this troublesome deformity cannot be corrected, amputation

EXCISE

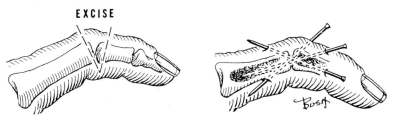

Figure 139. Diagram of technique for arthrodesis of interphalangeal joint in deep burns with pyarthrosis of the joint. The articular cartilages are excised and three Kirschner wires are placed through the finger and left in place until fusion occurs. This fixes the finger in a position of function and prevents deforming flexion contractures. Motion of metacarpophalangeal joints to stretch joint capsules is begun as soon as comfort permits.

may be the most satisfactory solution. This is particularly true, since metacarpophalangeal hyperextension and abduction occur along with proximal interphalangeal flexion in this digit even when other digits are normal.

In full-thickness burns of the hand, atrophy and fibrosis of muscles may occur, especially in the thenar region. The webbed space between the thumb and index finger is shortened unless special attention is directed toward maintaining the thumb in the appropriate position.

Third-degree burns of the palm of the hand are not common. When they do occur, immediate excision is indicated only if well localized. Even then, grafting should be delayed for 48 hours, since extent of necrosis cannot be accurately determined. In electrical injury, although tissue damage is localized, it is characteristically very deep, and ultimate healing often results in tendons immobilized by scar. If the full-thickness palm burn is extensive, the problem is almost technically impossible as an early excision exercise. If due to flame burn, the dorsum is usually so extensively destroyed that preservation of a mobile functional hand is impossible. As soon as a clean bed is obtained, it must be covered with thick split-thickness skin. After the grafts are healed, active physical therapy may be required for very long periods of time to achieve an optimal functional result.

The primary object in caring for burned hands is to maintain function. Skin coverage is secondary and is accomplished merely as a means of wound closure which facilitates functional activity. However, coverage must not be delayed, because delay impedes functional return.

BURNS INVOLVING BONE

Although tissue over bony areas may be thermally destroyed, if a viable periosteum remains, grafting is readily accomplished over it. One need not wait for granulations, but usually the burned soft tissue around the bone separates and leaves a granulating surface.

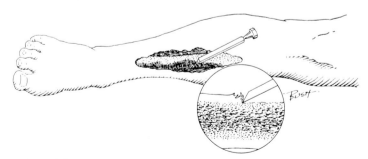

Figure 140. Diagrammatic illustration for removal of dead bone after a severe burn. When the periosteum is burned, the outer cortex of the bone down to the marrow cavity must be removed. If this is chiseled away, small granulating buds form from the marrow cavity and provide a surface upon which a graft may be placed.

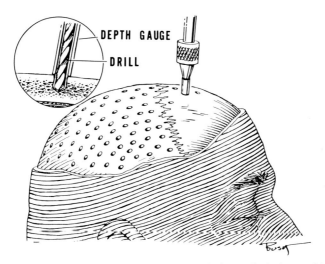

Figure 141. Diagrammatic illustration of the technique of placing multiple holes in the outer table of the skull after a deep burn of the periosteum. An electric bone drill is used. A depth gauge is placed over the drill to prevent the point of the drill from reaching the inner table. This procedure of putting multiple drill holes in the outer table is done as soon as the dead scalp is removed. A skin graft may be applied when granulation tissue is visible through these holes.

Sometimes a burn extends down to and includes the bone. The bone is dry and dead in appearance because of loss of periosteum. The aim of therapy is to achieve a viable granulating surface over which a skin graft may be applied.

When loss of periosteum is diagnosed, the surrounding eschar must be removed and graft closure of surrounding tissue is completed. The dead bone should be chiseled away (Fig. 140). Granulating buds will soon appear and a skin graft can be applied directly on the bone. The use of pedicle grafts in such cases as primary treatment is to be discouraged as it so often fails and is usually not needed.

In burns of the cranium, the electric bone drill is of value in making multiple small perforations (Fig. 141). If the injury is very deep, it may be necessary to remove the dead bone down to the dura. A split skin graft must then be applied directly to the dura. It is not necessary or advisable to wait for granulations to form. This gives immediate coverage to the area. Ultimate coverage by pedicle graft is necessary before reconstruction of the bony defect can be accomplished in full-thickness bone loss.

BURNS COMPLICATED BY FRACTURES

A burn is occasionally complicated by an underlying fracture. Such an injury should not be treated by the application of a cast, as this assures invasive infection of the burn wound. If it is a closed fracture, immobilization with bulky dressings is quite satisfactory for fracture stabilization but should be avoided for the same reasons as plaster. Also, with open fractures, bulky dressings must be avoided, as purulence or necrotic tissue is thereby trapped. The most satisfactory method is skeletal traction, which is utilized in both open and closed fractures. Debridement of nonviable tissue about the fracture is even more important in the burned patient than in the nonburned. Burns complicated by fractures usually do well if skeletal traction is used for immobilization of the fracture and the burned area is treated by exposure (Fig. 142). Such cases are ideally suited to topical antibacterial therapy with Sulfamylon or silver nitrate. Significant infection about pin tracts is unusual but the osteoporotic bone, due to immobilization, is associated with drifting of pins. Thus, these should be placed well into cortical bone. In deep burns, the eschar should be removed as rapidly as possible. As soon as the area is covered with a skin graft, it may be immobilized with plaster if necessary. Intramedullary fixation is never advisable as a means of immobilizing a fractured extremity that is burned. Infection is too prone to occur along the medullary nail tract.

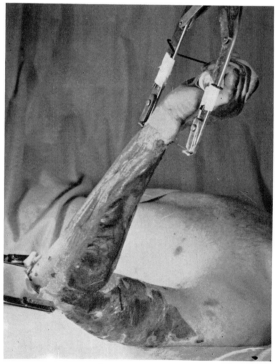

Figure 142. A deep dermal burn of the left hand and a fracture of the middle third of the humerus sustained in an airplane accident. The fracture was treated by skeletal traction and the burn was allowed to remain exposed. A hanging cast was applied during the fourth week, when the burn had healed. Burns complicated by simple fracture should be treated by exposure whenever possible.

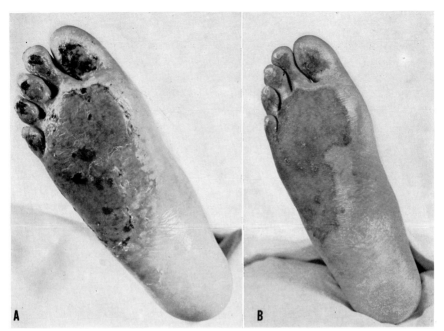

Figure 143. *A*, Deep third-degree burn of the sole of the foot treated by exposure. A thick, split-thickness graft was sutured in place after the eschar had been removed.

B, Photograph taken 3 months after injury. The thick, split-thickness graft served as a good cover for the wound.

BURNS OF THE FOOT

Burns of the sole of the foot are relatively uncommon. They occur occasionally when an individual walks through a burning area without shoes or sustains a contact burn or electrical injury. Burns of the sole of the foot usually do well when exposed. They should not be excised. As soon as the eschar sequestrates, the area should be prepared for grafting. A split-thickness skin graft (0.018 of an inch in thickness) is applied (Fig. 143). This procedure is much more satisfactory than pedicle grafts. The split grafts withstand weightbearing after initial protection and in contrast to pedicles are soon well innervated, do not require remodeling or revision and can be accomplished in one short procedure.

BURNS OF THE AXILLA OR NECK

Deep burns of the axilla are almost invariably followed by severe contracture. Such burns should ideally be splinted, with the arm in complete abduction until healing is complete. However, this is rarely possible because of burns elsewhere. Active exercise is instituted as soon as possible in the hope of minimizing contracture or severe webbing at the anterior or posterior axillary folds.

Grafting of axillary areas is greatly facilitated by utilizing open techniques without dressings or sutures (Fig. 115, Chapter Nine).

If functional impairment is severe in the early healed burn, release of contracture may be indicated before scar maturation is complete. Under such conditions, the area should be excised down to the fascia. It is important to excise beyond the anterior and posterior folds. These areas must be excised even though they are not burned. The grafts are placed transversely across the anterior fold, the axilla and the posterior fold and then sutured in place. If lines joining the grafts occur along the edges of the anterior and the posterior folds, these areas will contract and limit motion of the shoulder. This difficulty is eliminated if the grafts are placed transversely and extend well beyond both folds. As soon as the graft is applied, the area may be dressed or left exposed, but the arm must be held in abduction. Early motion and active physical therapy are encouraged.

Burns of the neck are a particularly frustrating problem because of the propensity for severe contracture to occur. While neck splints are of value in the reconstructive phases, when one is dealing with mature scar, the inflammatory scar of the healing acute burn inexorably draws the chin down. Of some assistance is the maintenance of a position of hyperextension of the neck by elevating the shoulders on pillows or an additional mattress. The mobile chin still moves down.

In the early treatment of burns of the neck, this hyperextended position prevents maceration of partial-thickness burns and obviates conversion by that means.

BURNS OF THE PENIS

When there is a burn of the penis, an indwelling catheter should be inserted initially, but if spontaneous voiding is possible the catheter should be removed after resuscitation is complete. Full-thickness burns in this area should not be excised. As soon as a clean viable surface is available, split-thickness skin grafts are sutured in place in a circular fashion. If the foreskin is intact, a dorsal slit and splitting of the layers will provide a surprising area of skin for coverage. In no instance should viable foreskin be removed during debridement. A firm dressing is difficult to apply, and grafts heal equally as well if exposed.

BURNS OF THE PERINEUM

Healing of burns of the perineum is usually delayed because of the surrounding moisture and infection. However, grafts applied without sutures and left exposed do quite well. Fortunately, the numerous deep hair follicles present in the area usually provide a source for spontaneous healing and actual grafting is seldom necessary. They heal more rapidly when they are exposed. Dressings in this area are most difficult and only make for a warm, moist environment which is conducive to infection.

In full-thickness burns, the recipient site is prepared by sitz baths or wet saline soaks. The colon is cleansed with multiple enemas before grafting. After grafting, paregoric should be used to inhibit bowel movements for 6 or 7 days.

In extensive burns, grafting of the perineum is postponed until most other areas are covered with skin. Remarkable spontaneous healing of the perineum occurs frequently, even though the burns first appear to be very deep. Because of difficulties with proper immobilization, grafts of the perineum often do not take as well as grafts in other areas. For this reason, it is better to use available grafts first in areas where a good take is more likely to occur.

REFERENCES

Artz, C. P., and MacMillan, B. G.: Treatment of burns of difficult areas. *Am. J. Surg.* **91**:517, 1956.

Aub, J. C., Pittman, H., and Brues, A. M.: The pulmonary complications: a clinical description. *In Management of the Cocoanut Grove Burns at the Massachusetts General Hospital.* Philadelphia, J. B. Lippincott Company, 1943, p. 34.

Epstein, B. S., Hardy, D. L., Harrison, H. N., Teplitz, C., Villarreal, Y., and Mason, A. D., Jr.: Hypoxemia in the burned patient: a clinical-pathologic study. *Ann. Surg.* **158**:924, 1963.

Epstein, B. S., Rose, L. R., Teplitz, C., and Moncrief, J. A.: Experiences with low tracheostomy in the burn patient. *J.A.M.A.* **183**:966, 1963.

Georgiade, N. G., Matton, G. E., and von Kessel, F.: Facial burns. *Plast. & Reconstruct. Surg.* **29**:648, 1962.

Jackson, D. M.: The treatment of burns: an exercise in emergency surgery. *Ann. Roy. Coll. Surgeons England* **13**:236. 1953.

Moncrief, J. A.: Complications of burns. *Ann. Surg.* **147**:443, 1958.

Moncrief, J. A.: Burns of specific areas. *J. Trauma* **5**:278, 1965.

Moncrief, J. A., Switzer, W. E., and Rose, L. R.: The treatment of hand burns. *Mil. Med.* **128**: 50, 1963.

Moncrief, J. A., Switzer, W. E., and Rose, L. R.: Primary excision and grafting in the treatment of third-degree burns of the dorsum of the hand. *Plast. & Reconstruct. Surg.* **33**:305, 1964.

Ross, W. P. D.: The treatment of recent burns of the hand. *Brit. J. Plast. Surg.* **2**:233, 1950.

Soderberg, B. N., Sichi, W. T., and Jennings, H. B., Jr.: Plastic repair of the eyelid. *U.S. Armed Forces M. J.* **4**:281, 1953.

Switzer, W. E., Jones, J. W , and Moncrief, J. A.: Evaluation of early excision of burns in children. *J. Trauma* **5**:540, 1965.

Taylor, F. W., and Gumbert, J. L.: Cause of death from burns: role of respiratory damage. *Ann. Surg.* **161**:497, 1965.

Taylor, P. H., Pugsley, L. G., and Vogel, E. H., Jr.: The intriguing electrical burn: a review of thirty-one electrical burn cases. *J. Trauma* **2**:309, 1962.

Vail, D.: Treatment of burns of the eyes. *Am. J. Surg.* **83**:615, 1952.

Chapter
Eleven

BURNS IN
CHILDREN

       Burns in children are tragic events resulting not only in injury or death of the victim, but also in disruption of family life and frequently permanent changes in plans for the future. Care of the burned infant or child (birth to 15 years) differs significantly enough from that directed toward the adult that a section on the subject is indicated.

       Although the older child rapidly approaches the adult and responds to injury and therapy in a correspondingly similar fashion, those in the younger age groups, particularly infants, pose quite different problems. Anatomic and physiologic differences, based primarily on growth patterns and gradually maturing body systems, require that therapy of the thermal injury be altered to conform to function as well as need.

       Physiologic as well as chronologic immaturity must be constantly considered in the resuscitation and later treatment of the burned child or infant (Table 18). At birth the anatomic lobulations of the infantile kidney reflect the immature functional ability, particularly of the tubules. The young kidney is unable to excrete sodium, chloride and other ions or to reabsorb water with any efficiency, thus producing hypotonic urine of relatively large volumes. Also, the kidney cannot rapidly excrete large volumes of ion-free water. This fixed volume and solute excretion makes the infant susceptible to problems of overloading and dehydration.

       The glomerulotubular function gradually matures so that by 24 months of age all normal infants have the ability to regulate their homeostasis by means of the kidney. Rate of maturation varies, however, and thus up to 24 months one must approach these little patients cautiously.

       The cardiovascular and pulmonary systems of the child are quite well developed and can withstand demands better than any age group. Prior to the age of 2 years in many instances and always prior to 1 year of age, however, there is a progressive reorientation of the cardiovascular system necessary in the adjustment from fetal to independent circulatory dynamics. This is most obviously noted in the progressive decrease in the size of the cardiac silhouette. The peripheral circulation is poorly developed and labile during infancy, its efficiency improving as the large abdominal

Table 18. PHYSIOLOGIC DEFICIENCIES OF INFANTS

SYSTEM	DEFICIENCY	CLINICAL IMPLICATION	AGE MATURATION
Temperature regulation	Labile system Surface area-body weight ratio greatly increased	Rapid shifts in core temperature with great tendency to equilibrate with ambient due to increased radiant and evaporative heat loss	10-12 years
Integument	Skin thin with dermal appendages (sweat glands and hair follicles) scant and close to surface	Heat penetrates more readily with resultant deeper burn Donor skin must be removed in thin layers	16-18 years
Renal	Glomerulotubular immaturity with inability to excrete ions actively or resorb water	Produce large volumes of dilute urine Fluids administered must be hypo-osmolar (e.g., 0.2-0.3 NaCl) but not electrolyte free to obviate water intoxication or hyperosmolality Very susceptible to overloading and dehydration	1-2 years
Cardiovascular	Peripheral circulation labile and most of volume in the relatively large abdominal viscera	Myocardium can function well but peripheral compensation is poor	1 year

viscera characteristic of this age decrease in size. Usually by 1 year of age, normal circulatory dynamics have been established.

The pulmonary system progressively matures with the aging of the patient. Gas exchange and ventilation are quite efficient shortly after birth, but the high metabolic demands of the infant require the continued functioning of this system with a small marginal reserve. As body size increases, particularly in relationship to surface area and metabolism, pulmonary area and capacity similarly increase so that a greater margin is provided. Prior to that time, however, atelectasis, pneumonia, interference with excursion of the thoracic cage, airway compromise or any encroachment upon this narrow margin can have a fatal result. With limited renal function, circulatory overloading may lead to a disastrous result.

The energy requirements of the infant are quite high and are gradually reduced as the body grows and its systems mature. This increased energy need is in great part due to poor peripheral circulatory dynamics, which preclude efficient heat conservation, and high body length–body weight ratio, which provides more surface area for heat loss. The addition of thermal injury may impose an insurmountable caloric burden on this already marginal system. By the age of 2, this situation is no longer a significant problem.

Children are subjected to thermal injury primarily through adult carelessness or innate childhood curiosity. The former often allows the latter to become quite deadly. While statistics from different clinics may vary in minor aspects, the general pattern is for the spill scalds (hot liquids and grease) to occur primarily among those below the age of 3 years. Above the age of three, more flame burns occur (Table 19). The male appears more curious in the younger age, for he pulls at coffee pot cords, pot handles and such; therefore, the male child sustains more scalds. However, the delicate, fluffy clothing of the young girl seems to attract flame, and it burns with incredible rapidity.

The distribution of burns over the body of children falls into a rather characteristic pattern. The scald is typically located on the side of the face and neck and the isolateral upper trunk and arm. The immersion scald, often due to a sibling caring for a younger one, usually involves the lower half of the body. Ignited clothing most often will result in a burn from mid-

Table 19. CAUSE OF BURNS IN CHILDREN — AGENT VERSUS SEX (SURGICAL RESEARCH UNIT)

AGENT OR MECHANISM	MALE	FEMALE
Scald	37	17
Gasoline	12	8
Hot grease	7	2
Conflagration	15	6
Clothing ignited	37	64
Contact	10	3
Electrical	1	0
Other (aircraft, fuel lamps, etc.)	8	2

thigh up, with deep burns on the anterior neck and lower face and the front of the trunk. Contact burns, of course, are well localized to the point of contact.

Thus, knowing the age of the patient and the causative agent, the physician can fairly well predict the extent and location of burn.

The occurrence of any burn other than the most trivial is a traumatic experience in the life of a child. The initial adjustment to the injury and prolonged treatment is a slow one, but once the child's confidence is gained and particularly after painful episodes are at least infrequent, the child adjusts quite rapidly and effectively. While it might be expected that a significant burn would leave deep emotional scars and hinder personality development in subsequent years, a review of the cases at the Surgical Research Unit reveals none of this, and in fact there are many instances of the development of outstanding personalities. Possibly this is an area of overcompensation.

Should the thermal injury occur in the late prepubertal or early pubertal years, a striking change occurs. During the severe catabolic phase no change is noted. When convalescence is well under way, however, pubertal changes rapidly accelerate and, in the case of the prepubertal, may occur 2 or 3 years prior to the usual time. No abnormal sexual changes have been noted, but deep burns of the breast in female children may impair breast development and lactation.

As in the adult, the skin of the infant and child varies greatly in thickness in different portions of the body. In infants and young children, the skin is so thin and has such shallow dermal appendages that full-thickness skin loss easily occurs upon exposure to heat. Similarly, conversion of a deep dermal burn to full-thickness loss is readily caused by contaminating organisms. In the adult male, the deep hair follicles of the beard area prevent any but the deepest burns from resulting in full-thickness loss, but it is different in children, and the face frequently sustains full-thickness loss.

The thinness of skin in these small patients must always be recognized in using such sites as actual or potential donor areas. As maturity approaches, the skin thickens and allows routine graft removal.

Following burning or graft removal, the involved area loses its ability to act as a barrier to evaporation of water. This is a significant problem in adults. In children with their relatively larger surface area per weight or height, the insensible water loss is of critical magnitude.

Respiratory complications in children may result from the circumstances of the injury, the location of the burn or a tracheotomy performed to overcome those difficulties. Should the child be burned under such circumstances that he is forced to inhale noxious combustion products, a severe tracheobronchitis with attendant bronchospasm results, which markedly impairs pulmonary ventilation. Symptomatology may not develop for 24 hours or more after the injury, thus leading to a false sense of security. Wheezing, prolonged expiratory phase of respiration, wet lungs and copious secretions are characteristic. The secretions are usually thick, and in severe cases, fragments of bronchial mucosa are present. On occasion, heavy coloring with carbonaceous material gives an appearance of soot. Cyanosis is ominous.

In such cases, clearance of the tracheobronchial tree may not be adequate without the aid of a tracheostomy through which gentle suction can be instituted. Heated water nebulization should be used through the tracheostomy, and mucolytic agents, such as acetylcysteine, administered to loosen the thick, tenacious secretion. On occasion, heavy sedation and a respirator may be necessary to overcome severe bronchospasm.

If a tracheotomy is done, it should be accomplished with the greatest care, since complications of this procedure are often fatal in children. The slim margin of respiratory reserve in these patients does not allow any tolerance for such complications as pneumothorax or obstruction of a bronchus by a long tracheostomy tube. Contrary to popular concepts, the tracheostomy stomas must be made as high as possible, at the second or third tracheal cartilage. The practice of positioning the patient with the neck hyperextended and entering the trachea near the suprasternal notch places the stoma at the fifth or sixth ring, a low position that is frequently fatal. The conventional Jackson tracheostomy tube is too long for children and must be shortened at least 2 cm. or a shorter one of different design used. Unless such precautions are observed, the tube impinges upon the carina and causes cough or bronchospasm. Even more important, the tube may pass the carina and go down one mainstem bronchus and completely occlude the other. To detect such possibilities, auscultation of the chest after tracheotomy is mandatory. The treatment obviously is correction of the situation by withdrawal of the tube.

In cases of deep burns of the chest, particularly those which involve at least the anterior two-thirds, severe restriction of the movement of the thoracic cage occurs secondary to the binding effect of the tight, inelastic eschar. Unless this is relieved by generous incision of the eschar down to the deep fascia, fatal hypoxia can result.

Among children, the mortality associated with thermal injury decreases with age and increases with extent and depth of burn. While no institution has a large enough series in children to delineate precisely this relationship, the experience at the Surgical Research Unit is likely to be representative (Fig. 144). This shows that in infants and children a burn of 20 per cent or less is well tolerated. Above the age of 3 years, the mortality is essentially that of adults, but below this age, resistance to thermal injury or its complications appears considerably lessened. The cause for this is unknown, but may be related to physiologic immaturity.

Other than those mentioned in Chapter Fifteen and those which are iatrogenic, such as tracheostomy and fluid overloading, complications encountered in infants and children are related primarily to the nature and location of the thermal injury. Deep burns due to contact or electricity are

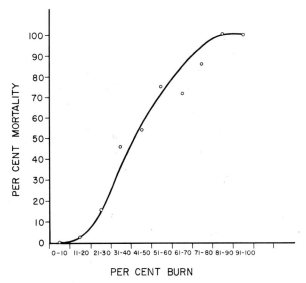

Figure 144. Per cent burn plotted against per cent mortality in children at the Surgical Research Unit.

quite common among the curious youngsters. Such burns are apt to be very deep and frequently involve vital functional structures such as flexor tendons, blood vessels and facial structures. Because of the high incidence of clothing fires, deep burns of the neck, with resulting contracture, are frequent among children.

Because of the child's reluctance to move if such results in pain or discomfort, stiffness of joints and flexion contractures are quite likely to occur. This can be readily prevented by proper splinting while the child is resting or asleep and active physical therapy while he is awake. Fortunately, the growing child is naturally active, and once pain is no longer a significant factor, he will move spontaneously and, unless involvement is severe, will completely overcome any limitation imposed by soft tissue contracture or joint ankylosis.

While not strictly a complication, changes in the growth pattern frequently occur, particularly in larger burns of older children. As in adults, hair growth and nail growth essentially stop during the catabolic phase. Bone growth likely does also, and weight loss is marked. When convalescence is well under way and the child is fully recovered, a spurt in bone growth and an overshooting of weight recovery occur. In the prepubertal child, there is often a rapid development of secondary sex characteristics. In the end, the child may far outstrip his siblings in growth and physical maturity. These changes are likely due to a prolonged and heavy production of growth hormone.

Resuscitation of the burned child is based upon estimation of extent and depth of injury and rapid replacement of fluids along with maintenance of an adequate airway. Estimation of the extent of burn in children is accomplished essentially as it is in an adult, but different percentages of surface area are ascribed to the anatomic divisions. This is necessary, since in the child the head and extremities comprise a greater proportion of the total surface area of the body. For practical purposes in an emergency situation, the Rule of Nines can still be used in infants and children.

The determination of the depth of burn in these cases, the infant in particular, is often quite difficult. The skin of the infant is so thin that it is readily destroyed by a burn of lesser severity, and yet the terrific powers of cellular regeneration allow for healing of many deep dermal areas in a short time. An additional difficulty is the fact that many of the burns are scalds, in which it is notoriously difficult to assess accurately the depth.

Once depth and area of burn have been ascertained, fluid therapy can be instituted rapidly, but it should be done carefully. While various tables of fluid requirements have been advocated, these contain so many numbers they serve only to confuse. The Brooke formula (Table 20) or the Evans formula can be used with much greater facility, and the ultimate fluid volumes are essentially the same.

There are, however, some precautionary measures which must be taken to prevent overhydration or imposing too heavy a load on the infant kidney. The salt solutions in patients below 2 years of age should be administered as 1:3 or 1:4 dilution of lactated Ringer's utilizing the requirement for nonelectrolyte-containing fluids as the diluent. This prevents hypernatremia during heavy sodium infusions and hyponatremia during administration of dextrose in water. The need for electrolyte-free water varies with the metabolic demands of the child or infant at different ages and with changing ability to conserve heat and evaporation from the body surface (Fig. 145). This evaporation is tremendously accelerated in the case of the burn and reaches a sustained maximum at about 48 hours post burn. In extensive burns, this may be as much as 300 ml./sq. m. body surface per hour but usually is in the range of 100 to 150 ml. Only close observation of the patient will prevent dehydration.

Table 20. Brooke Formula—Children[†]

Electrolyte*	1.5 ml./kg./per cent burn/24 hours ⟶			
Colloid	0.5 ml./kg./per cent burn/24 hours ⟶			
Dextrose/water	150 ml./kg.	100 ml./kg.	75 ml./kg.	50 ml./kg.
	(0–2 yr.)	(2–5 yr.)	(5–8 yr.)	(8–12 yr.)

*Diluted 1:3 with dextrose/water.

†Burns over 30 per cent are considered 30 per cent. Keep urinary output at 15–20 ml./hour. Administer one-half the above colloid and electrolyte the second 24 hours. Give same amount dextrose/water.

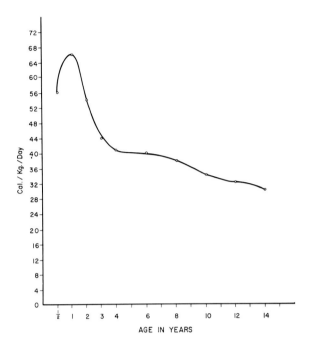

Figure 145. Graph of basal metabolic requirements for children of various ages.

Colloid requirements during the first 24 hours are met primarily with dextran or heat-treated plasma. Whole blood is delayed until the hemoconcentration is resolving and even then with caution in infants below the age of 2 years.

The care of the burn wound in the child varies little from that in the adult, but some aspects require even stronger emphasis. Escharotomy must be accomplished early and effectively in children to prevent ischemia of extremities and severe impairment of respiratory exchange.

Meticulous attention must be paid to the partial-thickness burn wounds and to donor sites. The normally thinner skin is readily converted by infection to full-thickness injury.

Closure of the burn wound is accomplished by skin grafting as early as possible. Timing is determined by an acceptable recipient site. Grafting techniques are the same as in the adult, but the open technique is more often appropriate in these cases. Skin is removed under brief general anesthesia, and the patient is immediately returned to the ward to recover. When the patient is fully awake, the recipient area is immobilized, and the donor skin is then placed over the area. No dressing is applied. As long as immobilization is effective, graft take is excellent. This technique is particularly effective on trunk, face, perineum and the proximal extremity area, which can be kept out of contact with other surfaces. The compressive dressing technique is equally good for distal areas of the extremities.

Physical rehabilitation of the child is not difficult, but emotional balance may be impaired if the parents, particularly the mother, wish to maintain a strong umbilical attachment. With the disappearance of pain every growing, happy child is active, and in fact, restraint and moderation are difficult to achieve. Under such circumstances, mobilization of joints and stretching of contractures is easily accomplished. If, however, the parents foster a dependent attitude on the part of the child, rehabilitation is unjustifiably difficult. As in many pediatric cases, most of the energy is then of necessity directed toward the healthy parent in order to aid the sick child.

REFERENCES

Abramson, D. J.: Curling's ulcer in childhood: review of the literature and report of five cases. *Surgery* **55**:321, 1964.

Abramson, D. J.: The care and treatment of severely burned children. *Surg. Gynec. & Obst.* **122**:855, 1966.

Batchelor, A. D. R., Sutherland, A. B., Kirk, J., and Colver, C. G.: Sodium imbalance in burned children. *In* Artz, C. P. (ed.): *Research in Burns*. Philadelphia, F. A. Davis Company, 1962, p. 89.

Becker, J. M., and Artz, C. P.: A study of the treatment of burns in children. *A.M.A. Arch. Surg.* **73**:207, 1956.

Conway, H.: Management of burns in children. *Am. J. Surg.* **107**:537, 1964.

Haynes, B. W., Jr.: Management of burns in children. *J. Trauma* **5**:267, 1965.

Sutherland, A. B., and Batchelor, A. D. R.: Nitrogen balance in children. *In* Wallace, A. B., and Wilkinson, A. W. (eds.): *Research in Burns*. Edinburgh, E. & S. Livingstone, Ltd., 1966, p. 147.

Welch, K. J.: Thermal burns. *In* Benson, C. D., et al. (eds.): *Pediatric Surgery*. Chicago, Year Book Medical Publishers, Inc., 1962, vol. 1, p. 53.

Chapter
Twelve

NURSING CARE
AND
PSYCHOLOGICAL
CONSIDERATIONS

The care of a severely burned patient demands the highest caliber of bedside nursing. The nurse is given more responsibility in such cases than in almost any other type of serious illness. It is extremely important that she be an integral part of the team of people caring for the burned patient.

Frequent conferences between the physician and the nurse are extremely important, particularly in the initial phases of treatment. The nurse must have some understanding of the burn problem. Part of this may be obtained by contact with the physician, but it is also important that she become acquainted with modern concepts in burn care by reading recent periodicals and textbooks. (See Chapters Three, Five and Six.) With an understanding of the burn problem, she should be able to anticipate the needs of the physician.

Materials required at the bedside at the time of admission of a severely burned patient are listed in Table 21.

Table 21. MATERIALS AVAILABLE AT BEDSIDE ON ADMISSION
OF A BURNED PATIENT

1. Masks, gowns and gloves
2. Tracheotomy set
3. Thermometer, blood pressure cuff
4. Selected dressing material
5. Several 10-ml. syringes and laboratory blood tubes
6. Intravenous set, with anticipated fluids
7. Venous cutdown tray with venous pressure manometer
8. Urinary catheter tray
9. Aspirating apparatus
10. Oxygen
11. Circular turning frame or Stryker frame
12. Nasogastric suction
13. Sterile basins for washing and cleansing

Role of the Nurse in Replacement Therapy

The nurse is responsible for adjusting the rate of administration of various fluids during the early phase of treatment in accordance with the physician's orders. She maintains a detailed, accurate record of intake and output, venous pressure and vital signs. These records must be kept up to date so that the physician may study them each hour if necessary. The physician makes his estimate of the amount and type of therapy needed on the basis of these records. Since the best sign as to adequacy of treatment during replacement therapy is urinary output, the type of therapy prescribed is often based on the record of the hourly output of urine. Usually the physician asks the nurse to adjust the rate of administration of fluid in accordance with the output of urine. Rate and character of respirations, adequacy of peripheral flow, sensorium and clinical evidence of state of oxygenation are also of great importance in monitoring response to resuscitation. Each must be carefully and frequently evaluated.

During the first week of therapy, burned patients may require intravenous vitamins, antibiotics and electrolytes. Generally, it is the nurse's responsibility to mix several solutions for simultaneous intravenous use. The orders for various intravenous solutions must be exact; they must be written by the physician with specific indications as to time to be started, duration and rate of administration. When a mixture of solutions causes a precipitate, infusion should be withheld until the physician is consulted. If several solutions are to be given at various times during the day, a nurse must plan for the entire 24 hours and make an even distribution for administering the fluids over that period. This procedure requires the close cooperation of physician and nurse to assure a clear understanding of the type of solution, the time of administration and the rate of administration. All bottles should be labeled clearly as soon as solutions are mixed (Fig. 146).

Management of intravenous catheters. All severely burned patients must have an intravenous lifeline in the early postburn period. This is established by using a cutdown cannula. Usually, a measured segment of a plastic catheter is inserted into the vein. It is the nurse's responsibility to see that there are no kinks in the catheter and that the extremity is properly anchored to prevent the catheter from being pulled out of the vein. A coil of tubing between the point of entry into the vein and the anchoring point assures some protection against accidental dislodgment. The dressing about the cannula should be changed as often as necessary to keep it clean and to prevent infection. In changing dressings, the nurse must be particularly careful not to cut the catheter at the skin edge and cause it to be lost in the vein. When the intravenous fluids fail to run freely through the catheter, the doctor should be notified immediately.

Care of urinary catheter. An indwelling urinary catheter is usually used in patients sustaining burns of more than 25 per cent of the body surface. This catheter should not be allowed to remain in place after the problem of replacement therapy no longer exists. The catheter should be

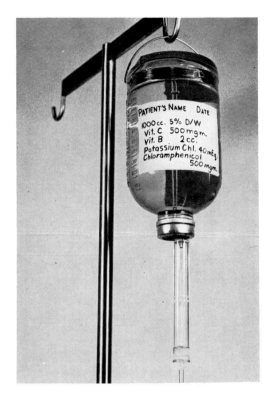

Figure 146. When several drugs are given in the same infusion, the bottle should be labeled. This prevents errors and simplifies the administration of complicated intravenous therapy.

irrigated with an appropriate solution every 6 hours. The amount of solution used is recorded on the intake sheet; generally about 100 ml. is sufficient. The type of solution used is important only from the standpoint that it not be irritating. While pH changes of the urine brought about by various solutions are theoretically beneficial, the clinical results are due almost entirely to frequent mechanical irrigation and maintenance of free flow. Instillation of antibiotics is not indicated. The use of externally attached urine collection bags in male patients obviates much potential difficulty. If the catheter is to remain in place for an appreciable period of time, a sterile irrigation set may be attached (Fig. 147). Complications of indwelling urethral catheters rise precipitously after 5 days. There are rare indications for maintenance of a catheter for more than 4 days, and thus it should be removed at least by then.

Catheters must be changed at least once a week if they must remain in place for long periods. It is the nurse's responsibility to position the catheter in such a way that it will remain free from tension. When tension is placed on the catheter, undue pressure may be exerted on the bladder neck, and this may cause necrosis of the bladder wall. The catheter should be kept clean to prevent contamination. Frequent observations must be made to detect any leaking about the catheter or any evidence of purulent drainage.

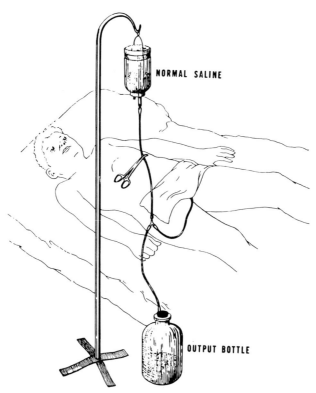

NORMAL SALINE

OUTPUT BOTTLE

Figure 147. Diagram of an acceptable method of urinary catheter irrigation. The urinary catheter should be irrigated about every 6 hours. The clamp is removed from the tubing attached to the bottle of irrigating fluid and applied to the tubing attached to the output bottle. This allows the bladder to fill. Then, as the clamp is removed and replaced on the tubing from the irrigation bottle, the bladder empties. This type of apparatus permits a closed, aseptic system and simplifies the irrigating procedure.

Use of Special Turning Frames

The circular electric bed and turning frames, such as the Stryker and the Foster, are very useful in the management of patients having extensive burns. A large burn wound is extremely sensitive, and these beds facilitate gentle handling and turning of a patient. They eliminate the need for lifting a patient when he uses the bedpan. They also make general nursing procedures easier. The linen may be changed on the posterior frame while the patient is resting on his abdomen; likewise, the linen on the anterior frame may be changed easily when the patient is lying on his back.

A patient who has extensive burns may have to spend a long period of time in bed and decubitus ulcers may develop. Patients can be turned easily four to eight times a day on the turning frame. Such care eliminates prolonged, undue pressure on any one area. When the patient is on the anterior frame, better nursing care may be given to the posterior portion of the body. A patient may be kept in one position on the frame for 4 or 5 days after grafting. This prevents shearing forces from dislodging grafts and allows constant observation and care both of grafts areas and the adjacent donor site.

When a patient sustains an extensive burn and large circumferential areas need to be exposed, he may be turned on the frame every 2 hours to allow drying of first one and then another exposed surface. Subsequent to position changes, the upper section of the frame must be removed to provide access to the patient and exposure of the wounds. Removal of linen adhering to the body surfaces can be traumatic and painful. This can be minimized by the use of Microdon nonadherent sheeting. See Figure 89, Chapter Six.

It usually takes two people to turn an adult easily on the Stryker frame (Fig. 148), but one person can quite readily operate the circular electric bed (Fig. 149). Small children are easily handled on a Stryker frame if it is properly padded, but the circular turning frames are too large for convenience. Usually a child is easier to care for than an adult because there is less strain in lifting and turning him.

The legs of a Stryker frame may be lengthened to elevate either the top or the foot of the frame. A patient lying on the frame may be restrained easily by placing a pillow and a strap over his knees.

With the electric circular beds, intermediate positions can be maintained with ease. Head-down positions for pulmonary drainage and positions of increasing upright posture are facilitated.

A patient is subjected to a great amount of discomfort when he is transferred from his bed to a cart to be taken to the operating room. Since

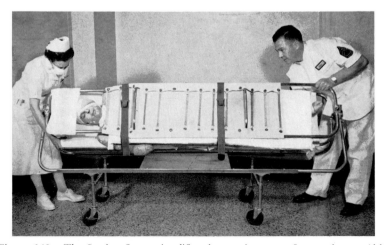

Figure 148. The Stryker frame simplifies the nursing care of severe burns. Although the patient may be turned by one individual, it is easier with two people. A strap should be applied around the frame to give support. A second strap may be applied around the arms so they will not dangle during turning.

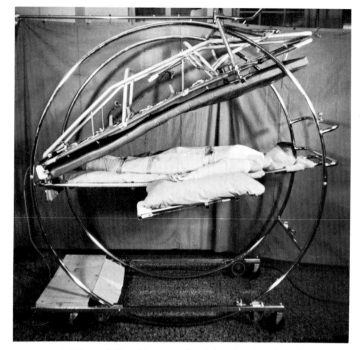

Figure 149.   Photograph of circular electric bed.

a Stryker frame is on wheels, a patient may be moved to the operating room without transfer to a cart. He may be anesthetized on the frame and then removed to the operating table under anesthesia. This not only decreases the amount of discomfort to the patient but also eliminates frequent lifting by attendants. The patient may be taken outdoors, to a recreation area or to the physical therapy area on the frame. A patient derives a psychologic benefit from being moved from place to place. While the circular beds are too bulky to be moved about routinely, changes of location are not difficult. With adaptive attachments, the patient can be moved from the circular frame to a litter or operating table with the same ease that he is turned.

Positioning for Exposure

The nurse's ability to care for a patient treated by the exposure method or one of its modifications requires an understanding of local wound care. The nurse must assist the physician in maintaining the proper position. Circumferential burns of large areas may be exposed by using a turning frame and turning it frequently. Partial-thickness burns of the hands do well when treated by exposure, but they must be kept in a position of function and used whenever possible to maintain motion. It is imperative that the nurse encourage a patient to use his hands in caring for himself. This not only provides excellent physical therapy, but also proves to the patient that he can use his injured hands.

When a burned surface is exposed, evaporation of water from the area results in cooling (580 kilocalories per liter of water evaporated). This can be a significant source of heat loss and is further aggravated by drafts. Exposed burned patients always complain of being cold. A sheet may be tented over them and warm air blown under the tent by the use of one or two hair dryers. Such a technique adds greatly to the patient's comfort, but evaporation of water is increased. This water loss must be corrected by fluid administration.

The nurse must observe the patient frequently and warn him against picking at the crust of an exposed burn. Fingernails must be kept closely clipped and filed, as the grafted and healing areas are readily traumatized by inadvertent scratching. Children quite frequently pick at a crust, and sometimes it is necessary to restrain their hands.

Wet Dressings

Wet dressings are of considerable benefit in treating burns, but they are time consuming and must not be allowed to dry completely. The important aspect of wet dressings is the frequent changing. The usual procedure is a change every 4 hours and sometimes more often. The wet dressing is occasionally changed only twice a day in dressings over large areas, such as an entire lower extremity, but it is kept wet between changes by frequent applications of normal saline. The underlying necrotic material adheres to the gauze and is removed with it. Since the interstices of fine-mesh gauze do not allow such adherence, the most efficient material for such dressings is the standard 4- by 4-inch or 4- by 8-inch gauze sponges. Antibiotics, enzymes or mucolytic agents do not increase the efficiency of such dressings.

A patient is usually apprehensive about the change of a wet dressing. These changes will not be painful if they are performed gently and painstakingly. Narcotics are of little value in preventing pain.

The nurse usually sets up at the bedside a sterile tray complete with wet dressings. She wears sterile gloves and a mask. The old dressings are removed as gently as possible. The gauze pads may be removed more easily and less painfully with the aid of an irrigating syringe (Fig. 150). Loose dead tissue is removed, but any firmly attached eschar is not disturbed. Loose strips of eschar may be cut off with scissors. Great care is taken to avoid pain and bleeding, but timidity should not be allowed to interfere with efficient removal of necrotic tissue.

Care of Tracheostomy

A tracheostomy is required in many severely burned patients, especially for those patients sustaining respiratory tract irritation or deep burns

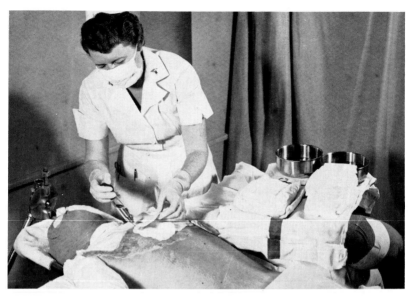

Figure 150. This photograph shows the typical arrangement for a nurse changing wet dressings. The sterile tray is at her left. Sterile gloves and a mask are worn during a change of dressing. The old dressing is removed with less pain if a bulb syringe is used to wet the dressing.

about the face and neck. Nursing care is extremely important following a tracheostomy.

A clean dressing must be kept around the tracheostomy tube to cover the tracheostomy wound until healing is complete. Humidification of the inspired air is required for all patients who have a tracheostomy to prevent drying of the mucous membrane, which favors infection and the formation of obstructing mucopurulent plugs. This may be accomplished by placing a damp sponge over the tracheostomy opening and keeping it moist if other methods are not available. A better technique is the use of some type of humidifying apparatus (Fig. 151). The heated nebulizing apparatus provides much more efficient moistening of the airway and should be used when possible in cases with significant pulmonary problems. Simple bubbling of oxygen through water does not provide any moisture. The rapid expansion of the compressed oxygen cools the gas so much that its vapor-carrying capacity is lowered below that of ambient air and actual drying occurs. Antibiotics or enzymes placed in the tracheobronchial tree do not reduce pulmonary infection or assist in liquefying secretions. However, acetylcysteine, which is a potent mucolytic agent, is very effective in loosening pulmonary secretions. It is mixed with the solutions passing through the nebulizer. The liquefaction of the sputum also causes an increased volume which must be actively cleared from the tracheobronchial tree.

The inner cannula must be removed and cleaned at least every 8

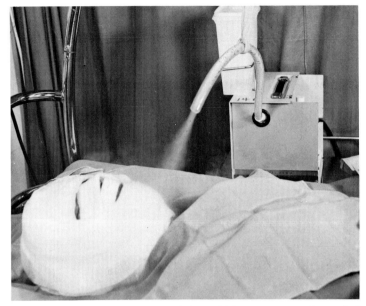

Figure 151.   Photograph of an acceptable humidifying apparatus to be used when there is a tracheostomy.

hours. The tracheostomy tube should be changed every day. This procedure is often accomplished when the burned patient is taken to the operating room for a dressing change or graft. The obturator must be kept strapped to the bed to facilitate reinsertion of the tracheostomy tube if it should come out. It is extremely important to make sure that the tracheostomy is functioning well before a patient is turned on his abdomen. Sometimes the curved tracheostomy tube abuts against the front of the trachea or slips out causing respiratory obstruction.

Unless suctioning is executed properly, the tracheal epithelium may be damaged, and tracheobronchitis, atelectasis and bronchopneumonia may occur. Excessively vigorous tracheal suction is the most frequent error in the management of a tracheostomy. A Y tube should be inserted into the suction line so that the vacuum may be released by fingertip control (Fig. 152). Usually a No. 12, firm rubber or plastic catheter is used. Ideally, the tracheal catheter must be kept scrupulously clean to prevent contamination and infection. However, from a practical standpoint this is difficult to accomplish. Gross contamination of the respiratory tree can be prevented, but unless a sterile catheter is used with each aspiration (a prohibitive cost), bacterial contamination is inevitable. Sterilizing solutions become so heavily impregnated with mucus that they are ineffective. Two separate trays, one for nasal catheters and the other for tracheal catheters, containing Zephiran or a 5 per cent sodium bicarbonate solution are kept at

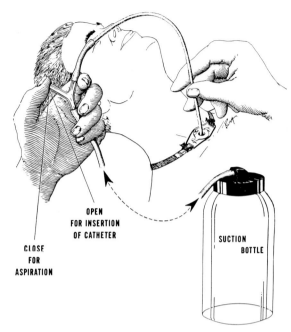

OPEN
FOR INSERTION
OF CATHETER

CLOSE
FOR
ASPIRATION

SUCTION
BOTTLE

Figure 152. The insertion of a Y tube into the suction line permits fingertip control of suction during aspiration of the trachea. The catheter should be inserted into the trachea without any suction. As it is withdrawn, the fingertip can be used to close the Y tube, and suction may be applied as the catheter is being removed. This procedure prevents irritation and trauma to the mucous membrane of the trachea.

the bedside. The tracheal catheter is never used for aspiration of the nose, because of the fear of cross contamination. The catheter should be inserted into the tracheostomy to the full depth desired, withdrawn approximately 1 cm. to remove the tip from the mucous membrane and then with the fingertip the Y valve is closed intermittently to obtain suction. Continuous aspiration is limited to 5 seconds. Unless secretions are extremely profuse, an interval of approximately 3 minutes is allowed between aspirations.

The head is turned to the right to aspirate the left bronchus; then it is turned to the left to aspirate the right bronchus. Gentle suction with the best possible aseptic technique decreases post-tracheostomy tracheobronchitis and hemorrhagic tracheobronchial secretions.

Because of the dangers and complications inherent in the presence of a tracheostomy, it should be removed as soon as possible.

Care of Eyes

In treatment of burns about the eyelid, keeping the cornea moist to prevent ulceration and infection is an important objective. The eyes should be irrigated with normal saline with a bulb syringe at least every 6 hours and sometimes more often. After irrigation, an ophthalmic ointment should be instilled. If the lids are not in apposition, a moist pad must be kept over the eye to prevent drying of the cornea. This is especially important at night. As she gives eye care, a nurse must be careful to reassure a patient that he will be able to see. Sometimes it is wise to pull the eyelids apart to convince a patient that he can see. Such strategy is quite impressive, especially if he has visitors. If some corrective measure on the eyelids is necessary, it is important to inform the patient before the operation about the type of procedure involved and that he will be unable to see for several days because his eyes will be bandaged. When patients have eyes that are closed because of edema or a bandage, it is advisable to speak to the patient before he is touched for any nursing procedure.

It is important to realize that burns of the skin about the eyes result in secondary infection which can readily involve the globe structures. It is imperative that these areas are attended to along with the eyes.

Care of Donor Sites

Donor sites may sometimes be treated with occlusive dressings or preferably by the exposure method. If the sites are treated by dressings, the nurse must be sure that the patient does not pick at the dressing and cause contamination of the area. If the donor site is treated by the exposure method, it must be kept completely exposed to the air. Immediately after skin has been removed, exposed donor sites are somewhat uncomfortable. Once the donor area is dry, pain ceases. Drying is hastened by exposing the area to a simple gooseneck lamp with a 100-watt bulb. Postoperatively a patient may require narcotics for the first 24 hours. The nurse must make sure that the exposed donor sites do not touch the bed clothing. A patient may have a tendency to pick at the crust as healing progresses, and this may lead to infection. The nurse may trim away any loose areas of crust as they appear; however, the crust must not be pulled away as long as it is attached. It should be allowed to fall off. See Chapter Eight.

Responsibility of Nurse in Nutritional Therapy

The survival of a severely burned patient may depend upon nutritional replacement. The regimen usually includes a high protein supplement given between meals. It is the responsibility of the nurse to make sure that the patient takes the full amount prescribed. See Chapter Thirteen.

When tube feedings are used, a patient must be observed frequently to insure that gastric dilatation does not occur. Usually such feedings are administered through a plastic nasogastric tube. The feeding apparatus must be changed with each feeding to minimize the amount of bacterial contamination of the residual feeding material. Unless this is scrupulously done, severe diarrhea will often result from overgrowth of organisms in the formula.

It is mandatory that nurses have an understanding of nutritional requirements of burned patients. Only by their close cooperation with the dietitian and the physician can proper nutritional therapy be achieved.

Emotional Factors in the Care of Burned Patients

When a severely burned patient is admitted to the hospital, he not only is in a state of physical pain, but he is also undergoing serious emotional disturbances. Many burned patients are difficult to manage because they are unable to adjust to their physical incapacity and to their surroundings. Emotional instability is reflected in abnormal behavior; some are noisy, loud and demanding and others are markedly depressed and sullen, often refusing to cooperate with the staff. The doctors and nurses responsible for the care of these patients must have some understanding of the problems and of the adaptive mechanisms that patients use in an attempt to cope with their situation.

Adaptive problems. The primary problems to which a recently burned patient must adapt are threat to survival, fear of disfigurement, prolonged physical discomfort, frequent anesthesia and surgical procedures and a long, tedious convalescence (Table 22).

In addition to these, others appear in varying combinations as secondary adaptive problems. These include separation from family and friends, feelings of inadequacy and rejection, emotional overtones associated with the accident, possible effect of the injury on future plans and conflicts engendered by a state of utter dependency (Table 22).

Sometimes a patient believes that the burn was caused by his own negligence or through the fault of a close friend. Patients may have strong feelings of guilt, especially if one of their loved ones was burned in the same accident. Separation of the patient from his family and friends deprives him of one of his main sources of emotional gratification at a time of great need. Sometimes a feeling of loneliness leads to depression and

Table 22.   ADAPTIVE PROBLEMS IN BURNED PATIENTS

PRIMARY	SECONDARY
Threat to survival	Separation from emotional gratification
Fear of disfigurement	Fear of rejection
Physical discomfort	Emotional pain from accident
Repeated operations	Effect of injury on future plans
Long convalescence	Conflict over dependency

self pity. Some patients are disturbed by the enforced extreme dependency on others. Many patients, particularly women, interpret their injury as a threat to their capacity to be loved. These patients are often hypersensitive to the slightest indication of personal rejection, and they need to be constantly reassured. One of the most important adaptive problems is the effect of the injury on the future plans of the individual. The patient whose livelihood depends upon the use of his hands is tremendously disturbed by burns of that area. Patients who have been active in athletics are particularly disturbed by burns of the lower extremities. Not infrequently, patients worry about the possible amputation of an extremity.

In addition, the previously healthy, independent individual suddenly becomes dependent upon others for aid. In the smaller burn, this is of short duration and of little significance. With extensive thermal injury, however, the victim is totally incapacitated and must depend on others for even the most elemental of body functions. Not only must he be fed, but he also must be helped in voiding and defecating.

Adaptive mechanisms. The multiple, severe psychologic threats involved in a nearly fatal injury cause a patient to be placed in the dangerous situation of becoming overwhelmed by physically and emotionally painful stimuli. The major initial responses are repression and suppression of unpleasant thoughts, feelings and sensations. The patient's attitude is that he will not think about these unpleasant things, and above all, he will not allow himself to have any feeling.

At times a patient may so completely shun the reality of his problems as to present a grotesque clinical picture. Hopelessly burned patients may indicate in their conversation that they consider their injuries trivial and that they expect to return home in a few days. Euphoria is not uncommon in the first 2 or 3 postburn days. It is often followed by a long period of disorientation that may be on a psychogenic basis in many instances, but it is more often a toxic manifestation of extensive sepsis and should be so considered unless proved otherwise.

Withdrawal from the reality of the injury situation may be so extreme as to be manifested by almost complete regression to childhood habits including immature speech patterns. Assumption of the fetal position at rest is often noted. Intolerance of even trivial annoyances, explosive verbal abuse, and need for physical restraint are not uncommon. Fortunately, reversion to the preburn personality almost invariably occurs with recovery.

Friendly personal contacts provide elements of hope that may aid the patient in giving up emergency repressive and constrictive techniques and in substituting mechanisms of constructive appraisal and planning, as well as direct action. Visitors and friendly patients diminish the feeling of separation and fear of not being loved. If a patient is encouraged to attempt some constructive activity early in his treatment, this may remove the conflict over his dependency and make him feel that he is contributing some direct action toward his future recovery. The physician and nurse must encourage a patient to think constructively about his future plans.

Prevention and Treatment of Emotional Disturbances

It is essential that the physician and the nurse understand the general nature of the patient's adaptive problems and assist him in the use of his adaptive mechanisms to achieve a psychologic adjustment. Effective burn therapy involves not only the management of the physical injury, but also a constant effort to make the situation less difficult for the patient and more bearable emotionally. The management of the patient's adaptive problems is closely related to his physical care. It is essential for a patient to have confidence in the competence of the staff. Many burned patients are deeply discouraged and see little prospect of recovery, but they do exhibit a form of primitive, childlike faith in the ability of the physician. This faith of the patient needs to be stimulated by an attitude of genuine interest on the part of all attendants. Each day the physician must sit at the patient's bedside, if only for a short time, and give assurance of his sincere concern.

Severely burned patients are better off in a ward than in a private room. Isolation reinforces the victim's impression that he alone is suffering, whereas exposure to the plight of others lessens the significance of his own wounds. While one cannot disregard obvious disability, the fact that others have something in some area which is worse has a peculiarly comforting effect. If several patients have been involved in the same accident, placing them in the same cubicle is particularly beneficial to group morale.

When a staff of several physicians is active on the ward, it is essential for one physician to assume primary responsibility in all phases of the care of a patient. It helps the patient to be able to refer to one of the physicians as "my doctor." This identification with a specific doctor often develops into a strong possessive feeling which upon complete recovery diminishes. This physician maintains close contact with the patient's family. He eases their apprehension, and in this indirect manner, he reassures the patient.

Visual evidence of the likelihood of uneventful recovery is particularly encouraging in the early phase of hospitalization. Contact with patients who have had similar burns and are almost recovered is an important source of encouragement. Many patients are reassured by seeing photographs of other severely burned patients showing burned areas at the time of injury and after recovery. Such photographs are particularly valuable for orientation of families and friends. The use of open wards gives the family and friends a good picture of the patient's own future progress and problems as reflected in other patients. This is of great value in their understanding.

It is interesting that patients who have recovered from severe burns often seem quite reluctant to help those who are acutely ill. Evidently they are striving to forget the physical and emotional suffering they have endured; any contact with others who are suffering from thermal injury reminds them of their own painful experiences. Nevertheless, their presence on the ward is helpful, as it reassures those who are just beginning to convalesce.

Isolation of patients should be avoided as much as possible. Early in the course of treatment diversional measures, such as reading, music and television, are helpful. Patients should be encouraged to manifest friendly relations with visitors, other patients and ancillary personnel, such as social and volunteer workers.

During the first 2 weeks, a patient is usually too frightened and bewildered to ask about his condition. After the acute effects of the injury have diminished, however, he begins to ask questions. It is most helpful at this time to explain what can be expected in the ensuing months. The physician should be as encouraging as he can be, yet he must be honest.

Anxiety on the part of a patient can frequently be avoided if the physician anticipates it. Usually a patient is most anxious about the expected length of hospitalization and the effects of the injury on his appearance and the functioning of the burned area. The possibility of permanent physical disfigurement may be particularly distressing to women.

Edema of the eyelids rapidly closes the eyes; patients who sustain facial burns are frequently terrified by the idea of the possible loss of vision. It is helpful to give emphatic reassurance on this point and usually this can be done truthfully.

The patient with a face burn that causes closing of the eyes due to edema of the lids, impairment of hearing due to fluid collection in the ears and edematous interference with smell and taste has had his sensory contact with his environment severely limited. He tolerates this for a limited period but soon begins to lose contact with reality and eventually is completely detached. If, in addition, bulky dressings enclose most of his body particularly the tactile surfaces, mental aberrations and loss of contact are swift in onset, profound and bizarre. Under such circumstances, it is mandatory that frequent contact be made with the patient by touch, loud talking, feeding or radio. The patients characteristically are totally disoriented unless brought back to reality by vocal and tactile stimuli. The balance is very delicate, however, and reversion to aberrant mental behavior rapidly occurs as isolation engulfs the patient.

Pain. Treatment of a severe burn is accompanied by some pain, and minor physical discomfort persists over a long period. Physical pain is considerably less severe, however, than is generally supposed. In contrast, emotionally induced pain is a much more serious problem. Frequently, patients do not distinguish between physical pain and emotional tension and, regardless of origin, report all discomfort as pain. The physician and nurse must realize that burned patients need not only relief from pain but also relief from fear. If all the complaints of a patient are treated with narcotics, he may rapidly become an addict, at least emotionally. In patients whose emotional needs are neglected, regressive behavior sometimes occurs as manifested by moaning, complaining and demanding.

Physical pain should be treated with narcotics; however, it is well to emphasize that pain is not severe or of long duration in the burned patient. The deep burn destroys sensory nerves and thus obliterates much pain.

The superficial burn, which is initially painful, feels better when drying of the surface occurs or an occlusive dressing is applied. When the patient is particularly fearful and tense, some type of relaxing sedation may prove highly beneficial. Pain and anxiety each compound and are often manifested by an exhausting hyperventilation. Sedation without respiratory depression will slow the rate of exchange to a more tolerable one.

Assisting the recovery mechanisms of a patient. Useful adaptive mechanisms should be encouraged as soon as possible. A patient's capacity for direct action is quite limited at first but increases progressively with time. Since the maintenance of nutrition is a crucial part of burn therapy, the patient is informed that eating the prescribed foods and protein supplements is one way in which he can hasten his recovery. As soon as a patient is convinced that he can take an active part in improving his situation, his adaptive problems become less terrifying. If he is inspired to help himself, his conflict over physical dependency upon others may be overcome. It is important for a patient to have a true evaluation of his limitations and a realistic appraisal of his potentialities. He must be given guidance and encouragement to plan and execute the required procedures for future vocational and nonvocational activities.

A most important and successful principle in recovery is demonstrating to the patient that he can function independently. This is most readily accomplished by having him feed himself, even though it may be quite painful at first. It is also good physical therapy.

The entire program of emotional rehabilitation is the direct responsibility of the attending physician. The need for expert psychiatric assistance is rare.

The special role of the nurse. There is no aspect in the therapy of burns in which a nurse can be more decisively helpful than in the promotion of a patient's emotional well being. The nurse must avoid attitudes of callousness, as well as of oversolicitude. If a nurse is somewhat unstable emotionally, she will tend to react to a patient's complaining with one or the other of these extreme modes of behavior. Callous treatment reinforces the patient's fear of rejection; oversolicitude may promote regression to childlike behavior. The good nurse, trusting in the intuition for which her sex is renowned, manages to be kind but firm. It should not be supposed that a kind, friendly, warm and sympathetic approach is incompatible with firmness.

REFERENCES

Artz, C. P.: Caring for the burn victim. *R. N.* **21**:33, 1958.
Artz, C. P.: Skin grafting for burns (part 1). *R. N.* **22**:33, 1959.
Artz, C. P.: Skin grafting for burns (part 2). *R. N.* **22**:39, 1959.
Colyer, B. L., Cox, J. J., and Vogel, E. H.: Principles of nursing care in the management of burns. *U. S. Armed Forces M. J.* **10**:1428, 1959.
Crasilneck, H. B., Stirman, J. A., Wilson, B. J., McCranie, E. J., and Fogelman, M. J.: Use of hypnosis in the management of patients with burns. *J.A.M.A.* **158**:103, 1955.

Davis, J. H., Artz, C. P., Reiss, E., and Amspacher, W. H.: Practical technics in the care of the burn patient. *Am. J. Surg.* **86**:713, 1953.

Hamburg, D. A., Artz, C. P., Reiss, E., Amspacher, W. H., and Chambers, R. E.: Clinical importance of emotional problems in the care of patients with burns. *New England J. Med.* **248**:355, 1953.

Hamburg, D. A., Hamburg, B., and de Goza, S.: Adaptive problems and mechanisms in severely burned patients. *Psychiatry* **16**:1, 1953.

Maher, M. L., and Davis, J. H.: The nursing care of burns. *Nursing World* **128**:33, 1954.

Plum, F., and Dunning, M. F.: Technics for minimizing trauma to the tracheobronchial tree after tracheotomy. *New England J. Med.* **254**:193, 1956.

Chapter
Thirteen

METABOLIC
RESPONSE
AND NUTRITION

Understanding a burned patient entails comprehension of his metabolic response. Many complex changes occur in the human organism after an overwhelming injury like a severe burn. These changes are most marked immediately after injury and continue decreasing in magnitude until the patient has recovered. The many complications that insult the burned patient have profound influence upon these changes. Much remains to be learned about the metabolic alterations in burns. Tremendous advances, however, have been made in this field in the last 30 years. The general metabolic response of the patient is extremely important to the surgeon who cares for him because rational supportive therapy is based upon the physiologic changes after injury and during convalescence. Generally, considerable emphasis is placed on replacement therapy during the first 2 or 3 days after a burn. A similar interest must be maintained in supporting the body's attempt to recover until the burn wound has been closed.

CHANGES IN BODY COMPOSITION

Water

During the early postburn period there is a rapid gain in total body water because of the therapy that is essential for prevention of burn shock. Most of the data obtained thus far indicate that the increase is limited chiefly to the extracellular fluid. The characteristic weight curve is shown in Figure 153. The rapid early weight gain is a reflection of water gain and obscures the fact that decreases in the fat and muscle mass occur simultaneously. Immediately following the maximum weight, the early descending limb of the weight curve usually has a more gentle slope than the ascending limb preceding the maximum. This is due to the delay in excretion of edema fluid. In a severely burned patient, several liters of

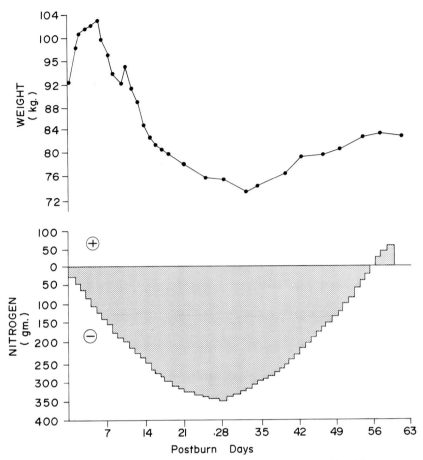

Figure 153. Weight curve and nitrogen loss data on a patient with a 70 per cent partial-thickness burn.

water may be given during the first 2 or 3 days. All well treated burned patients become edematous and thus have a marked weight increase. Sometime after the second day diuresis begins. The rate of diuresis depends upon the severity of the injury. In a relatively small burn, diuresis occurs early and requires only a short period of time. In a burn of more than 50 per cent of the body surface the diuresis may last until the twelfth postburn day. Losses in weight continue in spite of the finest nutritional support until the phase of wound closure. When all of the wound is closed, weight gain becomes rapid.

Protein Metabolism

Much of our knowledge concerning protein metabolism after injury has come from nitrogen balance studies. It must be remembered that 1 gm. of nitrogen represents 6.25 gm. of protein. Nitrogen is easily measured chemically and therefore is used as an expression of the amount of protein going in and out of the body. The normal adult is usually in protein equilibrium immediately prior to injury. In the early postburn period, however, strongly negative nitrogen balance is characteristic because of the large nitrogen losses and the low nitrogen intake.

Urinary excretion of nonprotein nitrogenous products is increased. This may not be evident in the first day or two after the burn, because of poor renal function. The high excretion of urinary nitrogen is nearly always evident in 3 to 5 days and reaches its maximum between the first and second postburn week. After this time the urinary nitrogen decreases progressively; it is often low after a month, sometimes extremely low. A normal adult ingesting an average diet excretes 10 to 15 gm. of urinary nitrogen per day. Approximately 90 per cent of this nitrogen is in the form of urea. In burned patients, however, urinary nitrogen excretion may increase to more than 30 gm. per day (Fig. 154).

The magnitude of urinary nitrogen excretion varies greatly and cannot be predicted in the individual patient, but a few generalizations can be made. (1) There is a rough correlation between the severity of the burn and the amount of nitrogen excreted; the more extensive the burn, the greater the nitrogen excretion. (2) Men generally excrete more nitrogen than women. (3) Most probably, nitrogen excretion is directly related to preburn body weight.

The amount of nitrogen lost through the wound exudate is highly variable and differs according to the type of local care. It does account in all burned patients for an appreciable fraction of total nitrogen losses. In second-degree burns, the nitrogen of the exudate tends to be high in the early postburn period but declines rapidly as the wound heals. In third-degree burns with extensive granulating wounds, the exudate nitrogen is well correlated with the amount of suppuration. Most of the loss of protein in burns is by way of the urine. The exudate is usually responsible for 15 to 20 per cent of the loss (Fig. 155).

In addition to increased losses, low protein intake contributes substantially to negative nitrogen balance. The duration and magnitude of negative balance is influenced by the severity of the burn as well as by the nutritional regimen used. An energetic nutritional regimen instituted 5 to 7 days after the burn may reduce substantially the duration of negative nitrogen balance.

In his classic studies, Soroff showed that the amounts of nitrogen per square meter of body surface per day necessary for equilibrium change in different phases after burning. Considerably greater quantities of nitrogen are required for equilibrium in the first 40 postburn days than thereafter (Table 23). In his studies, the nitrogen requirements of patients during the convalescent period (after 60 days) were similar to the requirements of the controls.

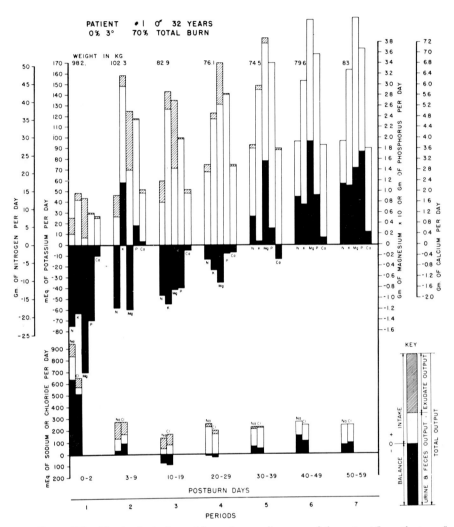

Figure 154. The intake is charted from the zero line up and the output from the top of the intake line down. Solid black areas indicate negative balance below the zero line and positive balance above it. The cross-hatched areas represent exudate contribution to the output. The relative contributions of urine and feces to the output are not shown. The data are charted on the basis of average per day. Four ordinate scales are applicable to the five elements charted in the upper portion. One gram of nitrogen is charted as equivalent to 3.3 mEq. of potassium and 1/15 gm. of phosphorus. Calcium and phosphorus are charted in a ratio of 2:1. "Magnesium times 10" and phosphorus are charted on the same ordinate scale.

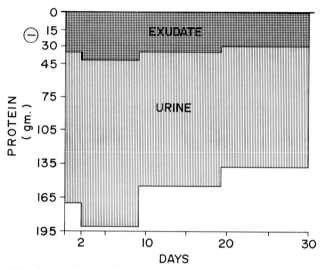

Figure 155. Composite protein losses typical of a 25 per cent second- and third-degree burn in an average adult male. The losses in grams of protein are plotted from the zero line down. During the first 8 days, the loss of protein approximates 190 gm. per day. Extensive losses continue for the first 30 days and then diminish as wound coverage is achieved. Most of the protein is lost in the urine, but the exudate is usually responsible for 15 to 20 per cent of the loss.

Table 23. NITROGEN REQUIRED FOR EQUILIBRIUM AT VARIOUS PHASES AFTER BURNING*

POSTBURN PERIOD	APPROXIMATE AMOUNT OF NITROGEN FOR EQUILIBRIUM IN GM. PER SQ. M.
7–17 days	20–25
30–40 days	13–16
60–70 days	3–9
90–100 days	3–7

*From Soroff et al.: *Surg. Gynec. & Obst.* **112**:159, 1961. By permission of *Surgery, Gynecology & Obstetrics.*

After the wound is closed, the patient given good nutritional therapy usually returns to nitrogen equilibrium or positive balance. Urinary excretion is generally low at this time, and nitrogen intake tends to be increasing. The changes are reflected in the detailed chart illustrated in Figure 156.

Marked changes in the concentration of plasma proteins occur as a result of two factors: the loss of proteins through the wound and alterations in the metabolism of plasma proteins. Mild hypoalbuminemia and hyperglobulinemia tend to persist until wound healing is complete. Large intakes of protein fail to increase the serum albumin to normal. Usually the extent of abnormal plasma protein concentration is directly related to the severity of the injury.

One of the most striking features of a severe burn is rapid muscle wasting. Figure 154 is constructed so that an approximate visual estimate can be made about intracellular changes. In the upper portion of the chart, nitrogen and various minerals are charted in their normal intracellular proportions. It should be recalled that calcium is found chiefly in bone and only in small quantities in muscle. On the other hand, phosphorus occurs in substantial amounts in both bone and muscle. The correlation between nitrogen and intracellular phosphorus balance may be obtained by visually subtracting the observed calcium from the observed phosphorus balance in an algebraic manner. For example, in Period 4, both the calcium and phosphorus balances are negative. The intracellular phosphorus balance is therefore represented by the small difference between the calcium and phosphorus balances, and this difference is noted to be less negative than the observed nitrogen balance. In Period 5, the phosphorus balance is positive, while the calcium balance is negative. Algebraic subtraction of a negative value from a positive value yields a large positive value. In this period it is seen that the intracellular phosphorus balance obtained in this way corresponds well with the observed nitrogen balance.

If all changes in nitrogen balance could be explained by muscle catabolism or anabolism, the correlation between nitrogen and mineral balances should be excellent. Some of the poor correlations are undoubtedly due to experimental errors.

The following conclusions seem valid on the basis of detailed nitrogen balance data in several long term studies of burned patients: (1) The sweeping changes in nitrogen balance are accounted for, in a large measure, by muscle catabolism and anabolism in the various phases of the natural history of a burn. Nitrogen losses and loss of muscle mass are far in excess of that due to muscle wasting from inactivity. (2) During the period of negative nitrogen balance usually a sizable nitrogen loss occurs over and above that which may be explained by the loss of other intracellular constituents. (3) One of the outstanding features of metabolic convalescence is that nitrogen retention does not cease when the nitrogen losses incurred during the early postburn period have been replaced. The

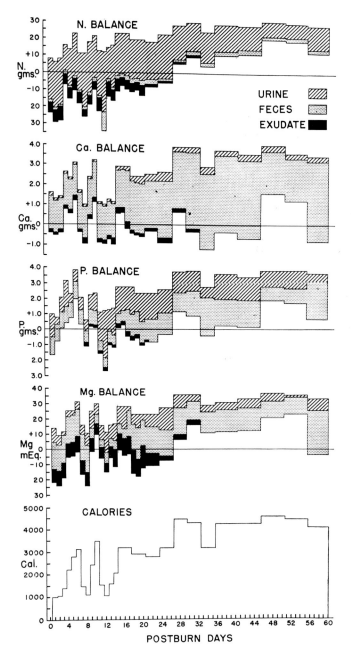

Figure 156. The intake is charted from the zero line upward and the output from the top of the intake line downward. Shaded areas below the zero line indicate negative balance; clear areas above the zero line indicate positive balance. The contributions of urine, feces and exudate to the output are indicated by different shading.

This 32-year-old man had partial-thickness burns of 70 per cent of the body surface. Nitrogen balance was strongly negative in the early postburn period because of the small intake and large excretion, both in the urine and the exudate. Gradually the appetite im-

Legend continues on opposite page.

patients may store nitrogen consistently for months after complete replacement of previous losses.

Fat

Extraordinarily large fat losses may occur. The magnitude of the estimated losses depends on the method used in determining the extent and the severity of the injury. In general, data based on periodic measurement of total body water and on comparison between observed weight changes and weight changes predicted by nitrogen balance are in agreement. In a severely burned patient, the early fat loss may average as much as 600 gm. per day. Minimal fat losses have been computed in smaller burns. The amount of body fat metabolized depends upon the nutritional regimen used. An energetic feeding regimen tends to diminish losses; it is doubtful, however, that any reasonable feeding program can completely prevent them.

Fat losses do not appear to cease when nitrogen balance becomes positive. Persistent fat losses in the presence of strongly positive nitrogen balance have been estimated to occur. This curious combination of findings indicates that negative caloric balance is not incompatible with highly efficient protein synthesis.

Potassium

Except for minor discrepancies, nitrogen and potassium balances are usually well correlated after the first 10 days (Fig. 154). The first 30 days may be divided into three distinct phases. (1) In the first 2 or 3 postburn days a striking outpouring of potassium occurs. During this time correlation with nitrogen losses may be good. In some patients the early urinary potassium losses may far exceed the amount expected by nitrogen losses. (2) Beginning about the fourth postburn day potassium retention commensurate with potassium intake is usually observed. At this time potassium and nitrogen balances are completely dissociated. The potassium balance is often positive, and the nitrogen balance is nearly always negative. In this phase of positive potassium balance the serum potassium concentration tends to be low. A marked shift of potassium from the extracellular fluid to the intracellular fluid undoubtedly occurs. (3) After the initial negative balance and the subsequent positive balance, potassium

Figure 156. *Continued*.
proved as evidenced by sustained high levels of nitrogen and caloric intake. The urinary nitrogen decreased. After a month, the wounds were almost completely healed. Nitrogen balance became positive after 28 days and remained so throughout the duration of the study. The degree of positive balance observed toward the latter part of the study was particularly striking when nitrogen retention rates reached a maximum of 20 gm. per day. During periods of strongly positive balance, the urinary nitrogen was often very low despite a large nitrogen intake.

balance usually becomes negative again in severe burns and then remains slightly negative until the nitrogen balance becomes positive. In this third phase, the level of potassium intake has little influence on potassium balance. The body behaves as though it were saturated with potassium and excretes an amount equivalent to the intake plus the amount of potassium liberated by protein catabolism. If the burn is of relatively small extent and nitrogen balance becomes positive shortly after injury, this third phase may not be observed.

ADRENOCORTICAL RESPONSE

The eosinophil count decreases rapidly during the first 12 hours after a burn. It is commonly reduced to a zero level in 12 to 24 hours and begins to rise the third to the seventh day. It may increase to exceptionally high levels during convalescence.

Some of the early studies in urinary corticoid excretion in burns were reported by Hardy. He found that the excretion of corticoids was sharply increased following a burn of significance and remained elevated or at normal levels throughout the course of the burn regardless of whether the patient eventually died or recovered. Some of the most meaningful studies come from the detailed work of Hume, who studied the victims of the Bennington disaster in 1954. He measured blood and urinary 17-hydroxycorticosteroids in 26 patients. The mean blood corticosteroid level for the fifth to the twentieth postburn day in patients with over 45 per cent body surface burns was 26.1 μg. per 100 ml. (range, 18 to 35). The mean level for those patients with less than 45 per cent of the body surface burned was 18.7 μg. per 100 ml. (range, 8 to 34). The mean level in the normal young male is 12 μg. per 100 ml.

The mean urinary corticosteroid excretion for the fourth to the sixteenth day in patients with over 45 per cent body surface burns was 15.5 mg. per 24 hours (range, 13.6 to 18.8). The mean excretion in those patients with less than 45 per cent burns was 8.3 mg. per 24 hours (range, 4.8 to 13.1). The mean excretion in the normal young male is 5.3 mg. per 24 hours. These figures suggest that a burn of 45 per cent of the body surface represents a very severe form of trauma and that adrenocortical secretion persists at high levels for a long time.

Haynes studied the adrenocortical function in 96 burned patients, utilizing measurements of 17-hydroxycorticosteroid, plasma corticoid response to exogenous ACTH, urinary corticosteroid conjugates, 17-ketosteroids and electrolytes. He found that during the second day after injury there is a direct relationship between the extent of second- and third-degree burn and the level of 17-hydroxycorticosteroids in the plasma. This appears to represent a direct relationship between the degree of trauma and the height of the adrenocortical response. Surviving patients showed moderately elevated plasma 17-hydroxycorticosteroid levels immediately after burn. This fell to normal levels with progress in healing. Nonsurvivors showed over-all higher plasma 17-hydroxycorticosteroid levels than the survivors, and these levels were usually sustained, owing presumably to extensive injury plus infection. Sustained high plasma corticosteroid levels are a grave prognostic sign. Urinary corticoids alone or with urinary 17-ketosteroids are unreliable as a means of determining adrenocortical insufficiency. After determining the steroid content of the adrenal glands in 22 patients who died, there did not seem to be any suggestion that adrenal exhaustion was a significant entity in extensively burned patients. Four patients dying of burns did show low or falling plasma corticosteroid levels suggestive of adrenocortical insufficiency. One showed no response to ACTH, and another died in spite of hydrocortisone therapy.

Adrenocortical insufficiency does occur in burns, but it is not common. Well documented studies on a 21-year-old man in whom adrenocortical insufficiency developed after a severe burn were made by Mandelstam. The patient responded well to hormonal therapy, and further medication was not required after skin coverage had been completed. When one suspects that adrenocortical insufficiency exists in a burned patient who is not doing well, an immediate eosinophil count along with plasma and urine sodium and chloride determinations should be done.

CATECHOLAMINES

Epinephrine is now generally accepted as being the principal hormone of the adrenal medulla. While norepinephrine is the neurohormone of the sympathetic nerves, both of these hormones are excreted in the urine, and the quantity excreted seems to parallel the quantity of these hormones produced by the adrenal gland and the sympathetic nerves. The fundamental studies concerning catecholamines in burns have been done by Goodall. He found that the normal 24-hour excretion in adult males averaged 15.7 μg. of epinephrine and 32.3 μg. of norepinephrine. All surviving burned patients have marked elevation of their epinephrine and norepinephrine output. The degree of elevation roughly parallels the severity of the burn. In severely burned patients, the urinary epinephrine output in Goodall's studies ranged from 25 to 260 μg. and the norepinephrine from 78 to 570 μg. for 24 hours. As recovery took place, there was a gradual return of the urine levels to a point within normal limits. In burned patients who die, about two-thirds show at the time of death subnormal epinephrine output and a low epinephrine content of the adrenal gland, a condition which appears to be commensurate with adrenal medullary insufficiency or depletion.

In a study with Moncrief, Goodall followed 12 severely burned patients who died. Daily 24-hour urine collections were bioassayed for epinephrine and norepinephrine. Shortly after death, the adrenals, lumbar sympathetic ganglia and axons were removed and bioassayed for epinephrine and norepinephrine. Goodall found that the thermal burn is a severe stress in which the sympathoadrenal medullary system is activated into releasing large quantities of both epinephrine and norepinephrine. One-third of the cases showed at the time of death a subnormal output of norepinephrine and a subnormal norepinephrine content of the sympathetic ganglia and axons, which points toward sympathetic nerve depletion. This absolute and relative depletion is probably a mechanism of dying rather than a cause of death.

BURN STRESS PSEUDODIABETES

In 1951, Evans and Butterfield described the syndrome of burn stress pseudodiabetes manifested by hyperglycemia, glycosuria without acetonuria, acute dehydration, shock, coma and renal failure. This phenomenon was a contributing factor in the death of two patients and was observed in less severe forms in other patients.

In most instances the syndrome develops during periods when there is a high carbohydrate, high caloric intake. The first sign recognized by the clinician may be an intense osmotic diuresis with severe dehydration. This syndrome is a potential threat in any burned patient given forced feedings. It is rare, but its occurrence may be more frequent than is generally recognized. The clinical and laboratory manifestations in order of importance are hyperglycemia, glycosuria without acetonuria, high urine specific gravity and a severe diuresis. This results in marked dehydration with elevation of the nonprotein nitrogen and hematocrit as well as an increase in the serum sodium and chloride. It is more common in patients who have a family history of diabetes. When it is recognized, it must be treated by vigorous water replacement and sufficient insulin to control the hyperglycemia. Recent well documented case studies have been reported by Arney.

THYROID AND PARATHYROID

Observations by Cope on patients having severe burns revealed a striking elevation of metabolic rate in normal protein-bound iodine concentration in the blood and a normal uptake of radioactive iodine by the thyroid gland. Since the latter two measurements are more or less specific tests of thyroid function, it must be concluded that thyroid hyperactivity is not responsible for the increased metabolic rate. In Cope's studies the metabolic rate was often +30 to +60 in extensive burns. It was roughly proportionate to the severity of the burn and tended to remain elevated until wound healing was almost complete. Harrison and Feller have described the coexistence of increased metabolic rate and evaluated free excretion of epinephrine and norepinephrine in burns. They found a significant correlation between the degree of metabolic rate increase and corresponding increases in free excretion of the catecholamines.

Although hypercalciuria and hyperphosphoruria are common, data on serum calcium and phosphorus levels indicate that they are normal in most patients (Fig. 156). The roentgenologic appearance of the skeleton is that of osteoporosis and not of osteitis fibrosa cystica. From these and other data, it may be inferred that marked alterations of parathyroid function do not occur. The hypercalciuria and the hyperphosphoruria are best explained by the effects of prolonged immobilization and high intake of calcium and phosphorus.

NUTRITION

Serious nutritional problems are unlikely to arise in the patient having burns of relatively small extent and in cases in which most of the burn wounds are predominantly partial thickness. If nausea and vomiting occur at all, these complications cease within a few days and the patient can then ingest increasing quantities of food. A degree of weight loss roughly proportional to the extent of the injury may be expected, but this is not clinically important. Excellent healing is the rule. Such patients do well if encouraged to take a high protein, high caloric diet. On the other hand, adequate nutritional support may make the difference between survival and death in a patient having severe burns. The more severe the injury, the more critical nutritional therapy becomes. Studies in energy metabolism show that the severely burned patients develop marked metabolic deficits, and when they die, they essentially "run out of gas." A major cause for caloric loss is evaporative water loss. Every effort should be made to minimize this. Control of ambient temperature is helpful. There is evidence that both Sulfamylon cream and silver nitrate soaks lower metabolic demands by control of infection and by diminution of evaporative water loss.

It is well known that excellent healing does occur in the presence of strongly negative nitrogen balance. It is also true that persistent negative nitrogen balance results in serious debilitation, increased susceptibility to invasive infection, poor granulation tissue, poor graft take and delayed healing of donor sites. These complications are often responsible for the death of a poorly treated patient. The burn wound itself initiates and perpetuates metabolic abnormalities. In the early phase, there is a marked outpouring of nitrogen. Later, nitrogen losses continue, and much is lost through the wound. Complicating infection increases these losses. When the patient's clinical condition is appraised, consideration must be given to both his nutritional status and the condition of the wound. They are inseparable, each contributing substantially to the other. The earlier the wound is closed, the quicker the patient returns to metabolic equilibrium.

The needs for protein and calories during the first 3 weeks after injury are great. With the present techniques available for nutritional support, it is doubtful that protein equilibrium can be achieved in this period by any means. Every effort should be made to encourage the greatest possible intake of protein and calories to maintain the patient in as good a nutritional status as possible. It is unwise to institute immediate forced feeding programs to offset all nitrogen losses. During the first 5 to 10 postburn days seriously burned patients often have nausea, vomiting and gastrointestinal atony as manifested by abdominal distention and decreased peristalsis. Acute gastric dilatation is not uncommon at this time. The essence of a proper nutritional program consists of good timing. The patient should receive increasing quantities of nutriments when his gastrointestinal tract is capable of accepting them and when reasonably efficient utilization can be expected. Good timing may be achieved if the patient's general metabolic response is understood, careful clinical observations are made and the need for adjustment of the individual requirements of particular patients is appreciated.

Nutritional Management

During the first 2 days after injury, it is best to rely on intravenous feeding altogether because nausea and vomiting are common. Thereafter, patients should be encouraged but not forced to ingest increasing amounts of food. Such a regimen will assuredly result in substantial tissue losses, but this condition is preferable to some of the complications of early forced feeding.

One of the greatest deterrents to an adequate nutritional intake is the use of narcotics. Few narcotics should be necessary. Initially after the burn injury one or two doses of a narcotic may be used intravenously. After this time narcotics should be used sparingly except in association with operative procedures. The use of these agents is followed by anorexia, nausea and constipation. Various tranquilizing drugs are ideal when prescribed intelligently.

The time when a high protein, high caloric intake becomes mandatory varies greatly. In a patient without complications, a good intake should be attainable in 7 to 10 days. As time passes, utilization of ingested nitrogen becomes increasingly efficient. This is indicated by decreasing amounts of nitrogen intake required for nitrogen equilibrium (Table 23).

The aim is to achieve a daily protein intake of 2 to 3 gm. per kg. of body weight along with an intake of 50 to 70 calories per kg. A healthy individual lying quietly in bed requires 1 gm. of protein and 30 calories per kg. of body weight per day to maintain protein equilibrium. Daily vitamin supplements are recommended as follows: ascorbic acid, 1500 mg.; thiamine, 50 mg.; riboflavin, 50 mg.; and nicotinamide, 500 mg. Usually two multiple vitamin tablets and additional ascorbic acid are sufficient. Although the protein and caloric needs in the burned adult are about twice those required in normal health, the needs of the burned child are not in excess of the normal, healthy requirements. Sutherland has pointed out that the normal child's caloric intake is expended in activity. The imposition of strict bed rest in the burned child reduces the caloric requirement. Thus, the maintenance of caloric intake of activity should provide a surplus capable of covering the high energy metabolism that follows thermal injury.

The routine serving of three standard hospital meals is totally inadequate for severely burned patients. To achieve an acceptable protein intake the patient should be put on a selective high protein, high caloric diet and given supplemental high protein liquid nourishment between meals. The physician and the dietitian must collaborate in planning a diet containing foods that the patient likes and excluding those he dislikes. Great care should be taken to explain to the patient the importance of an adequate nutritional intake. Many attempts have been made to manufacture intravenous protein and fat preparations to provide nutritional support. Unfortunately, satisfactory products have not been developed. One of the great needs in the treatment of burns and other serious injuries is the development of a safe and effective method of administering protein and fat intravenously.

Supplemental between-meal feedings. Since standard menus rarely suffice for the patient's protein and caloric needs, various supplements are used. Almost every hospital dietary department has a standard high protein supplemental feeding formula. Several excellent commercial preparations are available. It is extremely important that the supplementary feeding be a palatable liquid. Patients can be encouraged to accept almost any feeding for 1 or 2 weeks, but the burned patient must continue the high intake for several weeks or even months, and palatability therefore becomes a very important factor. An excellent between-meal feeding used in many burn units is a commercial preparation called Provimalt* mixed with milk and flavored with either strawberry Quik or chocolate syrup. When prepared according to instructions, a liter of this supplemental feeding provides 86.7 gm. of protein and 1080 calories. Most adult patients will take one liter or more of this formula in addition to a high protein, high caloric diet. Supplementary feedings should be served in 200-ml. amounts between meals and especially in the evening hours and during the night. The use of routine supplemental between-meal feedings should be standard practice in the management of all patients with major burns.

Tube feedings. It is difficult to give positive indications for the institu-

*Provimalt is manufactured by the C. B. Fleet Company. The use of this product by the authors cannot be construed as an endorsement by the Medical Corps, United States Army.

tion of tube feedings. An indwelling nasogastric tube is uncomfortable, and its use may be followed by complications such as aspiration, respiratory infection and gastric dilatation. Extreme care must be exercised in using tube feedings in burned children and seriously ill patients. They should not be attempted unless there is adequate nursing care to administer them without complications. In many extensive burns, however, tube feedings are necessary, and they may be life saving. Every effort should be made to provide a nutritional intake by other means before resorting to such feedings. If the patient has lost 15 per cent of his body weight and fails to maintain an acceptable intake, tube feedings should be initiated. It may be possible to use tube feedings for a few days and thus stimulate the patient to improve his oral nutrition.

A common tube feeding formula is a high protein diet homogenized in a blender with milk and supplemented with some type of commercial protein preparation. Two acceptable tube feeding formulas are shown in Table 24. Tube feedings should be started gradually. Before the feeding is initiated and during the first few hours thereafter, the abdomen should be examined for the presence of bowel sounds and to make sure that the gastrointestinal tract is not atonic. The most common error in tube feeding is to begin with an excessive volume. It is best to start with about 500 ml. and then increase the volume gradually over a 4-day period until the de-

Table 24.   Acceptable Tube Feeding Formulas

Formula A*

Evaporated milk	600 ml.	Total volume	1000	ml.
Light cream	120 ml.	Carbohydrate	134	gm.
Karo	80 ml.	Fat	88	gm.
Three eggs	150 ml.	Protein	64	gm.
Applesauce	50 gm.	Nitrogen	10.6	gm.
Salt (NaCl)	5 gm.	Sodium	123	mEq.
Elixir ferrous sulfate	8 ml.	Potassium	55	mEq.
Vitamin C	250 mg.	Calories	1580	
Vitamin B complex	1 tablet or 4 ml.			

Formula B

Commercial protein supplement†	5 oz.	Total volume	2000 ml.
Evaporated milk	8 oz.	Protein	100 gm.
Homogenized fat§	3 oz.	Fat	80 gm.
Karo syrup	5 1/2 oz.	Carbohydrate	2209 gm.
Water q.s.	2000 ml.	Calories	2000

---

*Adapted from F. D. Moore: *Metabolic Care of the Surgical Patient.* Philadelphia, W. B. Saunders Company, 1959.
† Provimalt, C. B. Fleet Company, Lynchburg, Virginia.
§ Lipomul (oral), The Upjohn Company, Kalamazoo, Michigan.

sired intake is achieved. Most patients can tolerate 2000 to 2400 ml. per day if the formula is not too concentrated. A continuous drip of 500 ml. may be given at intervals, or 50 to 200 ml. may be injected through the tube every 2 hours.

Diarrhea is the most frequent complication. It may be caused by too rapid an increase in the volume given, by bacterial contamination or by a mixture that is not suitable for the patient. When diarrhea occurs, the volume is decreased immediately. If it persists, the carbohydrate content is reduced. Some formulas are poorly tolerated because of an excessive fat content. Simple experimentation of these variables almost always results in an acceptable program. An adequate amount of water must always be given when tube feedings are used. It is usually wise to flush out the tube with water after a tube feeding has been given.

Androgens. These agents have anabolic activity, and because of this, they have been used in burns. Several preparations are commercially available. In most patients adequate concentration on the provision of large quantities of proteins and calories is sufficient. Usually the androgens have an anabolic effect for only 2 or 3 weeks. Few burned patients really require androgens. In some, however, when it is impossible to maintain an adequate intake, the use of one of the anabolic hormones for a period of 2 weeks may be of value.

REFERENCES

Arney, G. K., Pearson, E., and Sutherland, A. B.: Burn stress pseudodiabetes. *Ann. Surg.* **152**:77, 1960.
Artz, C. P.: Improving oral protein nutrition. *Postgrad. Med.* **43**:223, 1968.
Cope, O., Nardi, G. L., Quijano, M., Rovit, R. L., Stanbury, J. B., and Wight, A.: Metabolic rate and thyroid function following acute thermal trauma in man. *Ann. Surg.* **137**:165, 1953.
Evans, E. I., and Butterfield, W. J. H.: The stress response in the severely burned: an interim report. *Ann. Surg.* **134**:588, 1951.
Goodall, McC.: Adrenaline and noradrenaline in thermal burn. *In* Artz, C. P. (ed.): *Research in Burns.* Philadelphia, F. A. Davis Company, 1962.
Goodall, McC., and Haynes, B. W., Jr.: Adrenal medullary insufficiency in severe thermal burn. *J. Clin. Invest.* **39**:1927, 1960.
Goodall, McC., and Moncrief, J. A.: Sympathetic nerve depletion in severe thermal injury. *Ann. Surg.* **162**:893, 1965.
Goodall, McC., Stone, C., and Haynes, B. W., Jr.: Urinary output of adrenaline and noradrenaline in severe thermal burns. *Ann. Surg.* **145**:479, 1957.
Harrison, T. S., Seaton, J. F., and Feller, I.: Relationship of increased oxygen consumption to catecholamine excretion in thermal burns. *Ann. Surg.* **165**:169, 1967.
Haynes, B. W., Jr., Lounds, E. A., and Hume, D. M.: Adrenocortical function in severe burns. Unpublished data.
Hume, D. M., Nelson, D. H., and Miller, D. W.: Blood and urinary 17-hydroxycorticosteroids in patients with severe burns. *Ann. Surg.* **143**:316, 1956.
Levenson, S. M., Davidson, C. S., Lund, C. C., and Taylor, F. H. L.: The nutrition of patients with thermal burns. *Surg. Gynec. & Obst.* **80**:449, 1945.
Lund, C. C., Levenson, S. M., Green, R. W., Paige, R. W., Robinson, P. E., Adams, M. A., MacDonald, A. H., Taylor, F. H. L., and Johnson, R. E.: Ascorbic acid, thiamine, riboflavin and nicotinic acid in relation to acute burns in man. *A.M.A. Arch. Surg.* **55**:557, 1947.
Mandelstam, P., Goldzieher, J. W., Soroff, H. S., and Green, N.: The pituitary-adrenal axis: acute adrenocortical insufficiency and persistent occult dysfunction following thermal injury. *J. Clin. Endocrinol.* **18**:284, 1958.

Moore, F. D.: *Metabolic Care of the Surgical Patient.* Philadelphia. W. B. Saunders Company, 1959.

Pearson, E., Soroff, H. S., Arney, G. K., and Artz, C. P.: An estimation of the potassium requirements for equilibrium in burned patients. *Surg. Gynec. & Obst.* **112**:263, 1961.

Reiss, E., Pearson, E., and Artz, C. P.: The metabolic response to burns. *J. Clin. Invest.* **35**: 62, 1956.

Soroff, H. S., Pearson, E., Arney, G. K., and Artz, C. P.: An analysis of alterations in body composition in burned patients. *Surg. Gynec. & Obst.* **112**:425, 1961.

Soroff, H. S., Pearson, E., and Artz, C. P.: An estimation of the nitrogen requirements for equilibrium in burned patients. *Surg. Gynec. & Obst.* **112**:159, 1961.

Sutherland, A. B., and Batchelor, A. D. R.: Nitrogen balance in burned children. *In* Wallace, A. B., and Wilkinson, A. W. (eds.): *Research in Burns.* Edinburgh, E. & S. Livingstone, Ltd., 1966, p. 147.

Wilson, H., Lovelace, J. R., and Hardy, J. D.: The adrenocortical response to extensive burns in man. *Ann. Surg.* **141**:175, 1955.

Chapter
Fourteen
THE PROBLEM
OF INFECTION

Infection is the cardinal problem in the treatment of burns. It is a cause of pain, nutritional disturbances, conversion of second-degree burns to third-degree burns and failure of skin grafts to take, and it is by far the outstanding cause of death.

Widespread misconceptions exist concerning the importance of infectious complications. Most of those who have had abundant experience in the treatment of burns agree that infection is extremely important. Others think that infection is an avoidable, rare complication and therefore it should not pose a serious difficulty if a patient is treated properly. These contrasting points of view may be resolved if it is understood that the term infection may include diverse clinical entities ranging from simple colonization of a wound by bacteria of low pathogenicity to invasive infection that proves fatal. Unless the exact definition of infection is given, all statements about its incidence, seriousness and importance are meaningless. Appropriate definitions are essential for the evaluation of therapy. Systemically administered antibiotics, for instance, may be lifesaving in septicemia caused by group A beta hemolytic streptococci. They may be useless, however, in the treatment of localized suppuration on a granulating wound.

In various parts of the world the differences in climate, types of patients and methods of care have little influence on the etiology of burn infection, but these may compound the problem that exists. Some significant contributions on infection in burns have been made in several clinics in recent years.

DEFINITIONS

Infection may be classified broadly into two types, invasive and local. Invasive infection is further divided into locally invasive and generally invasive. Cellulitis, lymphangitis and regional lymphadenitis are common examples of the former and are in diverse surgical conditions as well as in burns. Burn wound sepsis may be locally or generally invasive, that is, spreading metastatically to other parts of the body. The important fact is that it is lethal in either form.

305

In this discussion, the term septicemia will mean a positive blood culture in combination with the signs and symptoms of sepsis as noted later in this discussion. In general, septicemia is associated with persistently positive blood cultures. A focus of infection is always present. Microorganisms enter the blood from this focal point either continuously or at very frequent intervals. After vigorous antibiotic therapy has been given, sometimes only the pretreatment blood culture is positive but clinical findings of sepsis persist. The diagnosis of septicemia is justified under this condition. Microorganisms may spread throughout the body from the burn wound or may arise from septic intravascular thrombi, most frequently associated with an infected intravenous infusion site.

Burn wound sepsis is a recent term originated to describe the massive invasive bacterial involvement of the burn wound and the adjacent tissues. Quantitative bacteriology routinely reveals 10^7 to 10^9 organisms in each gram of involved tissue. By definition, there must be in excess of 10^5 associated with invasion of adjacent tissue. Wound sepsis is predominantly due to a mixed flora of gram-negative organisms, but in many instances (50 per cent) is not associated with visceral involvement. The incidence of bloodstream involvement is somewhat higher, though variable, and except terminally, the number of organisms isolated from blood in gram-negative invasive sepsis is quite small—in the range of three to five colonies per milliliter of blood.

The frequent localization to the burn wound without visceral metastatic spread of the offending microorganisms makes the infection no less lethal and explains why it has been so universally misinterpreted until recent years. That it still is not recognized by many is because of failure to examine the burn wound, preferring to look only at the sterile viscera. The skin remains the largest organ of the body and extensive involvement of it can reasonably be expected to be fatal.

Local infection refers to the presence of microorganisms restricted to the wound. While some investigators have insisted that inflammation must be present as a sign of tissue reaction to the bacteria if the term infection is used, the present definition purposely includes instances without evidence of tissue response. The reason will be seen later. The term suppuration indicates that pus is present on a wound. It is the most common gross manifestation of local infection. Sepsis here means burn wound sepsis.

Obviously much overlapping occurs between these various forms of infection. Local infection may become locally invasive and finally generally invasive. Local infection, with or without suppuration, may also occur in combination with generally invasive infection.

SOURCE OF INFECTION

At one time it was thought that full-thickness burns were sterile initially and that they became colonized by bacteria only when inadvertent contamination occurred in the course of treatment. Studies in animal models and humans have refuted this viewpoint. The intensity of heat and duration of exposure to heat may be so great that the full thickness of the skin is rendered nonviable, yet bacteria may survive deep in the crypts of sweat glands and hair follicles. These bacteria are capable of rapid proliferation. Initially, only colonization of the wound occurs, primarily by staphylococci. This begins about the second or third postburn day. If conditions are good, and they usually are, rapid multiplication occurs with spreading invasive infection now including *Pseudomonas*, *Proteus* and other gram-negative organisms as well as staphylococci. By the fifth postburn day, invasive infection is well established and staphylococci are soon almost completely displaced by a gram-negative flora.

A second source of infection is contamination of wounds from the outside. Surface contamination may occur, particularly in the areas of the buttocks and inner thighs. In these areas, fecal flora abounds. Bacteria may gain access to the wound from unsterile dressings and instruments or from the respiratory or intestinal tract of the patient or of attendants. A distinct effort should be made to avoid cross contamination, as it is an added source of wound inoculation.

Although the therapeutic implications of these avenues of infection are described fully in Chapter Six, a few comments are pertinent. It is obvious that an effective, therapeutic approach to bacteria in the burn wound can be found only in local applications. The aims of therapy must consist of (1) protection from invasion of the bloodstream and (2) early establishment of a tissue barrier against invasive infections.

The avascular destructive nature of the burn wound with thrombosis of the vessels supplying the area precludes any effective systemic antibacterial therapy aimed at the burn wound. Such lesions also prohibit delivery of the normal cellular defense elements to the area of the wound. If, however, the magnitude of invasive infection is controlled by some means, granulation tissue with its rich neovasculature will be well established by 3 weeks and will act as a potent barrier to invasive infection. Topical therapy with highly diffusible, effective, nontoxic and rapidly eliminated substances appears the only logical solution. However, control of the bacterial flora, not total elimination, is the aim of present therapy.

Contamination from the outside appears to have an entirely different interpretation, depending upon whether early local care is by occlusive dressings or by the exposure method. If dressings are used, conditions are provided favoring an increase in the bacterial inoculum, which is harmful. When the exposure method is employed, successful treatment does not depend upon prevention of contamination—an utter impossibility—but on the fact that growth of contaminating bacteria is inhibited by the dryness of the wound. Because of drying, surface swab cultures are often sterile on an exposed burn wound, in spite of massive infection beneath the eschar, and lead to a false sense of security.

Invasive sepsis is initially spotty, however, and only late becomes universally confluent. Moisture greatly favors the process, as is seen in the dependent areas of a patient who is not turned and in the wet, constantly

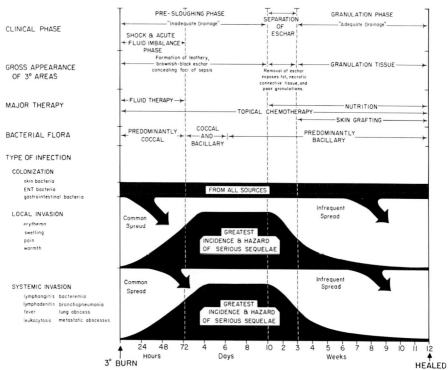

Figure 157. The natural history of a third-degree burn with survival. Note that the danger of invasive infection is greatest before separation of eschars has occurred. In the presence of granulating wounds, invasive infection is less frequent.

approximated upper medial thighs. In contrast, the anterior trunk, a usually dry area, may remain absolutely sterile for days.

Burn wound sepsis is most common in the early postburn period (Fig. 157). Its incidence is very low when the wounds have progressed to a granulating stage. The remarkable resistance of granulation tissue to invasive bacteria has long been recognized and is of crucial importance to an understanding of the rationale of burn therapy. The principal therapeutic problem is to prevent sepsis prior to the time when a granulating barrier is established.

Granulation tissue is an excellent example of local infection with suppuration. Invasive infection is very rare in the granulating stage, despite abundant suppuration.

BURN WOUND SEPSIS

Burn wound sepsis is probably the most serious complication in burns. In a recent survey of 81 deaths resulting from burns, 86 per cent of the deaths were caused directly or indirectly by invasive burn wound sepsis. This figure brings the magnitude of the problem into focus. It also emphasizes that prevention is a principal objective in the early care of a burned patient.

On reading the literature prior to 1950, the impression is gained that sepsis rarely occurred and that its high incidence at present is a recent development. This impression is only partially correct. In much of the earlier literature, data on blood and tissue were not given. Therefore, it is quite likely that sepsis was seldom diagnosed, for the simple reason that no cultures were taken to determine its presence. On the other hand, it is probable that recent improvements in fluid therapy have made possible longer survival of severely burned patients and, as a result, more patients now survive until such a time as sepsis is likely to occur.

The primary manifestations of burn wound sepsis are the typical appearance of the degenerating wound, the clinical appearance of the patient and the isolation of microorganisms from the blood. Such bloodstream isolation, or septicemia, is erratically accomplished, however, according to the nature of the invading bacteria. Staphylococci which invade the blood in large numbers or grow luxuriantly on septic thrombi are readily isolated in the magnitude of 1000 to 1500 per ml. of blood. *Pseudomonas*, on the other hand, primarily involves the lymphatics initially and though tissue destruction is great is seldom found in numbers higher than three to five per ml. of blood until late in the disease. Organisms such as *Aerobacter* occupy an intermediate position.

While not reflecting the true picture of the burn wound, septicemia as a term is well entrenched in the literature. As a means of determining onset of sepsis, it is of some value from a temporal standpoint.

Predisposing Factors

Burn wound sepsis occurs most frequently in patients who sustain extensive, full-thickness burns. It is a complication of partial-thickness burns only rarely but may be present when these burns are very extensive. When it does occur with second-degree burns, conversion to full-thickness loss is the rule.

Even the relatively small burn may terminate fatally when complicated by a septic phlebitis. This most commonly occurs secondary to long standing intravenous therapy and is usually staphylococcal though other organisms are sometimes isolated.

The extent and depth of burn are important factors affecting not only the incidence of sepsis but also the prognosis: the larger and deeper the burn, the less likely the success of therapy. Old age and a poor nutritional status are probably associated with an increased incidence and a less favorable prognosis. Data are not available on this point at present.

Source of Invading Bacteria

Most evidence favors the viewpoint that invading microorganisms originate at the wound and thence gain access to the bloodstream. Almost

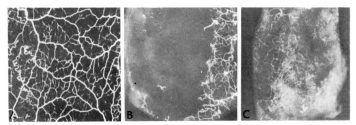

Figure 158. Demonstration of the arterial vascular network in the burn wound model (rat); mercury-barium injectate fills vessels of 10 micra or greater. *A*, Normal vascular pattern. *B*, At 24 hours post burn (third degree) there is essentially a complete obliteration of the arterial supply. The picture immediately after burn is only slightly better. *C*, Not until 3 weeks post burn is significant granulation tissue present, and thus until that time there is little effective barrier to invasive infection.

without exception, the same species of microorganisms are cultured from the blood and the wound.

There is no evidence that the type of sepsis differs in burned patients treated properly by dressings as opposed to patients treated properly by the exposure method.

The burn wound, particularly the avascular third-degree areas, is an excellent pabulum for bacterial growth (Figs. 158 and 159). Beneath an occlusive dressing the darkness, warmth and moisture favor a highly accelerated multiplication of organisms, and quantitative counts are in the range of 10^7 to 10^9 per gram of tissue. Under such circumstances, invasive burn wound sepsis readily occurs. Characteristically, with dressings the wound is grossly purulent and necrotic, and the eschar separates rapidly.

In the properly treated and exposed burn wound, drying rapidly occurs with cooling of the surface 2 or 3°C. below the temperature of normal tissue. The cool, dry environment inhibits bacterial growth, and quantitative counts may be as low as 10^3 to 10^5 per gram of tissue. The eschar may remain densely adherent for weeks. However, such efficiency is unusual and the ordinary course of events is proliferation at a mean rate in excess of 10^5 per gram tissue.

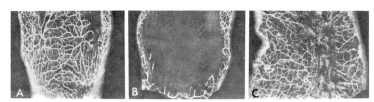

Figure 159. Infection studies of partial-thickness burn wound in the experimental model (rat); mercury-barium injectate. *A*, Vascular pattern of the area of burning 1 week after a partial-thickness burn. The normal network is readily re-established after initial disappearance. *B*, Complete loss of patency of arterial network in burned areas as the result of infection of the second-degree burn with *Pseudomonas aeruginosa*. This is conversion of a partial-thickness wound to full-thickness skin loss. *C*, This wound was infected as in (*B*), but local factors prevented conversion. Note the only slightly altered vascular pattern.

If the exposed patient is not turned or positioned in such a manner as to expose the burned areas for active drying, the wounds rapidly become macerated and microorganisms proliferate unchecked. The burned area which initially was properly exposed becomes, from neglect, tantamount to one treated by occlusive dressings, and invasive sepsis spreads rapidly.

Bacteriology

Precise bacteriologic information is essential not only for diagnosis but also for appropriate therapy. Although the clinical diagnosis of sepsis is frequently correct, a clinical diagnosis without bacteriologic data is a totally inadequate basis for rational therapy.

A blood sample should be taken from a carefully prepared, unburned site. If an unburned area is not available for venipuncture, the blood sample may have to be drawn by puncture through the burn. Such samples are meaningful only if they yield no growth, since it is impossible to be sure whether growth resulted from infection of the bloodstream or from contamination. Antibiotic sensitivity testing of isolated microorganisms is an essential part of the bacteriologic study.

Cultures of the burn wound, when properly done, may be of great value. The dry, hard surface of an exposed third-degree eschar is usually sterile. However, culture of deeper tissues or a macerated wound reveals a mixed flora of gram-positive and gram-negative organisms. The predominant growth is usually that isolated from the blood (Tables 25 and 26).

Over the last 15 years, the pattern of burn bacteriology at the Surgical Research Unit has displayed a distinct but changing design. Initially, staphylococci were the obviously predominant offenders with the gram-negative organisms a strong but somewhat distant second. Over the years, *Pseudomonas* and *Proteus* have increased in significance. By 1960, *Pseudomonas* predominated, with other gram-negative organisms and staphylococci comprising the remainder. This was prior to the advent of any of the

Table 25. Quantitative Bacteriology of Burn Mortality in the Absence of Topical Therapy*

SOURCE	ORGANISM	COUNT
Blood	*Pseudomonas*	1.6×10^4
Liver	*Pseudomonas*	9.8×10^4
Spleen	*Pseudomonas*	4.0×10^5
Kidney	*Pseudomonas*	8.6×10^6
Kidney pelvis	*Pseudomonas*	3.5×10^4
Bladder	*Pseudomonas*	1.0×10^7
Lung	*Pseudomonas*	2.3×10^8
Burn wound – A	*Pseudomonas*, staphylococci	1.0×10^7
Burn wound – B	*Pseudomonas*, staphylococci	1.0×10^8

*Predominant organism of wound is found in blood and many viscera.

Table 26. Quantitative Bacteriology of Burn Mortality*

SOURCE	ORGANISM	COUNT
Blood	No growth	0
Spleen	No growth	0
Liver	No growth	0
Kidney	No growth	0
Burn wound	*Pseudomonas*, staphylococci	
	Providence group	1.0×10^7

*This shows many organisms in the wound without systemic dissemination.

potent semisynthetic antistaphylococcal drugs and thus cannot be attributed to suppression of staphylococci. But the story does not end. At the time of this writing, *Pseudomonas* is being challenged for dominance by such gram-negative organisms as *Aerobacter*.

Immunologic Response in Burn Injury

Alteration of the immunologic capability of individuals following burn injury has been offered by some as the cause of the predominant role of infection of burn mortality. Studies in both human subjects and animals indicate that (1) any depression of immunologic response is proportional to size of burn and in general occurs in burns of 30 per cent or more; (2) if depression occurs, it is usually a depression of antigen administered after the burn; (3) there is an increased response to previously administered antigen such as tetanus toxoid; and (4) the depressed antigenic response is of a confusing nature but is probably more dependent upon the form of the antigen (i.e. cellular vs. noncellular) than any other factor.

Formation of antibody to *Pseudomonas* (either as the heat-killed organism or as a saline extract) is not depressed.

Clinical Features of Burn Wound Sepsis

1. Temperature response varies greatly. The large burn which is exposed evaporates water so rapidly that the attendant caloric demand impairs the usual febrile response to infection. In such cases, temperatures of 102°F. are the rule. Peaks above this level are not unusual, however. With inhibition of evaporation by occlusive dressings, temperatures of 105° to 106° are common.

In fatal cases, preterminal hypothermia of 93° to 95° is quite often seen, especially with the gram-negative infections.

2. The pulse is rapid and regular. It tends to be of good quality and becomes thready only when hypotension develops. The electrocardiogram shows a sinus tachycardia (rate 140 to 170 per minute). Carotid sinus stimulation produces only a transient slowing of the heart rate, and digitalis does not affect the rate significantly. For some reason, tachycardia is the rule in burned patients, and it does not in itself signify infection.

3. Hypotension and oliguria occur in severe cases.

4. Paralytic ileus is a common and most distressing finding. It prevents gastrointestinal feeding and thus contributes substantially to debilitation.

5. Disorientation occurs in a variable degree.

6. In severe cases, there is a bleeding tendency manifested by petechiae, ecchymoses and oozing from the wounds.

7. Mild jaundice may be observed.

The onset of sepsis may be insidious or acute. A gradual rise or drop in temperature may be the earliest manifestation; the complete burn wound sepsis syndrome then develops gradually within 2 or 3 days. Repeated blood cultures must be obtained. At times the clinical course of a patient may be quite satisfactory and then—suddenly and without warning —all the signs of sepsis become evident (Fig. 160).

Sepsis due to gram-negative organisms more characteristically is associated with a leukopenia, relative hypothermia and rapid wound deterioration. Hypotension, ileus and disorientation are usually more insidious in onset and less profound in degree than in those cases due to gram-positive organisms.

Although sepsis may occur at any time during the postburn period, a few generalizations may be pertinent. Burn wound sepsis is most common during the first 10 days following thermal injury, but quite rare after a month.

The peak occurrence in the early postburn period can be explained by the absence of local defenses against invading bacteria during this time.

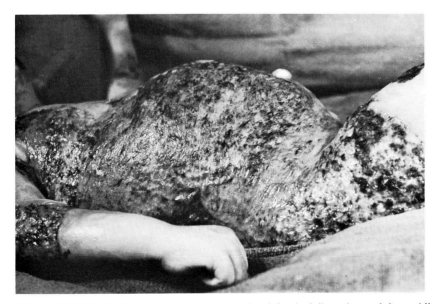

Figure 160.   Typical burn wound sepsis. Note the abdominal distention and the rapidly coalescing black punctate areas of disintegrating burn wound. This is almost never seen with effective topical therapy today.

As soon as granulation tissue appears, sepsis is controlled more easily. The time required for the growth of good granulation tissue varies. It depends upon the patient's metabolic response, the type of local therapy given, the adequacy of nutritional support and probably many other factors. Patients who develop sepsis after 3 weeks either fail to grow granulation tissue or experience destruction of this previously formed barrier. The sudden mysterious disappearance of apparently healthy granulations within a period of a few days is one of the most discouraging occurrences in the treatment of a severe burn. The disappearance of granulations and the onset of sepsis are almost simultaneous occurrences but it is possible to ascertain which is the cause and which the effect by careful tissue studies. Both animal and human studies indicate that somehow a fulminant invasive infection due to gram-negative organisms results in thrombosis of the neovasculature and necrosis of the granulating barrier. *This emphasizes the need for early wound closure with skin.*

Control of the Burn Wound Flora

The avascular nature of the burn wound completely precludes the successful use of systemic antibacterial therapy directed at the burn wound flora. Thus, any effective agent must be locally applied and capable of active penetration of the eschar in effective concentration, and because of the multiplicity of bacterial species existing in the wound, it must have a wide spectrum of activity. Preferably the agent should be nontoxic, both locally and systemically, readily excreted if absorbed in significant amounts, easy to use and cheap. Since 1964, two substances, both old drugs, have been found to possess many of the qualifications, and clinical use has resulted in remarkable success in the control of burn wound sepsis. These drugs are 10 per cent p-aminomethylbenzene sulfonamide (Sulfamylon) and aqueous 0.5 per cent silver nitrate. Others are being investigated, but results have been too scant or unimpressive to date to warrant comment.

It should be emphasized that complete eradication of the bacterial flora of the burn wound cannot be realized by present means. However, reduction of the bacterial population to a more manageable level can be readily achieved by either drug if the drug is used properly. If burn wound sepsis is defined briefly as active invasive infection by microorganisms existing in amounts exceeding 10^5 per gram of tissue, successful control would require reduction below this level. Indeed, such is the case, with the mean bacterial count being 10^4 per gram of tissue in responsive cases (Table 27).

Such reduction in numbers of microorganisms cannot be considered in itself as the only requirement for survival in the presence of infection. The bacterial population must be controlled at or below this level and the wound must be closed with skin grafts as soon as possible. If wound closure is not secured early, control of the wound flora is lost. This and the prolonged negative energy balance associated with the open wound result in a fatal outcome. Death does not come suddenly and dramatically

Table 27. Control of Burn Wound Flora by
Effective Topical Therapy

THERAPY	NO. CASES	NO. WOUND SAMPLES	ORGANISMS PER GRAM TISSUE	
			RANGE	AVERAGE
Without Sulfamylon	12	43	10^5–10^9	6.0×10^7
With Sulfamylon	9	38	10^2–10^5	8.4×10^4

but, rather, approaches insidiously with the gradual deterioration of all body systems.

The effective use of topical therapy demands that careful attention be paid to the method of application of the agents and that adjunctive measures be pursued with vigor, particularly skin closure. Topical therapy alone is not sufficient.

Silver nitrate. Silver nitrate is an ancient member of the drug armamentarium that is utilized with varying success in many local infections and was actually used for local application to the burn wound in the late 1920's. At that time it was used as 5.0 or 10.0 per cent solution with or without tannic acid. Even without the tannic acid such concentrations were tissue toxic, and its use fell into disrepute.

Moyer reintroduced topical silver nitrate therapy in burns but reduced the concentration to 0.5 per cent. At this strength, the substance is not toxic to local tissues and is effective against the wide spectrum of organisms inhabiting the burn wound.

Treatment with silver nitrate consists of covering the wound with 20 layers of coarse-mesh gauze which is saturated every 2 hours with the 0.5 per cent silver nitrate solution. The dressings are held in place with stockinette or circular bandages and changed twice daily. With each dressing change, the wound is progressively debrided, primarily by removal of gauze but also by instruments. The patient's dressings are covered with a light cotton blanket to reduce the rate of evaporation from the dressings.

As the silver nitrate must be applied in a distilled water vehicle, considerable absorption of electrolyte-free water occurs, resulting in dilutional reduction of serum electrolyte concentrations. In addition, sodium is leached from the wound and chloride is precipitated as insoluble silver chloride. Thus, an actual electrolyte deficit can rapidly occur. Other insoluble anion complexes (proteinate, carbonate) are also formed and significant decrements of potassium, calcium and occasionally magnesium occur.

To obviate these significant electrolyte abnormalities frequent monitoring of blood concentrations is mandatory. In children this may require checking electrolytes every 4 to 6 hours. Supplemental salt therapy given either intravenously as 5.0 per cent sodium chloride or, more commonly, as 20 to 30 gm. of enteric-coated sodium chloride orally is necessary. Success with the oral route is unpredictable, since irritation of the gastrointestinal tract often results in passage of much of the medication intact. Every effort must be made to keep the serum sodium above 130 mEq. per liter, but it is often much lower. Additional intake of magnesium and calcium and as much as 120 mEq. of potassium are necessary.

Absorption of the nitrate ion and its apparent metabolism to nitrite results in elevation of methemoglobin levels. This has been of no clinical significance, however. Silver levels in excess of 30 μg. per 100 ml. have not been measured, and argyria is no problem. Only trace amounts are found in the viscera.

The application of silver nitrate results in discoloration of the burn and the unburned skin. In 48 to 72 hours, the entire area is black or dark brown, and unless the surgeon is skilled in the use of this technique it becomes difficult to differentiate burned from normal skin (Fig. 161). The same black staining that discolors the skin and burn also affects linens, clothing of nursing personnel, floors and walls. This is both troublesome and expensive, but like all treatments the side effects must be balanced against the value of the method.

Sulfamylon. The clinical use of Sulfamylon was begun in January 1964 after extensive laboratory investigation (Table 28). Its use in burns was suggested by the successful application of a 5.0 per cent solution of Sulfamylon in the treatment of massive soft tissue injury in animals.

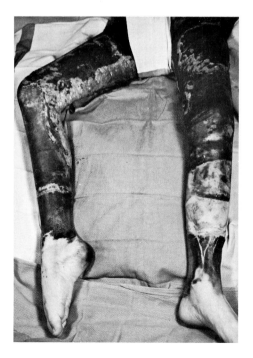

Figure 161. Burn treated with silver nitrate. Some of the eschar has begun to separate. The black-brown staining is evident and considerable experience is required in following progress of the burn wound under these circumstances.

Table 28. INFLUENCE OF TOPICAL THERAPY ON BURN WOUND SEPSIS

	PRE-SULFAMYLON 1962–1963	SULFAMYLON 1964–1966
Total patients	290	817
Number of deaths	111	160
Mortality	38.3 per cent	19.6 per cent
Incidence of burn wound sepsis among deaths	59.0 per cent	13.0 per cent
Incidence of pneumonia among deaths	10.0 per cent	70.0 per cent

Like silver nitrate, Sulfamylon has a wide spectrum of activity against the bacterial pathogens inhabiting the burn wound. Although primarily bacteriostatic, it can be bactericidal in high concentrations and is particularly effective against the clostridia. Used as a 10 per cent mixture in a water-soluble base, the drug actively penetrates the burn wound and exists in high concentrations in the deeper tissues. Its active penetration leads to high absorption rates, but the active form is enzymatically broken down rapidly on entering the blood. Blood levels of the active Sulfamylon usually run about 1.0 to 2.5 mg. per 100 ml. and the inactive p-carboxy salt breakdown product 3.0 to 7.0 mg. per 100 ml. The low blood level of the active form explains its lack of efficacy as systemic therapy.

Both the breakdown product and the active form are highly soluble in urine, even at a low pH. It is common to have urine volumes of 100 to 200 ml. per hour with a specific gravity of 1.030 when Sulfamylon therapy is used.

The large urine volumes are in part the result of diuresis associated with the strong carbonic anhydrase inhibition characteristic of this group of sulfonamide-like drugs. This interference with renal tubular transport results in excretion in the urine of large amounts of bicarbonate but very little ammonia and a selective retention of chloride. As a result of this there is a hyperchloremic acidosis which is intensified by the heavy load of the acid breakdown product, the p-carboxy salt. The use of an acetate salt of Sulfamylon rather than the hydrochloride salt initially utilized has resulted in some lessening of the acidosis.

The carbonic anhydrase inhibition interferes with renal tubular compensation for the acidosis and places the load directly on the pulmonary mechanism. For this reason, hyperventilation occurs with rates of 30 per minute as well as pCO_2 levels of 25 mm. Hg and CO_2 of 12 to 16 mEq. per liter. This pulmonary compensation results in an alkaline pH (7.50 to 7.60) which is maintained by easy breathing. If, however, the common complication of pneumonia occurs, the character of the respirations changes (24 to 48 hours prior to x-ray changes) to that of a ventilation requiring considerable effort.

After initial wound cleansing, institution of resuscitative therapy and complete evaluation of the patient, the Sulfamylon therapy is begun. As a 10 per cent concentration of the drug in a water-soluble base of glycerol, long chain alcohols and water, the substance is applied with the gloved hand to the entire burn wound. Application is at a thickness of 3 to 4 mm., which obscures the wound, and no dressings are applied. Total wound application is accomplished twice daily with immersion in the hydrotherapy tank and debridement of the wound preceding each morning application.

Recent experience would indicate that the acidosis can be lessened and bacterial control retained in the large burn wounds by once daily applications beginning at the second or third postburn day following initial twice daily administration.

Should a decompensated acidosis develop subsequent to Sulfamylon therapy, it is invariably due to the onset of pulmonary complications. This is with rare exception a rapidly advancing gram-negative bronchopneumonia. If such occurs, drug application must cease and buffering with sodium bicarbonate or THAM accomplished. More adequate pulmonary ventilation and alveolar exchange must be sought by means of endotracheal suction, bronchoscopy and ventilator support. Antibiotic therapy directed at the pneumonia is determined by identification of the predominant organisms on sputum culture. Control of the burn wound flora will persist for only 72 hours after cessation of topical therapy. Thus, to be successful the pulmonary lesion must clear in that time period. For some reason, pulmonary decompensation rarely occurs in children or infants.

The application of the Sulfamylon cream is associated with transient pain which varies in intensity from patient to patient. It is readily controlled with analgesics and rapidly diminishes so that it is rarely a problem after the first week. Allergic sensitivity in the form of a maculopapular rash is noted in 3 to 5 per cent of the patients. Use of antihistamines while continuing Sulfamylon leads to disappearance of the rash.

Daily debridement in the hydrotherapy tank and gradual closure of the large wounds by homograft and autograft are combined with the topical therapy, whether it be Sulfamylon or silver nitrate.

Results of successful topical therapy, although occurring throughout the burn population, are most striking in children. This is because burn wound sepsis as a cause of death is a much more prominent factor among children than adults.

It is unquestionably true that agents other than silver nitrate and Sulfamylon exist which would be equally if not more effective as a means of controlling burn wound sepsis. Indeed, topical gentamicin, silver sulfadiazine, silver acetate, colloidal silver and the subeschar instillation of antimicrobials show some promise, but data are too scant to allow clear appraisal at this time.

TREATMENT OF BURN WOUND SEPSIS

An accurate bacteriologic diagnosis is essential for proper treatment. Therapy is sufficiently difficult when detailed bacteriologic information is available, but it is virtually hopeless when it must be administered blindly. Therapy of established sepsis is rarely successful. *Prevention thus is the best treatment.*

Antibiotics

Prophylactic antibiotic therapy even in massive doses is of no value in eliminating or controlling burn wound sepsis. Systemic delivery into the avascular area is impossible, and the organisms residing there rapidly become resistant. However, bloodstream clearing of microorganisms and eradication of most satellite visceral lesions can be accomplished by appropriate therapy.

The frequency of pre-existing or concomitant upper respiratory or middle ear infections in infants or children is such that administration of penicillin for the first 5 postburn days is indicated. The existence of other injuries, such as an open fracture, may in itself be an indication for antibiotic therapy. Otherwise, antibiotic therapy is not indicated in the early phase of treatment. Sepsis cannot be prevented by systemic therapy. However, once established it may be controlled briefly by such measures until the source of sepsis is eradicated.

The burn wound is the source and thus the obvious target of any successful therapy.

Microorganisms isolated from blood cultures should be tested for sensitivity to several antibiotics. One or more antibiotics to which the invading microorganisms are sensitive *in vitro* should be given in large doses, preferably intravenously. If penicillin and streptomycin are given prophylactically during early therapy, invading bacteria are generally resistant to these agents. The tetracycline compounds and chloramphenicol may be effective against strains of coliform bacilli. Polymyxin B, colistimethate sodium and gentamicin are the drugs of choice against microorganisms of the *Pseudomonas* species. Sepsis due to *Micrococcus pyogenes* is most effectively treated with synthetic penicillins, methicillin, oxacillin and nafcillin. *Aerobacter* is most often sensitive to kanamycin. The aim in antibiotic therapy is to diminish the load of bacteria in the bloodstream and to prevent formation of abscesses in internal organs until wound care eliminates the wound as a feeding focus.

Wound Care

Wound management is extremely important but very difficult. The dry appearance of a burn wound frequently leads the inexperienced to conclude that no infection is present. However, dry and benign appearing eschars may actually obscure active bacterial proliferation and abundant suppuration that is often occurring beneath them.

Since the nature of the burn wound precludes successful systemic antimicrobial therapy, efforts are made to utilize the topical agents Sulfamylon or silver nitrate.

The care of a wound depends upon the status of the wound at the time sepsis develops. All efforts should be directed toward the elimination of eschar, followed by wound coverage in such a way that further insult is not added to the patient. Extensive surgical excision under general anesthesia produces more trauma than can be tolerated by a patient with burn wound sepsis. If the third-degree eschar covers less than 15 per cent of the body surface, excision may be justified. In more extensive burns, topical antibacterial agents or wet soaks may be used. As often as possible dead tissue should be removed with forceps and scissors in such a way that bleeding is minimal. This persistent approach to the elimination of dead tissue permits earlier coverage. If the eschars are boldly excised, further invasion of bacteria may occur via lymphatic and vascular channels.

Skin should be applied as soon as a suitable surface is obtained. Autografts may be applied if the burn is of moderate size and the patient is in good condition. In more extensive burns, homografts should be applied at the bedside without anesthesia.

Sometimes sepsis occurs when spontaneous sequestration of the eschar is well under way. Granulation tissue is being formed but it has not yet developed sufficiently to afford good protection against invasive infection. Profuse suppuration is characteristic of such wounds. If sepsis occurs at this stage, the prognosis is somewhat better than when the eschar is firmly attached, simply because wound closure can be accomplished rapidly when eschar is no longer present. Even at this stage topical applications of the

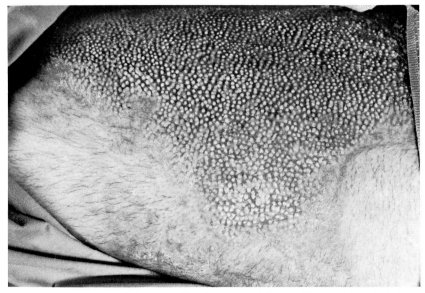

Figure 162. The result of controlling burn wound flora. With effective topical therapy, epithelial islands surviving the initial thermal insult are preserved and soon begin to proliferate. This photo, taken at 17 days post burn, shows early island proliferation. In 48 hours complete epithelial coalescence produced a smooth, healed wound. Herein lies the reason for the lessened mortality associated with effective topical therapy, for without topical therapy this deep dermal burn would have been converted to full-thickness skin loss by bacterial autolysis.

highly diffusible antibacterial agents may control the bacterial population on the wound, and the number of microorganisms gaining access to the bloodstream may be reduced sufficiently to enable body defenses to cope with them (Fig. 162). Such therapy is successful for limited periods, however, and can ultimately be overwhelmed. Thus, during this period of control, every effort is made to debride the wound and obtain wound closure as soon as possible with autograft or homograft.

Supportive Therapy

Oxygen is indicated in patients who have marked tachypnea and tachycardia. This is usually due to pulmonary pathology associated with septic visceral lesions or pneumonia in late stages. Necrotic tracheobronchitis in the early postburn period is usually nonseptic and due to inhalation of noxious combustion products. Administration of oxygen by mask is seldom practical, nor is a tent. Delivery by catheter or a nebulized system is best.

Nasogastric suction should be used if abdominal distention is marked.

Aspirin and other antipyretics are recommended when the temperature rises to 103°F. or higher.

Digitalis is indicated in the presence of heart failure. Acute left ventricular failure with pulmonary edema is a common terminal event. If pulmonary edema occurs, rapid digitalization is indicated, but successful relief is rarely obtained. The drug has been shown to be effective in the normal myocardium. The demonstration of many nonspecific as well as septic myocardial lesions post mortem at the Surgical Research Unit has been used as the indication for prophylactic digitalization in most burns over 50 per cent in that installation.

Corticosteroids in pharmacologic doses are indicated for the management of shock due to overwhelming sepsis.

Blood transfusions may be lifesaving. Transfusion requirements vary greatly; the amounts of blood required during sepsis depend upon the hemolytic properties of the offending microorganism. One or two daily transfusions may be necessary to maintain an adequate hemoglobin concentration.

Fluid and electrolyte administration is important. Since the problems of burn wound sepsis following thermal injury are critical, any gross errors in fluid therapy must be avoided. Frequent measurements of plasma electrolyte and nonprotein nitrogen concentrations are essential guides to therapy. If large volumes are lost, gastrointestinal fluids should be measured and analyzed for sodium, potassium and chloride content. The losses of these ions must be replaced quantitatively. The water requirements, often quite high in uncomplicated extensive burns, may be extraordinarily high if sepsis is present. The increased need for water in the hyperthermic stage of sepsis, in addition to massive evaporative losses in extensive burns, necessitates great volumes of replacement fluids. Five to seven liters of electrolyte-free water are not an unusual daily requirement to maintain adequate clinical hydration.

Nutritional supportive measures are of utmost importance. Effective nutritional support is often prevented by gastrointestinal atony that precludes oral and intragastric feeding. Intravenous feedings must then be relied on, but this procedure is far from adequate. Vitamins should be given in large doses.

From a nutritional standpoint successful topical therapy is important because it not only lessens metabolic demands but also prevents impairment of caloric intake.

To recapitulate, it appears likely that appropriate antibacterial therapy and judicious wound care are the most important factors in the prevention of wound sepsis following thermal injury. However, all of the supportive measures mentioned may play decisive roles under special circumstances. It is well to remember that more patients are recovering whose condition once appeared to be hopeless. Regardless of how desperate the clinical picture may appear, a defeatist attitude is never justified.

PROGNOSIS IN BURN WOUND SEPSIS

There is ample evidence that the magnitude of the burn injury is the dominant factor influencing prognosis. Experience at the Surgical Research Unit has shown more specifically that magnitude of injury is determined by both extent and depth of the burn wound. Survival is rare in patients having third-degree burns covering 50 per cent of the body surface.

The following hypothesis is proposed as an explanation of the problem of wound sepsis in burns. When the cumulative case fatality rate is plotted as a function of the extent of burn, an S-shaped curve is obtained. By appropriate transformation, it can readily be shown that this curve has the essential features of a dosage-fatality curve commonly encountered in bioassays. Some of these curves have a characteristically rapid rise in mortality in the central portion. Thus, only a small increase in dosage may result in an enormous increase in the case fatality rate. From the similarity of the extent of burn-fatality function and the dosage-fatality function in bioassays, it may be reasoned that extent of burn acts in a manner analogous to dosage.

When it is recognized that death following burns is frequently due to sepsis, it is reasonable to assume that the dosage phenomenon is related to the number of pathogenic microorganisms invading the burn wound. If large numbers of bacteria invade the burn wound, even though bloodstream involvement is minimal, host defenses become exhausted and eventually they are overwhelmed. If the number of invading bacteria is not too large, host defenses can cope with them successfully providing both specific and nonspecific therapy is utilized until local barriers are formed against invasive infection. From laboratory and clinical observations, it appears that the body can withstand a bacterial population in the burn wound of 10^5 or less organisms per gram of tissue over large areas for a considerable period of time. However, extensive spread of higher population rates is poorly tolerated even for short periods. Quantitative counts of 10^8 microorganisms per gram of tissue are common in deaths due to burn wound sepsis. The viscera may be quite sterile in such cases, indicating that bloodstream invasion is not a necessary prerequisite for a fatal outcome.

Although this concept may be somewhat oversimplified, it forms an effective basis for the planning of therapy. Efforts are directed not only at ridding the bloodstream of invading microorganisms but also at reducing the bacterial inoculum causing persistence of burn wound sepsis. Reduction of the inoculum is the chief aim not only in removal of the eschar but also in the use of topical therapy and in grafting. Since only a slight margin may exist between the body's successful defense against invading microorganisms and its failure, supportive measures must be viewed not as minor adjuvants to other therapy but as an essential component that may make the difference between survival and death.

BACTEREMIA

From clinical observations, bacteremia is frequently suspected in burns, but it can rarely be substantiated bacteriologically. Bacteremia is often suspected if a sudden, transient increase in temperature occurs after a dressing change. In considering the definition of bacteremia, a high incidence of bacteriologic confirmation would not be expected because body defenses rapidly clear the bloodstream of the small showers of invading microorganisms. Bacteremia may occur in third-degree burns even after the formation of a good granulating barrier. If this condition occurs, it is usually caused by unduly rough treatment of the granulations. Microorganisms may gain access to the bloodstream when the integrity of granulations is impaired by mechanical trauma.

The bacteremia noted in thermal injury is primarily of two types: gram positive, predominantly *Staphylococcus,* and gram negative, predominantly *Pseudomonas.* The staphylococci inhabit the bloodstream in characteristically large numbers (1000 to 1500 per ml. of blood) and often are associated with metastatic visceral abscesses. The source is originally the burn wound but with effective antistaphylococcal therapy presently available, persistent residence of these microorganisms in the blood is almost invariably due to a septic intravascular locus, usually a septic thrombus.

The gram-negative microorganisms (particularly *Pseudomonas*) initially invade primarily by way of the lymphatics.

Quantitative counts of organisms residing within the bloodstream in these circumstances are usually limited to two or three colonies per ml. of blood. Thus, positive cultures appear late. Later, involvement of the perivascular lymphatics sets the stage for invasion of the vessel wall. This is ordinarily limited to penetration as far as the internal elastic membrane, but late in the disease complete involvement, with intravascular septic thrombosis and embolization, occurs. While metastatic septic foci have been identified in every organ of the body, in such cases the viscera are often sterile until late in the stage of the disease process.

LOCAL INFECTION

Local infection is manifested by clinical signs such as cellulitis, lymphangitis and regional lymphadenopathy. Fever and leukocytosis are generally present. Group A beta hemolytic streptococci and staphylococci are the causes of this type of infection in most instances.

In contrast to invasive sepsis, a primary problem in extensive full-thickness burns, local infection often complicates partial-thickness burns of minor extent. This type of infection was a very serious problem prior to the availability of antibiotics that are highly effective against streptococci. Uncontrolled streptococcal sepsis proved fatal in many instances.

Local infection can be effectively controlled by careful wound hygiene with removal of devitalized tissue when possible and judicious use of topical and systemic antibacterial agents. Penicillin is particularly effective against streptococci, and the newer semisynthetic penicillins against the staphylococci. However, each must be combined with local care. Uncontrolled infection results in prompt conversion of partial-thickness burns to full-thickness loss. Close observation and immediate treatment are indicated.

Partial-thickness burns are often surrounded by a halo of edema and erythema due to first-degree burns. This erythema may be confused with cellulitis and, conversely, cellulitis may be mistaken for a first-degree burn. The presence of an unexpected degree of fever, leukocytosis, pain or regional lymphadenopathy favors a diagnosis of cellulitis. At times, it is impossible to differentiate between cellulitis and a first-degree burn. Then it is best to give large doses of penicillin on the assumption that a streptococcal cellulitis is present.

Streptococci may be present on wounds and destroy viable epithelium long before there is any clinical indication of streptococcal infection. This is an important reason for taking cultures of a burn wound when suspicion exists.

The clinical implications of local infection are quite different from those of generally invasive infection. Local infection does not threaten survival except in isolated and preventable instances. Nevertheless, local infection has very serious consequences that contribute substantially to the patient's discomfort, metabolic derangements and length of time required for healing.

Partial-thickness Burns and Donor Sites

In wounds of this type, infection may cause partial-thickness skin loss to become converted to full-thickness skin loss. If the burn is of the deep dermal type, even a small amount of local infection may destroy the remaining viable epithelium. One advantage of the exposure method over occlusive dressings seems to be a more frequent, spontaneous healing of deep dermal burns as a result of better control of infection. As a consequence, the need for skin grafting is decreased. Even more important, since the conversion to full-thickness loss is minimized the magnitude of burn injury is not increased. This is one of the most significant aspects of successful topical antimicrobial therapy.

It should be noted that an inevitable feature of treatment by exposure is the contamination of wounds by all bacteria in the patient's environment. Various microorganisms may be cultured from the surface of the crust, but have no consistent relationship to the flora deep in the wound. As long as invasive sepsis is prevented or controlled, surface contamination is of little consequence.

The size of the contaminating inoculum is probably important in determining whether or not suppuration may be avoided. If suppuration occurs by either method of local care, there is great danger of full-thickness skin loss. Meticulous wound toilet and frequent observation can greatly minimize the incidence of this, and appropriate topical Sulfamylon antibacterial therapy is of aid.

Extensive infection of donor sites may be a catastrophe. Infection of donor sites may convert a relatively small third-degree burn into very extensive, full-thickness skin loss. For this reason an essential aspect of treatment is detailed attention to donor sites. (See Chapter Eight.)

Granulating Wounds

Controversy exists over the significance of infection of granulating surfaces. However, when there is a dearth of specific information, controversy is to be expected. The important fact is that the granulations are never sterile and grafting should proceed when the wound appears healthy and free of nonviable tissue.

Many different types of streptococci may colonize a granulating wound. However, only group A beta hemolytic streptococci cause widespread destruction of grafts (Fig. 163). The emphasis on group A is important. Streptococci that cause beta hemolysis on blood agar plates but do not belong to Lancefield's group A are apparently no more harmful than other microorganisms that may colonize a wound. Streptococci that produce alpha hemolysis and nonhemolytic streptococci do not appear to affect graft takes. Even though these microorganisms are present, good graft takes occur, provided the inoculum is not overwhelming. The granulating surface does become rapidly sterile following grafting because of the very effective phagocytosis that occurs beneath the graft. Viable homograft accomplishes the same result.

Ps. aeruginosa frequently colonize burn wounds and rarely affect the take of grafts unless the inoculum is unusually heavy. In fact, the pre-

DISTRIBUTION OF GRAFT TAKES

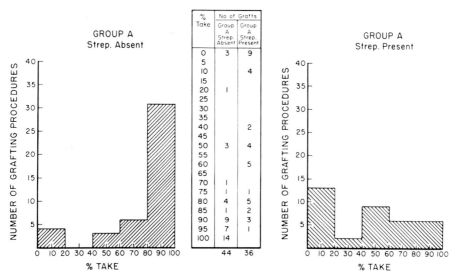

Figure 163. Distribution of graft takes on burn wounds colonized by group A beta hemolytic streptococci and on burn wounds not colonized by streptococci. Variation in takes is strikingly different. The deleterious effect of these streptococci on graft takes is unique.

ferred method for eliminating *Ps. aeruginosa* is to apply a skin graft. Acetic acid soaks are of no value against *Pseudomonas* as the acid does not kill the microorganism but only decolorizes it.

It is reasonably certain that grafts would take better on bacteria-free granulations than on contaminated surfaces. If the bacterial species colonizing the wound are not of critical importance, however, what aspect of local infection of granulations is responsible for some of the graft failures? This may be answered, at least in part, by clinical experience. Wounds on which suppuration abounds are poor recipient sites for grafts, whereas wounds that are largely free of suppuration generally are good recipient sites. Suppurative granulations are always boggy and edematous with poor circulation. The very factors favoring bacterial growth also mitigate against successful grafting. A crucial factor in determining the take of a graft may be the size of the bacterial inoculum and the rate of bacterial growth rather than the particular microorganisms involved.

These considerations greatly simplify the preparation of granulating surfaces for grafting. Clinical criteria are the primary basis for determining the readiness of a wound for grafting. The only essential bacteriologic information concerns the presence or absence of group A beta hemolytic streptococci. Grafting must not be performed if these microorganisms are present. If other bacterial species are present, it is of no special importance provided the wound clinically appears ready for grafting.

Antibiotic therapy for granulating wounds. Systemically administered antibiotics are of value during the grafting procedure only because they afford protection against streptococci. They are probably of no value in the treatment of wound suppuration caused by other microorganisms. There is no conclusive evidence that systemically administered antibiotics alter the wound flora qualitatively or quantitatively except with respect to streptococci.

If a wound becomes infected by group A beta hemolytic streptococci, vigorous treatment must be instituted to eliminate these microorganisms. They can spread from wound to wound with amazing rapidity and, unless the staff is vigilant, an epidemic of streptococcal wound infection may occur. If streptococci suddenly appear on wounds, it is wise to obtain nose and throat cultures from the attending personnel, visitors and other patients to determine whether anyone is a carrier. Vigorous penicillin treatment of carriers is indicated.

Although group A beta hemolytic streptococci are always sensitive to penicillin and the drug diffuses freely into the exudate of granulations, elimination of streptococci is not always achieved by means of penicillin. In some instances, the failure of penicillin therapy appears to be due to its inactivation by penicillinase that is produced by other microorganisms present on the granulating surface. Also, the presence of nonviable tissue enhances the bacterial growth. The most efficient method of eliminating streptococci from a burn wound is by a combination of systemic and local therapy. Penicillin should be given intramuscularly for this purpose and/or one of the semisynthetic penicillinase-resistant antistaphylococcal drugs administered. Systemic therapy should be continued for 2 days after a graft has been applied. At least one negative culture for streptococci should be obtained prior to grafting. Contrary to a common misconception, clinical evidence may not suggest wound infection by streptococci. It is therefore essential to make a careful bacteriologic study of all burn wounds. Streptococci may prevent the take of grafts even when their presence is not suspected.

The value of antibacterial substances applied locally to granulating surfaces is difficult to assess. Results similar to those with local antibiotic therapy can be achieved by reduction in the bacterial population by means of more frequent attention to the burn wound and meticulous mechanical cleansing. Many antibacterial agents are currently on the market and others are sure to come.

Some general conclusions may be formulated in regard to local antibacterial therapy. To be effective, topical antibacterial therapy must be (1) effective against the existing major wound pathogen; (2) not toxic to tissues; (3) highly diffusible into tissues; (4) broken down in blood or excreted rapidly so that toxic blood levels do not occur; and (5) readily applied in an effective concentration which can be easily maintained.

It must be emphasized that granulation tissue is desirable in a graft recipient site, but the only characteristics necessary are a clean bed and adequate circulation. The delay of grafting until granulations appear may prove fatal in large burns if in fact a clean wound was ready earlier.

Poor graft takes are usually the result of poor wound care, inappropriate timing, inadequate immobilization with dressings and mechanical dislodging. With proper care, infection is an insignificant problem.

REFERENCES

Aldrich, R. H.: The role of infection in burns: the therapy and treatment with special reference to gentian violet. *New England J. Med.* **208**:299, 1933.

Alexander, J. W., Brown, W., Mason, A. D., Jr., and Moncrief, J. A.: The influence of infection upon serum protein changes in severe burns. *J. Trauma* **6**:780, 1966.

Alexander, J. W., Brown, W., Walker, H., Mason, A. D., Jr., and Moncrief, J. A.: Studies on the isolation of an infection-protective antigen from Pseudomonas aeruginosa. *Surg. Gynec. & Obst.* **123**:965, 1966.

Alexander, J. W., and Moncrief, J. A.: Immunologic phenomena in burns. *J.A.M.A.* **199**:257, 1967.

Baar, S.: Serum and plasma proteins in thermally injured patients treated with plasma, its admixture with albumin or serum alone. *Ann. Surg.* **161**:112, 1965.

Best, R. R., Coe, J. D., and McMurtrey, G. B.: Effect of soaps containing hexachlorophene on wounds and burned surfaces. *A.M.A. Arch. Surg.* **62**:895, 1951.

Cason, J. A., and Lowbury, E. J. L.: Prophylactic chemotherapy for burns. Studies on the local and systemic use of combined therapy. *Lancet* **2**:501, 1960.

Colebrook, L., Duncan, J. M., and Ross, W. P. D.: The control of infection in burns. *Lancet* **1**:893, 1948.

Contreras, A. A., Evans, B. W., Moncrief, J. A., Lindberg, R. B., Villarreal, Y., and Mason, A. D., Jr.: Some aspects of cyanide-producing capabilities of *Pseudomonas aeruginosa* strains isolated from burned patient infections. *J. Trauma* **3**:527, 1963.

Jackson, D. M., Lowbury, E. J. L., and Topley, E.: *Pseudomonas pyocyanea* in burns; its role as a pathogen and the value of local polymyxin therapy. *Lancet* **2**:137, 1951.

Jackson, D. M., Lowbury, E. J. L., and Topley, E.: Chemotherapy of *Streptococcus pyogenes* infection of burns. *Lancet* **2**:705, 1951.

Liedberg, N. C.-F., Kuhn, L. R., Barnes, B. A., Reiss, E., and Amspacher, W. H.: Infection in burns. II. The pathogenicity of streptococci. *Surg. Gynec. & Obst.* **98**:693, 1954.

Liedberg, N. C.-F., Reiss, E., and Artz, C. P.: Infection in burns. III. Septicemia, a common cause of death. *Surg. Gynec. & Obst.* **99**:151, 1954.

Moncrief, J. A., Lindberg, R. B., Switzer, W. E., and Pruitt, B. A., Jr.: Use of topical antibacterial therapy in the treatment of the burn wound. *A.M.A. Arch. Surg.* **92**:558, 1966.

Moncrief, J. A., and Teplitz, C.: Changing concepts in burn sepsis. *J. Trauma* **4**:233, 1964.

Moyer, C. A., Brentano, L., Gravens, D. L., Margraf, H. W., and Monafo, W. W., Jr.: Treatment of large human burns with 0.5% silver nitrate solution. *A.M.A. Arch. Surg.* **90**:812, 1965.

Order, S. E., Mason, A. D., Jr., Switzer, W. E., and Moncrief, J. A.: Arterial vascular occlusion and devitalization of burn wounds. *Ann. Surg.* **161**:502, 1965.

Order, S. E., Mason, A. D., Jr., Walker, H. L., Lindberg, R. B., Switzer, W. E., and Moncrief, J. A.: Vascular destructive effects of thermal injury and its relationship to burn wound sepsis. *J. Trauma* **5**:62, 1965.

Price, P. B., Call, D. E., Hansen, F. L., and Zerwick, C. J.: Histologic changes in experimental thermal wounds. *Surgery* **36**:664, 1954.

Pruitt, B. A., Jr., Tumbusch, W. T., Mason, A. D., Jr., and Pearson, E.: Mortality in 1,100 consecutive burns treated at a burns unit. *Ann. Surg.* **159**:396, 1964.

Teplitz, C., Davis, D., Mason, A. D., Jr., and Moncrief, J. A.: Pseudomonas burn wound sepsis. *J. S. Res.* **4**:200, 1964.

Teplitz, C., Davis, D., Walker, H. L., Raulston, G. L., Mason, A. D., Jr., and Moncrief, J. A.: Pseudomonas burn wound sepsis. II. Hematogenous infection at the junction of the burn wound and the unburned hypodermis. *J. S. Res.* **4**:217, 1964.

Zaroff, L. I., Mills, W., Jr., Duckett, J. W., Jr., Switzer, W. E., and Moncrief, J. A.: Multiple uses of viable cutaneous homografts in the burned patient. *Surgery* **59**:368, 1966.

Chapter
Fifteen

COMPLICATIONS
OF BURNS
AND BURN THERAPY

The road to recovery from a severe burn is beset with many complications. The seriousness of the injury, the frequent administration of anesthetics and operations, the large wounds, the prolonged period of bed rest and the large number of other procedures required in therapy all predispose to the occurrence of a wide variety of complications. Many complications are really complications of essential therapy.

Most of the serious complications of burns are related to infection. (See Chapter Fourteen.) In this chapter, some noninfectious complications are considered. The most difficult problem in the management of burned patients is often the treatment of some of these complications. Recognition of the more common complications aids in the institution of effective prophylactic measures.

COMPLICATIONS INVOLVING THE
RESPIRATORY TRACT

Respiratory derangements complicating burns occur during two rather distinct time periods post burn. While there are some notable exceptions, the complications occurring during the first 2 to 5 postburn days are primarily due to inhalation of noxious combustion products which irritate the tracheobronchial mucosa. For some reason, however, unless the involvement is overwhelming and rapidly fatal, the signs are delayed in appearing (Fig. 164). The characteristic rales, ronchi and wheezing respiration usually are first noted 24 to 48 hours after injury. The respiratory impairment becomes progressively worse and, unless vigorous methods are utilized, may result in enough of a deficit of gas exchange to precipitate a fatal episode of hypoxia.

A weird assortment of blood gas alterations may exist, and it is often

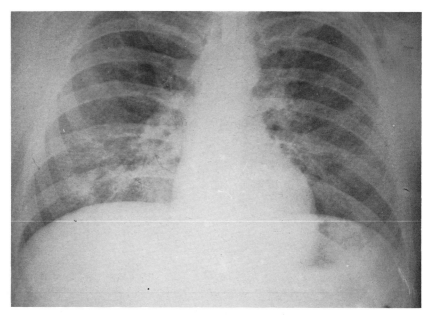

Figure 164.   X-ray showing heavy bronchial markings and scattered areas of pneumonitis at 10 days after inhalational injury. Much clearing had occurred radiographically in the preceding week, but severe ventilatory problems still existed with a pO_2 of 65 mm. Hg.

necessary to have pO_2, pCO_2 and pH determinations if a realistic interpretation is to be made. Metabolic or respiratory acidosis or alkalosis either compensated or uncompensated may occur. Usually the respiratory compensatory mechanisms are adequate and prominent clinically, though terminally they may fail along with everything else. Some decrease in pO_2 is common, but frank hypoxia is rare in the absence of obvious respiratory irritation.

The pathology (Chapter Two) noted in such circumstances consists of congestion of the bronchial arteries, edema and sloughing of the bronchial mucosa. In the early stages, inflammatory response is minimal. If involvement of the mucosa is extensive, the reparative processes are necessarily prolonged. Symptoms thus persist longer. During this period, the patient may cough up carbonaceous or bloody sputum with tissue fragments present.

During the first 24 to 48 hours post burn, the fluid resuscitation may result in overloading the vascular tree with resultant pulmonary edema. This also occurs as a complication of vigorous support of the circulation during terminal episodes of septic hypotension. It is not the primary cause of death under such circumstances, however.

Of great importance is the recognition of the tight, constricting effect of a third-degree eschar of the chest. This must be released rapidly or death will ensue within a few hours (Fig. 165). This is a particularly lethal complication in children.

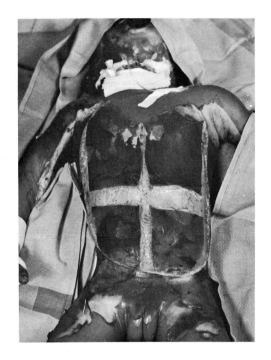

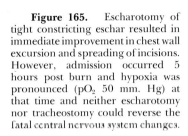

Figure 165. Escharotomy of tight constricting eschar resulted in immediate improvement in chest wall excursion and spreading of incisions. However, admission occurred 5 hours post burn and hypoxia was pronounced (pO$_2$ 50 mm. Hg) at that time and neither escharotomy nor tracheostomy could reverse the fatal central nervous system changes.

Near the end of the first postburn week and for the next 5 to 7 days, the respiratory complications are due primarily to the generalized immobility and serious disability of an injury of great magnitude. Atelectasis, pneumonia and aspiration are ordinarily seen during this period. Impaired ventilatory exchange secondary to prolonged immobilization, aspiration of vomitus or inspissated tracheostomy crusts, traumatic aspiration of tracheobronchial tree by nursing attendants and introduction of infection by the same route all predispose to pulmonary complications. However, one must be cognizant of the fact that these events are not due to the burn, but rather due to being burned. There is a distinct difference. *The former cannot be reversed, the latter can be prevented.*

The serious pneumonic processes which are seen with such frequency in cases of extensive thermal injury have a peculiar temporal pattern in relation to injury. Strong suspicion of such a development is generated by the appearance of carbonaceous sputum, but problems usually do not appear for at least several hours post burn unless due to severe inhalation injury and often are delayed 2 to 3 days.

The pneumonic processes are generally of two types: a rapidly confluent bronchopneumonia or a metastatic pneumonia. The latter is characterized by septic metastatic abscesses secondary to bacterial spread from the septic burn wound. The foci are located subpleurally in the peripheral portions of the parenchyma and like the skin lesions of ecthyma gangrenosa consist of a central mass of bacteria surrounded by the pneumonic reaction. Microscopically the capillaries of the area are engorged with organisms.

The radiographic appearance is one of miliary lesions throughout the lung fields.

Unfortunately these metastatic lesions are a part of the fatal process of a burn wound sepsis which has extended to the viscera. No known therapy exists at present.

The bronchopneumonic process as its name implies originates in the peribronchial areas but may rapidly become confluent and effectively obliterate all functioning pulmonary parenchyma. It is so commonly seen in those individuals requiring tracheostomy that a causal relationship has been suggested but none is demonstrable.

Early recognition of the bronchopneumonia is essential to successful therapy. Suspicion of the impending likelihood is strong when carbonaceous sputum is produced, the patient has difficulty clearing thick, tenacious sputum, and rales and ronchi are prominent. That bronchopneumonia does exist is certain when respiratory effort increases and acidosis or hypoxia occurs. These rapidly progressive events can occur far out of proportion to the roentgenographic changes demonstrated.

Antibiotic therapy is utilized on the basis of sputum cultures and sensitivities of the predominant organism. However, such therapy is to no avail unless adequate respiratory exchange can be established. Pulmonary dead space can be reduced by tracheostomy, which also serves as a means of improving tracheobronchial toilet. In clearing excess mucus, inspissated plugs and sloughing mucosa, which are common in the immediate and early postburn period, the endotracheal suction catheter is of great value. However, its use can often perpetuate these problems or initiate new ones. The margin of success or failure is very slim and the trauma of the suction catheter often exceeds the benefits of use.

Vigorous suctioning with the endotracheal catheter may lead to temporary improvement but ultimately is disastrous and is to be avoided. The primary objective is to stimulate coughing which forcefully expands pulmonary parenchyma and delivers mucus and debris to more proximal areas of ready access by the suction tube. Should simple procedures of this type fail, bronchoscopy, which is readily accomplished through the tracheostomy stoma, should be utilized to force coughing and clear the airway. Bronchial lavage may be required.

Mucolytic agents are of great assistance in loosening secretions, but the associated increase in volume is a hazard if unrecognized. Intermittent positive pressure breathing can be quite effective in maintaining or reinstituting expansion of parenchyma. In the cooperative patient a mouthpiece is used, but in most burned patients it is necessary to administer intermittent positive pressure breathing by way of a tracheostomy. The same portal must be utilized for assisted ventilation and the volume control type of controlled respiration. In the latter, an expired positive pressure may be of assistance in overcoming atelectasis.

Recovery from the pneumonic complications is often slow, with gas exchange impaired in the lung and bronchiectasis resulting from the destructive infection (Fig. 166).

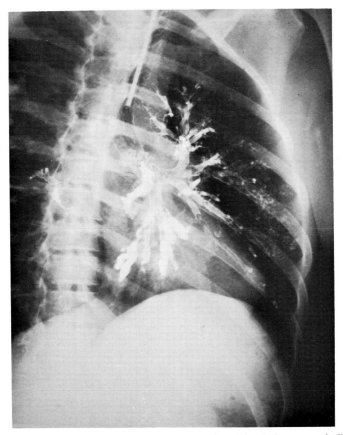

Figure 166. X-ray taken at 4 months post burn. The subject is the same as in Figure 164. The bronchogram shows extensive lower lobe bronchiectasis. Copious foul sputum was diminishing and blood gases were normal at this time.

Endotracheal suction in the burned patient undoubtedly introduces bacteria into the tracheobronchial tree, but this is probably only a bit sooner than they would spontaneously find their way there. While use of sterile catheters with each suctioning is theoretically desired, the logistical load can be staggering when it is realized that the burned patient requiring suctioning usually needs it over 200 times a day. Trauma to the tracheo-bronchial mucosa must be the paramount factor.

While a tracheostomy is of great aid in many instances it can also be a source of serious complications. The most dramatic are those associated with improper performance or care. All too often the stoma is made too low so that the tracheostomy tube either rides on the carina or slips down one mainstem bronchus occluding the other. Poor ventilation, coughing and bronchospasm result. In addition, the apical pleura are often opened, with resultant pneumothorax. Failure to provide adequate moisture to the inspired air is a well known fault. (See Chapter Twelve.) Because of frequent suctioning and constant abutment of the tube on the anterior tracheal wall, erosion of the area with invasive infection is common and actual perforation can occur.

In children and elderly individuals, acquired pneumonia is not uncommon. It usually follows a prolonged period of bed rest with the patient lying in one position. Changes of position, particularly by the use of the Stryker frame, may prevent the development of pneumonia. Sometimes pneumonia follows the use of a gastric feeding tube in children. Deep burns around the chest prevent adequate coughing. In some seriously burned patients the cough reflex is diminished. When the patient is unable to remove secretions from the tracheobronchial tree, tracheotomy should be performed.

Tracheostomy itself predisposes to serious complications and should not be undertaken without full consideration of the possibilities. (See Chapter Ten.)

Atelectasis may develop after anesthesia or following aspiration of gastric contents as a complication of tube feedings. Aspiration of gastric contents is more common in children than in adults. When patients are receiving tube feedings, care should be taken that the stomach is not over-distended and that the patient has adequate opportunity to cough, particularly when he is turned from side to side. Aspiration of gastric contents is apt to occur when a patient with a full stomach is turned on his abdomen.

COMPLICATIONS INVOLVING THE GASTROINTESTINAL TRACT

Acute dilatation of the stomach may occur at any time during the entire course of the burned patient. It is more common than is usually recognized. It may occur during the first week after injury and is not uncommon as a complication of tube feedings. It frequently accompanies septicemia. Acute distention of the stomach may develop during oxygen therapy if the oxygen is administered by a nasal catheter. In the elderly, particularly the kyphotic, aerophagia with respiratory exertion is a common cause of gastric dilatation.

The stomach may be enlarged because of simple gaseous distention or it may be acutely dilated with fluid. Acute dilatation of the stomach is characterized by regurgitation of fluid, upper abdominal distress, dyspnea, dehydration and, if untreated, circulatory collapse. The early symptoms are expectoration of small mouthfuls of fluid. The patient does not vomit but merely spits out the overflow. Anorexia and nausea occur but pain is rarely severe. A persistent hiccup may accompany eructation and regurgitation.

The exact mechanism of acute dilatation remains obscure. However, it is generally believed that dilatation is caused by reflex inhibition of the gastric motor mechanism. Gastric atony appears to be a part of the generalized ileus that develops under many different circumstances. In addition, patients with severe burns may be unable to control the epiglottis properly, and may thus swallow large amounts of air. This leads to gaseous distention and progresses to acute dilatation.

Unfortunately, gastric dilatation occurs in the burned patient often with little or no change in the contour of the abdominal wall because of the tight eschar over the abdomen. A change in the character of the respirations may be the only sign, and the index of suspicion should be high during the first postburn week.

The nasogastric tube aspirate often has the appearance of coffee grounds. This does not usually mean significant hemorrhage from a Curling's ulcer unless it is of large volume. More characteristically[5] the volume of fluid is small, though large amounts of air are present, and represents bleeding from congested capillaries in the gastric mucosa. One must be aware that acute hemorrhage from a Curling's ulcer can often follow such findings, however, and the patient must be watched very closely.

Paralytic ileus is a common complication of burns. In most burns of more than 45 per cent of the body surface, peristaltic activity is absent during the first few postburn days. For this reason, extensively burned patients should not receive food by mouth until there is evidence of good peristaltic activity. When peristalsis becomes audible, feeding may be started cautiously. In general, it is not safe to begin tube feeding during the first postburn week.

Paralytic ileus after burns often appears to be a nonspecific manifestation of severe injury. It may, however, be the only prodrome of Curling's ulcer. Usually the ileus persists only a short time and disappears as the patient's condition improves. Persistent paralytic ileus is commonly associated with septicemia, particularly that due to staphylococci, but the precise relationship, if any, is unknown.

Prolonged immobilization predisposes to the occurrence of fecal impactions. Too often the physician is so busy attending to the many urgent facets of burn care that he neglects routine management of the bowels. In seriously burned patients, it is advisable to do a rectal examination at the time the patient is under anesthesia for grafting or a dressing change. Generous amounts of presently available water-binding stool softeners effectively eliminate the problem of impactions of inspissated stool. However, the general debilitation of the patient may be of such a degree that weakness of abdominal muscles may prevent expulsion of even a soft stool. Frequent digital examinations must be done, and the use of a mild enema is often of great assistance.

Esophageal stricture, a rare complication, may follow prolonged use of an indwelling nasogastric tube for feeding purposes (Fig. 167). Such strictures are usually benign and respond to esophageal dilatation. They usually manifest themselves several weeks after the patient is completely healed.

The burned patient also may develop acute appendicitis or other

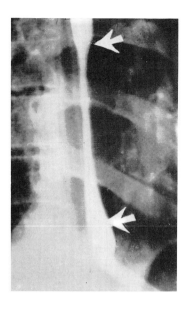

Figure 167. Roentgenogram of a patient who developed a stricture of the esophagus. The stricture, seen between the two arrows, developed after a rubber intragastric feeding tube had been in place for a period of 6 weeks. This is an unusual complication. The patient had a very extensive burn complicated by Curling's ulcer and septicemia. He required supportive nutritional therapy for a long period of time. The stricture was corrected by means of repeated dilatation.

intra-abdominal problems during the postburn period. It is imperative to observe closely the electrical burn for abdominal complications; they occur with greater frequency in such cases for reasons not known but are likely associated with vascular thrombosis initiated by the electric current. Necrosis of the colon is the most common lesion.

In burned patients who have lost great amounts of weight and who vomit frequently, obstruction of the third portion of the duodenum should be suspected. This is likely a long standing problem, as the patients give a history of early childhood vomiting, and an upper gastrointestinal series at this time reveals a superior mesenteric artery syndrome with almost complete duodenal occlusion. Duodenojejunostomy is the treatment of choice.

Curling's Ulcer

In 1842, Curling reported 12 cases of gastrointestinal ulcerations complicating thermal burns. There are numerous theories as to the cause of this type of ulceration. Factual data are scarce and theoretical considerations are controversial. Although it has been demonstrated that there is an increase in the blood histamine level in burned animals, there is no evidence that elevated levels play any part in the formation of Curling's ulcer. Some investigators have reported an increase in gastric secretion and acidity following burns in a small series of dogs. Studies in humans, however, fail to reveal any consistent increase in uropepsin excretion or 24-hour gastric acid secretion, and the presence of numerous bacteria in the bed of the ulcer crater is evidence against hyperacidity as a major factor. Recent studies by O'Neill reveal that the absolute quantity of gastric mucus formed is decreased, but the composition is normal.

Two hundred and twenty-five cases of Curling's ulcer (about two-thirds of the total recorded in the literature) have been reported from the Surgical Research Unit at Brooke Army Medical Center and form the basis for the most comprehensive understanding now available (Table 29). The incidence of gastrointestinal ulcer in burned patients admitted to the Surgical Research Unit during the 13-year period 1953–1966 was 13.3 per cent. The autopsy incidence of acute ulceration following burns is 65 per cent when examination is not delayed until autolysis of the gastro-intestinal mucosa has occurred. However, as autopsies are now accomplished within 2 to 4 hours of death, the smaller lesions are recognized and the true over-all incidence approaches 25 per cent.

Curling's ulcer may develop in a patient with any size burn, having occurred in the Surgical Research Unit series in patients with burns as small as 10 per cent and as large as 93 per cent. Most cases are concentrated in those with a burn index of 30 to 65. Of the 225 cases, there were only 44 survivors.

It is conceivable that a larger number of patients with Curling's ulcer survive. This is particularly apparent when it is noted that the Surgical Research Unit series contains a 40 per cent incidence of autopsy cases of Curling's ulcer with no symptoms other than abdominal distention or discomfort. It is difficult to diagnose the lesion unless some type of catastrophe, such as massive bleeding, occurs. Frequently there are no signs or symptoms of ulcer formation. The patients may complain of some abdominal discomfort and, if a gastric tube is in place, small amounts of blood may be seen. The first sign is usually related to acute hemorrhage

Table 29.   CURLING'S ULCER (SURGICAL RESEARCH UNIT, 1953–1966)

Total cases		225
Died	155	
Died of sepsis	109	
Survived	44	
Site		
Stomach		86
Multiple	68	
Duodenum		63
Multiple	18	
Stomach and duodenum		25
Other areas		8
Treatment		
Active nonsurgical		56
Rebled	21	
Stopped bleeding	35	
Surgical		24
Died	14	
Survived	10	

or perforation. Not infrequently ulcerations develop and are completely unrecognized until discovered as an incidental finding at autopsy. Ulcers may develop as early as the first or second postburn day, but the usual time for manifestation of hemorrhage is near the end of the first week. Some occur as late as 9 weeks post burn.

A drop in hematocrit in the early postburn period presents a difficult problem in differential diagnosis to the attending surgeon. Should significant hematemesis or melena accompany the drop in red blood cell mass, active bleeding is obviously occurring. However, at the time of initial hematocrit drop no gross evidence of bleeding may be present, and it often coincides with the period of diuresis and mobilization of edema fluid which is associated with hemodilution. The latter can be sudden and of significant magnitude. The hemodilution does not require blood replacement but the hemorrhage does. Use of venous pressure response to infusion is of great aid in clarifying this situation. Pulse rate is of no value, as tachycardia is present in all the patients.

The ulcer was most frequently located in the duodenum in the previous reports, but the early autopsy studies now completed show the gastric location as the most common. The ulcers may be multiple. Severe hemorrhage is usually caused by large single ulcers on the posterior wall of the first part of the duodenum or the eroding of a large gastric vessel.

Since the ulcerations occur in very extensively burned patients, the cause of death is usually something other than a complication of the ulcer. In some instances, however, severe hemorrhage or perforation with peritonitis is the primary cause of death.

Usually only the more severely burned patients (greater than 35 per cent of the body surface) and those with burns complicated by other injuries or systemic infection develop ulcers which are recognized clinically. All patients with major burns must be carefully questioned about abdominal complaints if gastrointestinal ulceration is to be diagnosed. Minor complaints of epigastric pain are frequently overlooked while caring for the more obvious needs of a severely burned patient.

Since many extensively burned patients may develop Curling's ulcer, prophylactic treatment of all patients in this category has been recommended. However, antacids and anticholinergic drugs have not been found to be of any significant benefit clinically. In fact, massive hemorrhage has occurred while patients were on heavy therapy with both medications. If hemorrhage occurs the patient should be treated energetically with blood. The indications for operation should be the same as for any bleeding duodenal ulcer. Experience has shown that severely burned patients withstand gastrectomy well followed by per primam healing of anastomoses. Poor or delayed healing of the abdominal wall is not unusual, however. Although death may ensue from other causes, surgery is well tolerated.

When possible, the ulcer should be removed or excluded from the alimentary continuity, as continued progressive ulceration may occur. The surgical experience has not been extensive in any clinic, but results to date indicate vagotomy and hemigastrectomy as the procedure of choice. Vagotomy with pyloroplasty has been disastrous and is to be avoided.

Of the 225 cases reported from the Surgical Research Unit, 24 required surgical intervention; there were 10 survivors. Conservative non-surgical management is to be attempted originally, but significant uncontrolled hemorrhage responds only to surgery. Of those patients having a single significant hemorrhage, one-third rebled if not operated upon, and if the individual bled twice, he had a 50 per cent chance of bleeding again. While only 10 of 24 survived after surgery, nine of the remaining tolerated the surgery well and were being maintained on oral alimentation at the time of death from 3 to 54 days postoperatively from a variety of causes. Three of the deaths were the result of inadequate surgery – pyloroplasty and vagotomy. One of the three perforated through the pyloroplasty, and two exsanguinated from the original ulcer site.

COMPLICATIONS INVOLVING THE GENITOURINARY TRACT

The most common complication referable to the genitourinary tract in burns is cystitis. A certain degree of cystitis always follows the routine use of the indwelling catheter. Frequent irrigations can eradicate or greatly minimize this problem. Rarely is it necessary to have a catheter in the bladder for a prolonged period of time to prevent soiling of the burn wound, as urine has no deleterious effect on an open wound. Dressings should be changed frequently or protected from repeated soiling. The catheter should be removed as soon as practicable. Careful attention should be paid to frequent irrigation of the catheter and change of catheters every 5 days. (See Chapter Twelve.)

After prolonged use of indwelling catheters in males, a periurethral abscess may form. This follows irritation by the catheter and contamination of the urethra by bacteria from the burn wound. Such abscesses require drainage. The trauma of a catheter may soften the urethral wall by inflammation leading to the formation of a urethral diverticulum. Acute epididymitis and orchitis sometimes occur. Urethral stricture may follow prolonged use of the catheter with constant inflammation of the urethra. This can usually be prevented by proper care of the catheter and early removal. Presently available plastic collection devices for external application have completely eliminated the need for catheters in male patients.

Urinary calculi are not uncommon complications. They may be present in the renal pelvis or in the bladder. Bladder calculi are more frequent than renal calculi. Recumbent posture made necessary by prolonged illness causes stasis in the urinary tract and leads to stone formation. Infection in the urinary tract adds to the stasis factor. Prolonged bed rest is frequently followed by osteoporosis and withdrawal of calcium from the bony skeleton. In addition, dietary imbalances and increased calcium excretion in the urine are factors favoring stone formation.

THROMBOEMBOLIC COMPLICATIONS

Deep venous thrombosis and gross pulmonary embolism are not common complications of burn injury. This is rather surprising in view of the predisposing factors that are present in a burn, such as a severe injury, infection and immobilization.

Most of the thromboembolic complications are related to therapy. Superficial thrombophlebitis is common following prolonged intravenous therapy and frequently is the site of a septic focus, most likely due to staphylococci. Other organisms also are involved, though less frequently. This complication can be prevented if the polyethylene tubing is left in place for only 2 or 3 days. However, in extensively burned patients, this intravenous lifeline may be required for longer periods of time. Thrombotic complications are seen with much less frequency in the upper extremities than in the lower. Superficial peripheral veins should be utilized whenever possible so that complications of prolonged intravenous therapy can be readily detected and treatment instituted. If the deep femoral vein is used, thrombosis is recognized only after it is well established and often beyond correction. Septic phlebitis of superficial veins is most often seen in the long saphenous vein. It can be rapidly fatal. The only effective

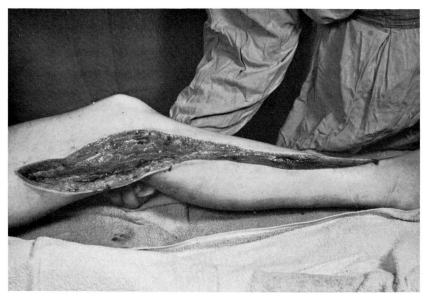

Figure 168. Septic or purulent thrombophlebitis is often seen in superficial veins and can be rapidly fatal. It does not usually respond to antibiotic therapy. The only effective treatment is radical excision. The wound is closed secondarily in 5 to 7 days.

therapy is excision of the vein to well above the area of involvement (Fig. 168).

Sometimes it becomes necessary to insert a segment of polyethylene tubing through the femoral vein into the vena cava. If this tubing is left in place more than 5 days, thrombi may form in the iliac veins and the vena cava. Occasionally fragments of thrombi in these large veins break off and cause pulmonary infarction. In some instances, thrombi in the iliac veins become infected, and septic thrombophlebitis may occur. The only really effective therapy is thrombectomy, but ligation may be accomplished with benefit if the more major procedure cannot be tolerated by the patient.

CONTRACTURES

The most common complication interfering with musculoskeletal function in the burned patient is contracture. Contractures may occur around any joint but are most common in the neck and axilla and about the elbows. Contracture occurrence can be minimized by proper positioning of the affected parts and early skin coverage. In some areas contractures are almost inevitable, but the severity of deformity may be considerably lessened by judicious early therapy. Full-thickness burns of the

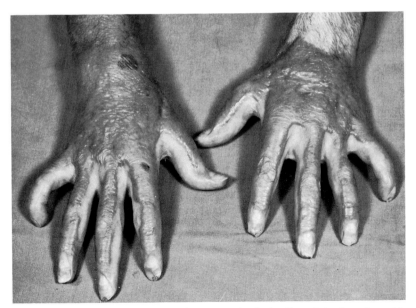

Figure 169. Hypertrophic scarring is common in the healing of the deep dermal burn. In time (12 to 18 months) maturation of scar tissue results in a soft, pliable, flattened scar. Because of functional impairment, surgical correction may be required prior to scar maturation but best results are obtained after maturation.

hands are frequently complicated by contractures. Deep dermal burns may be followed by hypertrophic scars (Fig. 169). Most third-degree burns in the axilla and in the anterior portion of the neck are followed by contracture. Such complications are best managed by reconstructive plastic procedures which are performed months after initial skin coverage has been achieved. In some instances, however, it is not possible to wait for scar maturation, as functional impairment may dictate early correction with the likelihood of having to repeat the procedure. Such is the case particularly in ectropion, everted lower lip and some major joints.

Ectropion

Contracture of the eyelids leads to ectropion formation due to eversion of the lid (Fig. 170). As the skin of the lid contracts it slides over the underlying tarsal plate drawing the ciliary margin and palpebral conjunctiva with it. Thus, eversion of the ciliary border occurs first and not until very late does eversion of the tarsal plates occur. Since the skin of the upper lid is normally more redundant than the lower, significant ectropion is less common there. When it does occur, it is more often in the lateral third.

Though not involving the lids directly, burns of the face, especially the malar area, often are associated with an ectropion of the lower lid. This is due to tightening of the skin of the face and drawing down of the adjacent lid. If an ectropion develops and is not corrected, the cornea

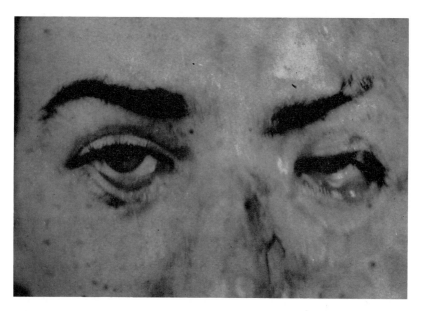

Figure 170. Bilateral ectropion. This is a common complication of burns of the eyelid. It can be lessened by tarsorrhaphy and early grafting. Once ectropion develops, the contracture is released with overcorrection of the lid and a split-thickness skin graft is applied.

dries and becomes ulcerated and infected. Panophthalmitis may occur with loss of the eye. Corneal ulcers can be prevented by proper eye care, tarsorrhaphy and early grafting. (See Chapter Ten.)

MISCELLANEOUS COMPLICATIONS

Chondritis

Of unknown etiology and distressing frequency in facial burns is chondritis of the ears. The painful, tender, swollen ear standing out from the head demands attention. Incision and removal of the necrotic cartilage is the only treatment to date. (See Chapter Ten.)

Infection of Donor Sites

One of the most frequent and troublesome complications in burns is infection of the donor sites with conversion of the area to granulating surfaces. Careful attention must be paid to the donor sites because infection may destroy the remaining viable epithelium. Occasionally when the donor site is taken too deeply, the area fails to heal, and a granulating surface

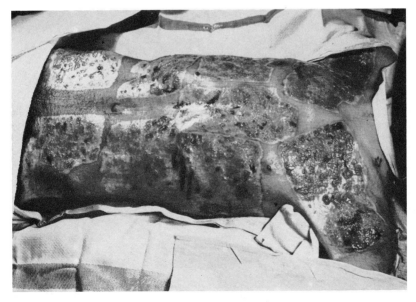

Figure 171. Photograph of the body of a patient whose donor sites became converted to granulating surfaces following infection. Several drums of skin had been removed from the body of the patient in an overseas hospital. The patient was transferred before the donor sites had healed. During transportation the areas became infected and converted to granulating surfaces. Prolonged transportation of patients with fresh donor sites is contraindicated. These areas were grafted, and the patient recovered.

results. These areas must then be grafted. Less infection occurs when donor sites are exposed than when dressings are applied. (See Chapter Eight.) Occasionally patients are seen whose burned surfaces are practically healed but whose donor sites have been converted to granulating wounds (Fig. 171).

Constricting Eschars

One of the most disastrous and tragically underestimated complications of thermal injury is the constricting effect of a circumferential eschar of the chest or extremities. In the arms and legs, the edema forming rapidly beneath the unyielding eschar produces pressure sufficient to occlude first the venous circulation and then the arterial, resulting in ischemic necrosis. Even unburned portions of extremities distal to the eschar may be lost in such a fashion (Fig. 172).

Escharotomy. Circulatory embarrassment can be recognized by early congestion with poor capillary flow in nail beds. Later, pallor and pain are prominent. Treatment is simple and effective—merely incise the eschar.

Decubitus Ulcers

In some extensively burned patients it is most difficult to prevent the development of decubitus ulcers. These may occur in the sacral regions,

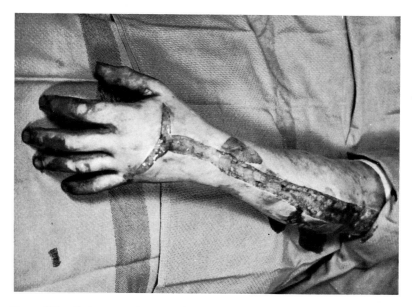

Figure 172. Escharotomy is accomplished without anesthesia, as the wound is essentially anesthetic. Practically no bleeding occurs and the wound spontaneously spreads widely as soon as the eschar and subcutaneous fascia are divided. It is not necessary to incise muscle fascia. As soon as any hint of circulatory embarrassment appears, the eschar must be split. Delay is often disastrous.

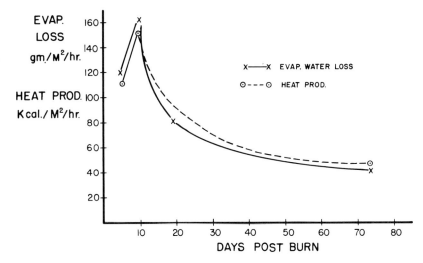

Figure 173.   Evaporative water loss reaches its peak at about 10 days post burn and gradually diminishes with the aid of wound closure. Vapor loss is greatest through the areas of third-degree burn but is still of great significance in second-degree areas, being 50 to 76 per cent of the rate through third-degree areas. (From J. A. Moncrief: Management of burns. *Monogr. Surg. Sci.* **3**:175, 1966.)

over the anterior superior iliac spine, on the posterior aspect of the head, and on the back of the heel. In most instances the decubitus ulcer can be prevented by proper positioning of the patient, particularly with the aid of the circular electric bed. Pressure points must be observed frequently and every effort made to prevent the breakdown of skin in these areas. While many devices such as air mattresses, water flotation beds and silicone pads have been developed to prevent this, it still occurs in the long term debilitating patient.

Evaporative Water Loss

The burned patient's metabolic response (Chapter Thirteen) is determined to a great extent by his loss of water through the burned area. The dry, exposed second- and third-degree burned skin has essentially lost its ability to function as an effective barrier to the evaporation of water. Most individuals treated by the exposure method will lose about 150 ml. of water per M². per hour (Fig. 173). The very large burns, particularly in children, may lose almost twice this amount. Unless this is replaced, severe hypernatremia may insidiously result and such dehydration significantly contributes to a fatal outcome. Since the severe outpouring of nitrogen produces an osmotic diuresis, urine volume remains respectable until very late and cannot be used as an index of hydration.

REFERENCES

Arturson, G., and Ponten, B.: Burns: their causes, mortality and preventability. *Acta chir. scandinav.* **124**:483, 1962.

Best, R. R., Coe, J. D., and McMurtrey, G. B.: Effect of soaps containing hexachlorophene on wounds and burned surfaces. *A.M.A. Arch. Surg.* **62**:895, 1951.

Birke, G., Liljedahl, S.-O., and Linderholm, H.: Studies on burns. V. Clinical and pathophysiological aspects on circulation and respiration. *Acta chir. scandinav.* **116**:370, 1958.

Epstein, B. S., Rose, L. R. Teplitz, C., and Moncrief, J. A.: Experiences with low tracheostomy in the burn patient. *J.A.M.A.* **183**:966, 1963.

Griswold, M. L., Jr.: Extra-articular bone formation as a burn complication. *Plast. & Reconstruct. Surg.* **32**:544, 1963.

Harrison, H. N., Moncrief, J. A., Duckett, J. W., Jr., and Mason, A. D., Jr.: The relationship between energy metabolism and water loss from vaporization in severely burned patients. *Surgery* **56**:203, 1964.

Moncrief, J. A.: Complications of burns. *Ann. Surg.* **147**:443, 1958.

Moncrief, J. A., and Mason, A. D., Jr.: Evaporative water loss in the burned patient. *J. Trauma* **4**:180, 1964.

Moncrief, J. A., Switzer, W. E., and Teplitz, C.: Curling's ulcer. *J. Trauma* **4**:481, 1964.

Taylor, F. W., and Gumbert, J. L.: Cause of death from burns: role of respiratory damage. *Ann. Surg.* **161**:497, 1965.

Teplitz, C., Epstein, B. S., Rose, L. R., and Moncrief, J. A.: Necrotizing tracheitis induced by tracheostomy tube. *A.M.A. Arch. Path.* **77**:14, 1964.

Teplitz, C., Epstein, B. S., Rose, L. R., Switzer, W. E., and Moncrief, J. A.: Pathology of low tracheostomy in children. *Am. J. Clin. Path.* **42**:58, 1964.

Wilson, J. S., and Moncrief, J. A.: Vapor pressure of normal and burned skin. *Ann. Surg.* **162**:130, 1965.

Chapter
Sixteen

MUSCULOSKELETAL CHANGES SECONDARY TO BURNS

by E. Burke Evans, M.D.

In most thermal burns the skin alone is affected by the initial trauma. Occasionally, muscles or tendons are exposed and are actually altered by the heat. Rarely, bone is likewise exposed. As a rule, however, the alterations of the musculoskeletal system that are observed in the severely burned occur after the acute injury and are not a direct result of the thermal insult.

Histologic examination of muscle, tendon, bone, cartilage and synovial membrane from autopsy and amputation specimens of extremities with severe or even circumferential third-degree burns shows little or no alteration of these structures except for occasional evidence of chronic inflammation. Even this finding cannot be ascribed to the acute burn. Thus the significant musculoskeletal alterations observed in thermal burns are largely sequential in nature.

In 1959 the bone and joint changes following burns were classified according to their roentgenographic appearance. In 1962 this classification was restated and expanded. Other reports have dealt with skeletal alterations descriptively or in general. The following classification includes all alterations of the musculoskeletal system that may occur as a result of severe burns.

CLASSIFICATION OF MUSCULOSKELETAL CHANGES SECONDARY TO BURNS

ALTERATIONS LIMITED TO BONE
  Osteoporosis
  Periosteal new bone formation
  Irregular ossification
  Diaphyseal exostoses

Acromutilation of fingers
Pathologic fractures
Osteomyelitis
Necrosis and tangential sequestration
Epiphyseal arrest

ALTERATIONS INVOLVING PERICAPSULAR STRUCTURES
Pericapsular calcification
Heterotopic para-articular ossification
Osteophytes

ALTERATIONS INVOLVING THE JOINT PROPER
Septic arthritis
Spontaneous dissolution
Ankylosis
Dislocation

ALTERATIONS SECONDARY TO SOFT TISSUE CONTRACTURE
Muscle shortening
Malposition of joints
Scoliosis

ABNORMALITIES OF GROWTH

NONVIABILITY OF EXTREMITY LEADING TO AMPUTATION

Certain of the listed changes can be prevented or reduced in severity. Others can be corrected. It is the awareness and recognition of the changes over which there is a degree of control that are important in the prevention and correction of deformity and in long term rehabilitation of burned patients.

PHYSICAL THERAPY

Physical therapy should begin on the day of the burn or very soon thereafter. Even if the general state of the patient precludes any active measures, there is distinct value in having as part of the burn team a therapist who, from the outset, is aware of the extent of the burn and of the general prognosis.

One of the most formidable obstructions facing the physician and the therapist is the patient's fear of pain or fear of moving a burned extremity because of anticipation of pain. If a patient learns early that he can move his limbs without causing extreme discomfort, he is better able to cooperate with the therapist. After even a few days or a week of absolute immobility following acute trauma, the severely burned patient will be extremely fearful of and resistant to any passive or active motion.

The goals of the therapist are relatively simple. They are (1) prevention of contracture, (2) maintenance of joint motion and (3) maintenance of muscle tone. These goals are accomplished through the recognized measures of positioning and of active, passive, resistive and isometric exercise.

Positioning

In positioning of the acutely burned patient, special attention is given to all major joints, namely, ankles, knees, hips, shoulders, elbows, wrists and hands.

Ankles are supported at 90 degrees of dorsiflexion. Knees are straight but not hyperextended. Hips are in neutral rotation and symmetrically abducted to 10 to 15 degrees (Fig. 174A). Shoulders are abducted at least 60 degrees and are alternately externally and internally rotated; elbows are flexed no more than 30 to 40 degrees; wrists are supported in slight extension. At the metacarpophalangeal joints, fingers are allowed to drop

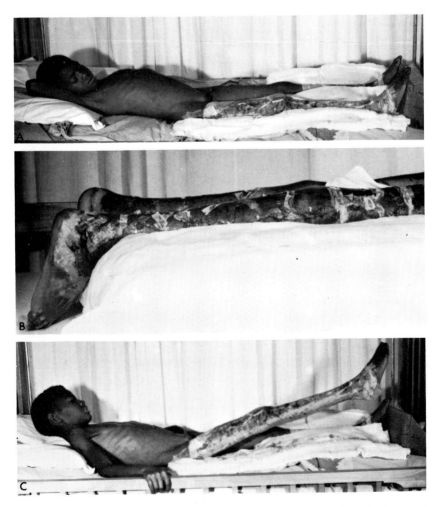

Figure 174. *A*, Positioning of lower extremities showing symmetric abduction of hips and use of footboard. *B*, When the patient is treated prone, a short mattress placed on top of a regular mattress allows the feet to fall into dorsiflexion. *C*, Active exercise of lower extremity with total circumferential third-degree burn. Hip, knee and ankle motion were retained throughout the course of burn treatment.

into flexion, and the thumb into an abducted and slightly flexed position. In burns of the neck, the head is positioned so that there is slight extension of the neck but no more than that amount which will allow the patient to close his mouth easily.

Ankle. Ankle equinus can be prevented by proper posterior splinting when the distribution of burn permits it or by the use of footboards when the patient is recumbent (Fig. 174A). In all lower extremity dressing and wrapping, the ankle should be positioned at 90 degrees or neutral. When a patient is to be treated in the prone position, a short mattress will allow the feet to project over the end and to fall into dorsiflexion (Fig. 174B).

Hip. As in any painful condition of the lower extremity, it is the tendency of the burned patient to bring the thigh into flexion, adduction and internal rotation. In the period before a contracture has developed, it is reasonably simple to maintain the hip in abduction and extension. Once the position of adduction, flexion and internal rotation has become established, particularly in the severely burned patient, there is increasing tendency for this position to become exaggerated and for the head of the femur actually to become laterally displaced in the acetabulum. From this position dislocation may easily occur (Fig. 188). Skeletal traction is a secure means of correcting hip and knee deformity. (See Skeletal Suspension, p. 358.)

Shoulder. When the axilla has been burned, the shoulder is placed

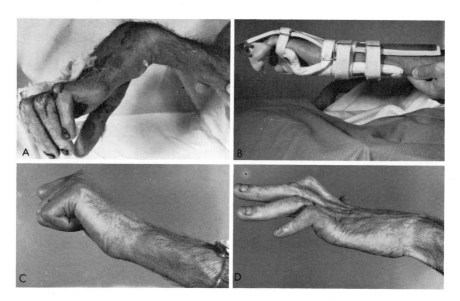

Figure 175. *A,* The typical deformity in an adult hand which was not severely burned. The fifth digit and the second digit (under gauze) show a greater degree of metacarpophalangeal extension and correspondingly more flexion at the proximal interphalangeal joints than do the third and fourth digits. *B,* The malleable aluminum corrective splint designed for use before and after complete skin coverage. *C,* and *D,* The final result 5 years after acute burn. Note the persisting greater deformity of the second and fifth digits.

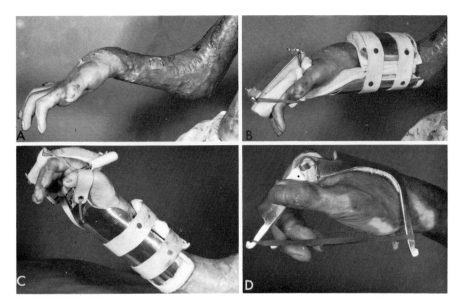

Figure 176. *A,* The typical hand deformity in a 10-year-old girl with 18 per cent third-degree burn 3 months after acute burn. *B,* Corrective splinting was begun while there were still open granulating areas. The specially designed splint was first applied with the palm support and the dorsal plate flat. Note the thick foam rubber padding. *C,* As correction proceeded, the palm support was bent to support the wrist in dorsiflexion, the dorsal plate was curved to maintain flexion at the metacarpophalangeal joint and a thumb strap was added. *D,* This final dynamic splint was used to increase functional range. Dorsal incisional release and split skin graft had been performed to correct the extension-adduction deformity of the thumb. Total time for correction to this stage was 3 years.

in 60 degrees of abduction. The position of comfort for the patient is that with the shoulder adducted and internally rotated. Static abduction of the shoulder is uncomfortable for a healthy person, and it is certainly poorly tolerated by those who are burned. Once an axillary contracture has become established, there is little that can be done beyond maintaining as much abduction as possible through the use of active contraction of the shoulder abductors. It is especially important throughout all phases of treatment to maintain abductor muscle power. Skeletal traction through radius or olecranon provides a means of prevention of contracture should ordinary positioning fail and a means of partial correction once a contracture is established.

Hand. The typical deformity in the neglected burned hand is one of flexion at the wrist, extension at the metacarpophalangeal joints, flexion at the proximal interphalangeal joints and flexion or extension of the distal interphalangeal joints (Figs. 175A and 176A). The thumb is adducted and extended, and there is loss of web space. The transverse palmar arch is flattened. It is more or less the clawhand deformity or that of the intrinsic minus hand. The deformity occurs early in the postburn period if the wrist is allowed to drop slightly into flexion. This is probably the position of greatest comfort for the acutely traumatized hand. Following the slight drop of the wrist, because of the normal reciprocal tenodesing effect, the fingers will be drawn naturally into extension at the metacarpophalangeal joints, just as they would fall into flexion if the wrist were dorsiflexed. The little finger and the index finger, because of their relative functional freedom from the rest of the hand, will tend to go into a greater degree of extension than the other fingers; thus, the transverse arch is lost. All

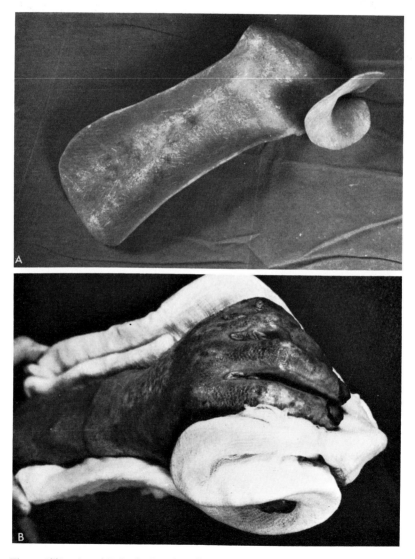

Figure 177.   *A,* and *B,* In the Brooke splint shown here the wrist is supported at about 30 degrees of dorsiflexion, the metacarpophalangeal joints are flexed less than 90 degrees and the fingers curve gently. The thumb assumes a position which is natural with this degree of wrist extension.

of the features of the deformity become exaggerated if the hand rests unsupported on the flat surface of the bed.

The deformity is often made worse by the destruction of the long extensor tendon over the proximal interphalangeal joint. In the later stages, burn scar or graft contracture accentuates the deformity. Hand burns are almost always of the dorsum, and although the deformity would seem, initially at least, to be positionally imposed, contracture of dorsal skin is also a major factor.

The hand should be positioned, as much exposed as possible, in a splint which will accomplish the following: (1) hold the wrist straight or in a few degrees of extension; (2) allow the fingers to drop into as much as 90 degrees of flexion at the metacarpophalangeal joints and remain slightly apart, which will allow the interphalangeal joints to remain straight or to fall into very slight degrees of flexion; (3) support the thumb in fairly wide abduction and in a few degrees of flexion but not bring the thumb into opposition. Splints of the type used at Brooke General Hospital, the University of Michigan and currently at the University of Texas Medical Branch will support the hand properly (Figs. 177, 178 and 179). The Brooke splint allows interphalangeal flexion, whereas the Michigan splint keeps the fingers straight. The UTMB splint combines features of the two and incorporates Velcro straps.

Pressure dressings can be applied in such a way as to hold the position described. Such dressings are often not necessary if attention is paid to elevation of the hand and if the patient is allowed to move the fingers. A pressure dressing can be harmful if it is left in place over a period of several days because it inhibits joint motion. Furthermore, it is quite difficult to maintain the hand in good position within a soft dressing unless the dressing incorporates a supporting splint (Fig. 180). Miller and co-workers have shown a simple polyester resin splint for maintaining what they call the modified position for burn dressing.

Strict immobilization is not essential to the recovery of the severely traumatized hand; elevation, immobilization and pressure are by no means better than elevation and motion for mobilizing fluid and for reducing edema.

Exercise

The therapist begins by having the patient move those parts which are free of burn. The patient must be made aware of the extent to which these parts can be moved without disturbing the burned areas (Fig. 174C). The therapist then determines how much active motion is possible in the burned extremities and which joints are bridged by unburned skin. If the patient refuses to move independently, the therapist begins passive assistance. If an extremity is so severely burned that there is no area which will allow support, the therapist looks for a point which will take resistance and begins to teach the patient how to contract his muscles without moving the part.

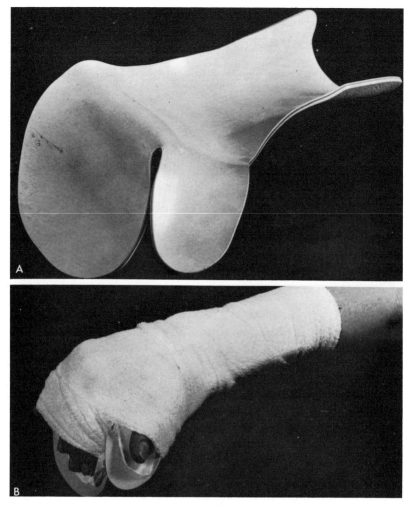

Figure 178. *A,* and *B,* In the Michigan splint the wrist is almost straight, the meta-carpophalangeal joints are flexed almost 90 degrees, and the fingers are straight.

By the use of points of resistance and by repeated instructions, even small children can be taught the use of isometric contraction. Thus, when a part may not be moved, muscle setting can still be accomplished.

Joint motion. A slight degree of joint motion is better than no motion. If only a few degrees of motion are tolerated at a given joint because of pain, crust or restriction of adjacent new grafts, this joint is taken regularly through this permitted range. Because of skin restriction, passive motion may not exceed that which the patient could obtain with active motion. Motion is much better tolerated if extremities are in moist dressings or if they are liquid supported. A Hubbard tank may be used as soon as the patient's general state will allow it. Drying or crusting should be assiduously avoided. Skeletal suspension frees an extremity of bed contact and makes joint motion less painful and thus easier for the patient.

Occasionally tendons are exposed by the burn. These structures require coverage with a moist dressing and early skin coverage, or as often as not they will not survive. As long as the tendons are intact, however, they will continue to move the part to which they are attached; there probably is nothing to be gained by restricting or forbidding motion because of the exposure. Tendons most often exposed are those about the wrist and ankle and on the dorsum of the foot.

The hand merits special attention from the physical therapist. On the day of the burn or as soon thereafter as possible, the therapist begins a hand program by asking the patient to identify all of his fingers and to move each separately. If the hand is in a pressure dressing, the patient should be aware of the position and should be asked to hold the wrist in

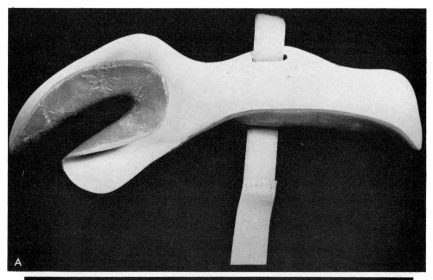

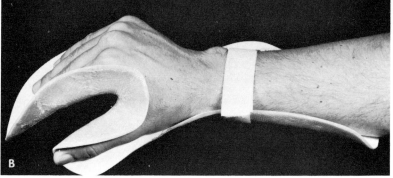

Figure 179. *A,* and *B,* In the UTMB splint the wrist is in dorsiflexion and the metacarpophalangeal joints are flexed approximately 90 degrees.

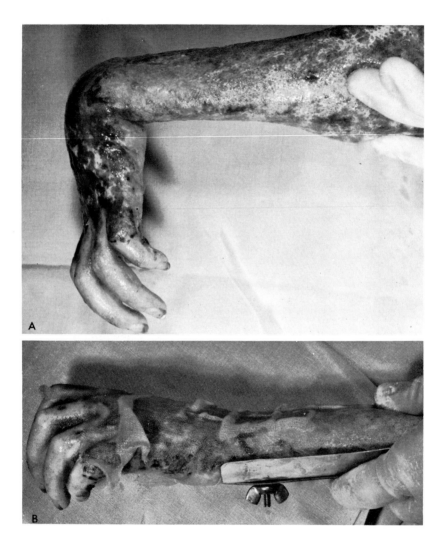

Figure 180. *A*, With the wrist unsupported, this hand showed the typical deformity. *B*, Supporting the wrist with a simple adjustable aluminum spoon splint corrected much of the deformity. The splint was incorporated in a pressure dressing.

extension and the fingers in flexion at the metacarpophalangeal joints. The patient should be taught how to effect isometric contractions of the flexors and extensors, and how to move his fingers slightly without taking the joints through measurable excursion. This trick is particularly useful when the hand is being grafted.

If the patient is unable to cooperate with active motion, the therapist must take the fingers through full allowable passive range at least once a day. Even in the most severe burns, attempts at finger motion should never be stopped.

If contractural deformity is already established, physical therapeutic measures are used to maintain the existing range of motion and to prevent further contracture. Passive periodic stretching of scar tissue is harmful and is scrupulously avoided, but stretching is used when the contracture is muscular. When contracture seems inevitable, it is practical occasionally to construct special splints which can be, with proper padding, applied even in the period preceding full skin coverage (Figs. 175B and 176B,C). These splints, constructed of malleable aluminum and styled to the individual need, may be used to prevent further contracture and actually to achieve a degree of correction. Dynamic splinting is occasionally helpful (Fig. 176D).

Muscle tone. Muscle atrophy progresses relentlessly in the catabolic phase following a severe burn; although this cannot be prevented, a degree of muscle tone can be retained. In the five patients studied by Reiss and his co-workers, the period of negative nitrogen balance varied from 15 to 28 days following the acute burn. If the early negative nitrogen balance was considered as a reflection of the whole tissue catabolism, the patients lost between 8.2 kg. and 11.7 kg. of lean body tissue during the catabolic phase. In this catabolic phase, which in most patients roughly corresponds to that period preceding skin coverage or wound closure or the formation of healthy granulating surfaces, no measures, dietary or otherwise, will bring the patient into nitrogen equilibrium. The nitrogen loss through exudate, but principally through the urine, far exceeds any realistic dietary intake.

The therapist, thus, cannot have as a goal the retention of muscle bulk. It is nevertheless imperative, throughout the catabolic phase, that every effort be made to retain muscle tone and muscle awareness. The patient should contract daily all of the muscles in the involved parts and use actively all uninvolved parts. In this circumstance isometric or resistive exercise is particularly useful. Once the catabolic phase is passed and the patient is in nitrogen equilibrium or positive balance, weight gain and the restoration of muscle bulk are usually rapidly progressive.

Grafting and exercise. When split skin grafts are applied to an extremity, motion is restricted. Motion need not be prohibited, however, if grafts are placed so as not to bridge a joint. Thus, grafts placed on a forearm should not prevent supervised motion in the wrist, hand or elbow; neither should grafts placed on the back of the hand preclude slight motion at the wrist. When the graft bridges or closely approximates a joint, however, there is imposed a 5-day period during which no active or passive motion of that joint can be allowed. In such a period of immobility, isometric contraction of the muscles in the restricted area can be of great value in retaining function of that part.

Stretching exercises. Stretching has very limited use in a physical therapy program for burns in any stage. It is to be avoided when there are active granulations or when there is red and indurated scar tissue overlying the joint. Stretching of a burn scar results in further damage and probably increases the amount of scarring. Once the scar is mature and soft, stretching of persistent muscle contracture may be permitted. By the time the burn scar has softened sufficiently, however, the patient has often regained full range of motion of the joint. When muscle contractures affect joints that are not involved in the burn, stretching of the muscles through these joints is permissible.

Exercise and osteoporosis. It is tempting to assume that the routine programmed exercise of severely burned patients impedes skeletal demineralization. In practice, this assumption cannot be supported. Immobility is only one of the causes of bony atrophy in severe burns, and considered alongside protein deficit and hyperadrenalism, it could easily be the least important. It remains, however, as the one factor which can be to some extent controlled from the outset; it is safe to assume that exercise affects favorably the degree of local atrophy in burned extremities, whereas its effect on generalized demineralization is probably negligible.

SKELETAL SUSPENSION

Skeletal suspension is a useful and realistic adjunct to burn treatment. When extremities are burned circumferentially, suspension by means of Steinmann pins facilitates debridement and grafting. These pins may be inserted directly through the burned area. The distal femur and tibia, the calcaneus, the metatarsals, the metacarpals, the olecranon and the distal radius have been used for this purpose.

Skeletal traction cannot be totally recommended. Some surgeons will not use it because they have a profound fear of bone infection caused by the transport of organisms from contaminated skin. This complication can be avoided if the pin sites are kept open and free of crust. It is usually an advantage to use threaded pins.

There is some hazard, however, with the placement of pins. The lower extremity should not be suspended by a single pin placed either in the distal tibia or in the calcaneus because of the tendency of the knee to fall into hyperextension. Such a position could lead to the double encumbrance of knee extension contracture and peroneal palsy. If the lower extremity is to be suspended, it should be by means of a pin through the distal femur or proximal tibia and the distal tibia, calcaneus or metatarsals. With this type of suspension, the patient is comfortable and retains free motion of ankle and knee (Figs. 181A, B and 182B).

The upper extremity may be suspended through the second and third metacarpals, through the radius or through the olecranon. The metacarpal pin is best inserted diagonally (Figs. 183 and 184). If this type of suspension is used, the wrist will be held at 180 degrees or in slight extension. If radial suspension is used, the hand must be extrinsically supported. The radial pin should be inserted at least 1 inch proximal to the epiphysis. It is frequently desirable to utilize a second pin through the olecranon to allow flexion at the elbow. This second pin facilitates motion of both the elbow and the shoulder while the extremity is suspended. If the suspen-

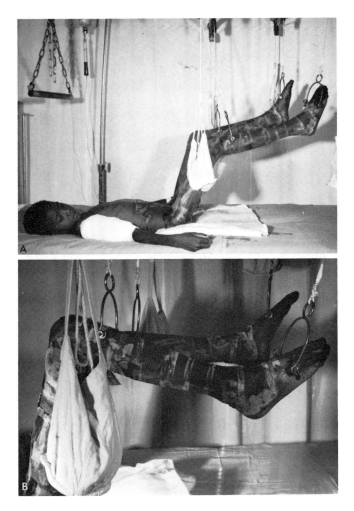

Figure 181. *A*, and *B*, Skeletal suspension through tibiae and metatarsals used to facilitate circumferential split skin grafting of legs. The patient moved freely and painlessly. The pins were removed as soon as the grafts had taken. (Same patient as in Fig. 174.)

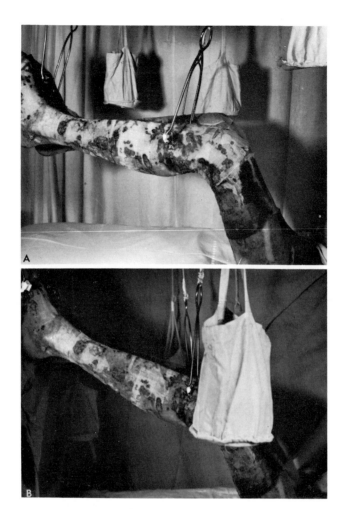

Figure 182. *A*, and *B*, Skeletal suspension of circumferentially burned lower extremities used to facilitate debridement. The patient, a 22-year-old man, exercised his extremities freely and painlessly.

sion pin for the hand is inserted through any part of the extensor mechanism of the third digit, it will restrict motion of all four fingers.

It is occasionally useful to employ skeletal traction in the severely burned lower extremity for the correction of knee and hip flexion contractures. In such a situation the pins are inserted as for suspension, and the Russell or split-Russell type of traction is applied.

In small children, if feet and ankles are free of burn, hip and knee flexion can be corrected by the use of shoe traction; or shoes may be used for simple suspension (Fig. 185). This type of suspension may not be tolerated for more than a few days at a time because of heel pressure, but this short period is often sufficient to correct a contracture or to allow a graft to take.

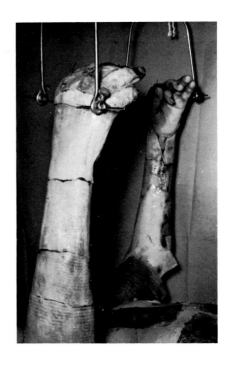

Figure 183. Bilateral skeletal suspension of circumferentially burned upper extremities used to facilitate grafting. The pins were inserted through the second and third metacarpals. The wrists are straight and the metacarpophalangeal joints are in flexion. The wraparound split-thickness grafts are clearly shown.

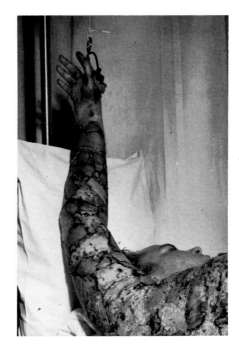

Figure 184. Skeletal suspension through the second and third metacarpals facilitated grafting the arm and axilla and secured postgrafting shoulder abduction.

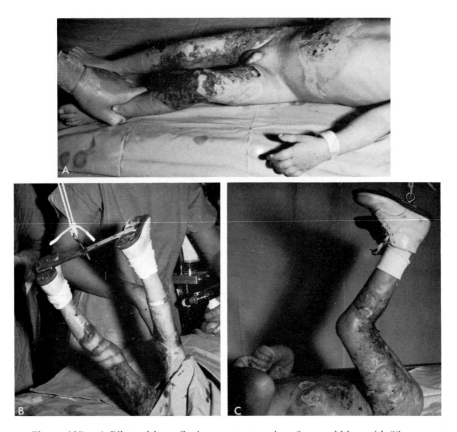

Figure 185. *A*, Bilateral knee flexion contracture in a 3-year-old boy with 23 per cent third-degree burn. The burn extends just below the knee. *B*, Shoe suspension corrected the deformity and made circumferential grafting possible. *C*, Suspension was well tolerated by the patient, and it was thus continued until the lower extremities had healed.

FRACTURES

Two types of fractures are associated with burns: acute fractures, or those which occur at the time of the acute burn and pathologic fractures, or those which occur later in the course of the burn as a consequence of bony atrophy and slight trauma.

Acute Fractures

Fractures occurring at the time of the burn are treated in the standard, conservative manner. Open fractures are meticulously debrided. Skeletal traction is used as necessary, the pins being inserted through areas of burn if proper placement requires this procedure. Occlusion of burned skin with circular bandaging or plaster is undesirable and can be avoided if skeletal traction is properly employed. In most instances, fracture treatment in severely burned patients is of secondary importance; definitive fracture care, except for such splinting as may be needed to reduce motion at the fracture site, is often postponed until the patient's general condition will allow it. Open reductions are never performed in acute burns.

Pathologic Fractures

During the period of protein deficit, atrophy of the bone is occasionally of such severity as to lead, with small insult, to pathologic fracture. A fracture may occur with routine handling during burn dressing changes, in physical therapy (Fig. 186) or as a result of relatively minor trauma after the patient has begun to walk (Fig. 187). Such fractures, likewise, are treated in a standard manner. If skin coverage is complete, occlusive supporting splints or casts may be used. The inactivity and immobility imposed by such support simply exaggerates the degree of atrophy. Granulations or crusts prevent open reduction.

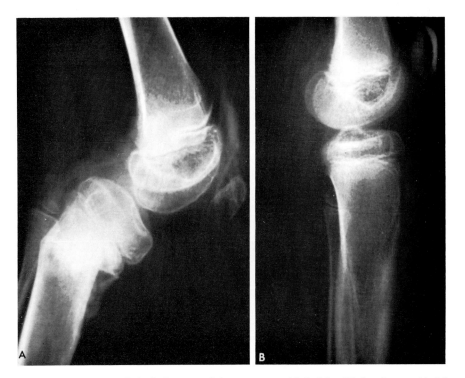

Figure 186. *A,* Pathologic fracture of the upper one-third of the tibia in a 5-year-old girl with 11 per cent third-degree burn. The fracture occurred 6 months after acute burn, apparently as a result of overzealous manipulation of knee flexion contracture during dressing change. *B,* The appearance 4 years after fracture. Range of knee motion was normal. Leg lengths were equal. The fracture was treated for a short period with a posterior splint.

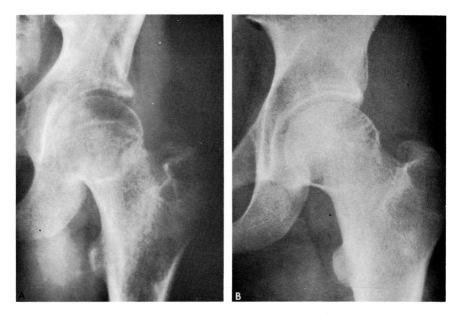

Figure 187. *A*, Pathologic fracture of the neck of the femur in a 13-year-old boy with 22 per cent third-degree burn. The fracture was the result of a minor fall in the physical therapy department. The patient had been bed confined for 5 months. *B*, The appearance 2½ months after injury at the time weight bearing was resumed. The fracture was treated for 6 weeks with skeletal traction.

DISLOCATIONS

Acute dislocations are treated as in patients who are not burned. If positioning with external support or skeletal traction is essential, the burn is ignored.

Spontaneous dislocations may occur at the hip in a patient who has been confined to bed for several weeks if positioning has been faulty or if the joint is put under additional stress during dressing change or grafting while the patient is asleep (Fig. 188). Although dislocations are most common at the hip, they may occur at other joints as well.

Septic dissolution of a joint accounts for dislocations of a distinct type. Whereas the positional or traumatic dislocation can be treated by simple manipulative reduction and postreduction positioning, septic destruction usually precludes satisfactory reduction because of the degree of alteration of articular surfaces.

ANKYLOSIS

In severely burned patients, it is likely that all intra-articular ankylosis occurs on the basis of septic destruction. Ankylosis secondary to heterotopic extra-articular osseous bridging and that due to intra-articular septic destruction have not been observed to occur at the same joint.

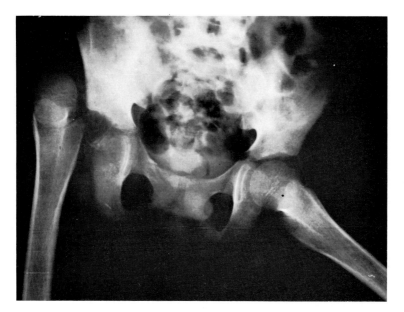

Figure 188.   Spontaneous dislocation of the right hip in a 6-year-old boy with 40 per cent third-degree burn. There was severe flexion adduction contracture on the right, and the dislocation occurred during routine dressing change 2 months after acute burn. The hip was reduced by manipulation and reduction maintained by strict positioning only.

The diagnosis of septic arthritis is made on the basis of clinical manifestations and roentgenographic appearance. All patients in which this type of destruction has been observed have had recognized bacteremia or long standing, open, infected granulations. Needle aspirations of affected joints may fail to yield bacteria-containing material, perhaps because these patients are already being treated with high doses of broad spectrum antibiotics. Tidrick, nevertheless, reports positive cultures of *Staphylococcus aureus* in all joints subjected to aspiration.

Abrupt and total dissolution of a joint in burned patients subjected to long confinement suggests some process other than septic destruction. In addition, in burn autopsy and amputation specimens, the occasional presence of a hemorrhagic pannus in otherwise normal appearing joints suggests that there may be some mechanism for articular destruction other than that of a pyogenic nature.

Septic joints in burns may become ankylosed (Fig. 189A) or may simply undergo derangement. According to Tidrick, ankylosis invariably occurs if the infective organism is *S. aureus*. When a septic joint becomes ankylosed, the final position may be functionally unsatisfactory. It may thus be necessary to perform osteotomies to restore extremity alignment (Fig. 189B, C). No reconstructive procedures of this sort should be performed until the patient is free of hypertrophic scarring. Septic ankyloses have been observed in all major joints.

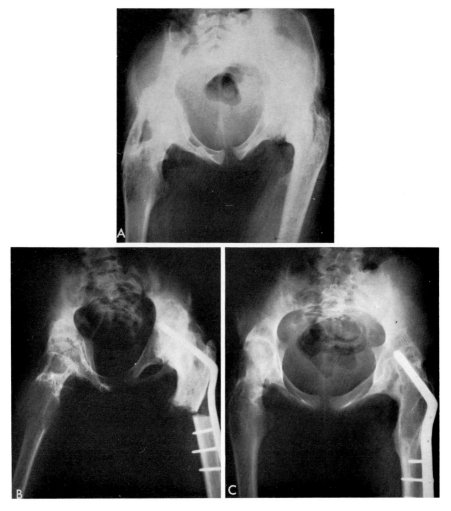

Figure 189. *A*, Heterotopic osseous bridging of the right hip and intra-articular septic ankylosis of the left hip in malposition in a 7-year-old girl with 50 per cent total burn. Roentgenogram taken 5 years after the acute burn. *B*, The right hip was mobilized by means of surgical excision of the heterotopic bone. The adduction deformity on the left was corrected by means of a subtrochanteric osteotomy. There was a fixed lumbar lordosis. *C*, The final result, with satisfactory alignment on the left and a good range of motion on the right.

HETEROTOPIC OSSIFICATION

Heterotopic periarticular calcification or ossification is observed in approximately 2 per cent of the patients burned severely enough to require hospitalization. Of the 1460 burned patients treated at the University of Texas Medical Branch from August 1955 through August 1964, only 29 showed some degree of periarticular calcification or ossification. Of these patients, 24 had alterations of sufficient severity to limit joint function.

Eleven had similar change at more than one joint. Heterotopic ossification has been observed at elbow, hip, shoulder and knee, in order of frequency. It has not occurred at the ankle or wrist. The knee is rarely involved.

Etiology

Among burned patients there are recognizable factors which may or may not be related to heterotopic bone formation. In the affected patients at The University of Texas Medical Branch, the per cent of third-degree burn varied from 10 to 50, with an approximate average of 20 per cent. In a study undertaken at the University of Michigan, it appeared that

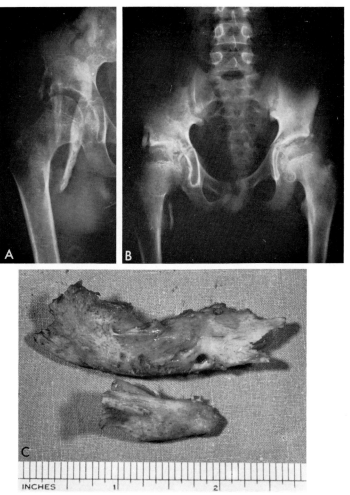

Figure 190. *A,* Heterotopic bone as it appeared one month after spontaneous dislocation (Fig. 188) of the hip of a 6-year-old boy. Bridging was not complete. There were still a few degrees of hip motion. *B,* The appearance 2 years after resection of heterotopic bone. There was full range of motion. *C,* The operative specimens consisted of two mature struts of bone with cortex and medullary cavity.

heterotopic bone occurred most often in patients with 22 per cent or more full-thickness skin loss.

The period of confinement is probably as significant a factor as the percentage of burn. Among the UTMB patients, heterotopic bone was detected after bed confinement of 2 or more months. What seemed of even greater importance, however, was the rather extreme immobility of some of these patients and their resistance to all efforts of physical therapy. Superimposed trauma may determine the location and extent of the heterotopic deposit (Figs. 188 and 190).

The anatomic distribution of burn does not dictate the location of osseous deposits. Although most heterotopic bone occurs about joints which underlie areas of burned skin, it has been observed in joints at a distance from areas of burn.

In patients showing heterotopic bone there is no significant alteration of serum calcium, phosphorus or alkaline phosphatase or urine calcium. The Michigan study shows that most of the extensive burns are accompanied by elevation of serum alkaline phosphatase levels and slight depres-

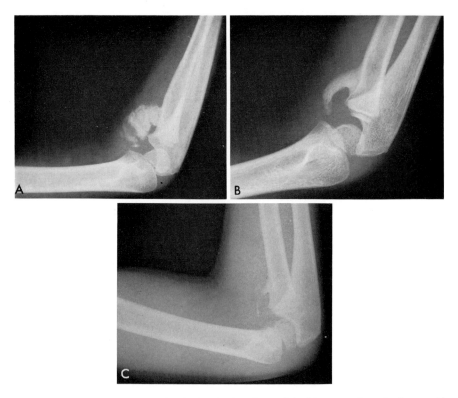

Figure 191. An exostosis developing in the plane of the biceps tendon of a 6-year-old boy with 47 per cent total body burn. From a relatively shapeless outcropping seen 2 months after the burn *(A)*, it matured to a well defined exostosis 4 months after the burn *(B)*. Following healing of the burn, it gradually decreased in size after 1 year to a mere nubbin *(C)* and finally disappeared. (Same patient as Figs. 188 and 190.)

sion of serum calcium and phosphorus levels as early as the first hours after the burn. However, these elevated levels are not observed at the time of detection of heterotopic bone.

The heterotopic bone observed in burns is not unlike that observed in patients with lesions of the spinal cord or with paralytic encephalomyelitis. These three states have in common certain features, such as progressive bony atrophy, muscular atrophy and general wasting of connective tissue, local hyperemia and varying degrees of superimposed trauma.

Both in the burn and in the paralytic disorders the new bone first appears radiographically as an amorphous, cloudy mass which gradually assumes limit and contour and linear orientation with the capsular, fascial or muscle planes about the affected joint (Fig. 191A, B). The final product is mature bone with cortex and medullary cavity (Fig. 190C).

In the burned patient heterotopic bone may continue to increase in size so long as there are open granulating areas or areas of active proliferating scar tissue. If the new bone bridges a joint from bone to bone, it becomes a permanent strut which remains quite solid after the patient has recovered from the burn (Fig. 189A). On the other hand, heterotopic bone which does not establish this structural continuity will begin to diminish in size once skin lesions have healed and nitrogen equilibrium has been restored (Figs. 191 and 192). In adults the exostoses will become significantly smaller; in children, they may disappear (Fig. 192). This phenomenon is likewise observed among patients with paralytic disorders of a transient nature.

It seems reasonable to suggest, because of the periarticular distribution of the heterotopic bone, that in burns these deposits develop spontaneously or are caused by unrecognized local trauma. The trauma is significant because of the compromised state of the tissues. The chemical milieu at the site of trauma supports bone formation, and increased mobilization of mineral salts may help to trigger the process. The fact that there is resorption after clinical improvement underscores the importance of local and humoral alterations. The character of these alterations may differ from patient to patient, or patients may respond differently to alterations of identical character. At any rate, it seems likely that among human beings there is some degree of individual predilection to the formation of heterotopic bone, since, of the great numbers of persons similarly involved by disease or similarly traumatized, only a very small percentage is known to develop it.

Anatomic Location

Anatomically, heterotopic bone has been seen to lie in the plane of the gluteus medius and minimus, on the lateral aspect of the hip, and in the plane of the iliopsoas anterior to the hip. At the shoulder it has bridged the joint from acromion to humerus, and has been observed in the substance of the subscapularis. At the elbow it has been observed in the plane

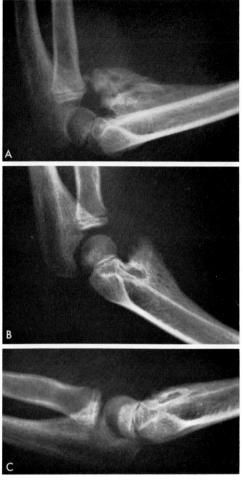

Figure 192. *A*, This large heterotopic exostosis lay in the plane of the brachialis. The patient was a 5-year-old girl with 25 per cent total burn. The opposite elbow was bridged posteriorly by heterotopic bone. The roentgenogram was taken 4 months after acute burn. *B*, After skin healing the exostosis began to diminish in size. This is the appearance 1 year after the acute burn. *C*, The appearance 3 years after burn.

of the brachialis and biceps muscles anteriorly and along the medial border of the triceps, extending from the humerus to the olecranon posteriorly.

Treatment

Physical therapy. There is little evidence to indicate that physical therapeutic measures bring about reduction in the size of established calcific deposits or heterotopic bone. It seems, however, that routine physical therapy has significantly reduced the incidence of these complications.

Surgical excision. Heterotopic bone occurring in burned patients is amenable to resection. Surgery is postponed until surrounding skin is soft and all granulating areas are healed. It is not performed if there is skin infection in any area or if there is proliferating scar tissue. Adequately removed heterotopic bone will not regenerate to its original dimension. Excision should restore a useful or even normal range of motion.

In children, resection is usually unnecessary if the heterotopic bone

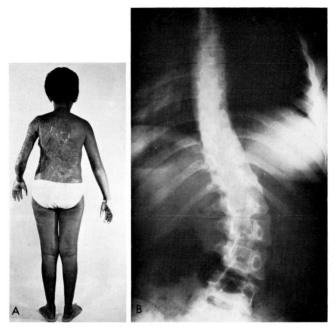

Figure 193. *A* and *B*, A 15-year-old girl with lumbar scoliosis secondary to scarring of the trunk. Photograph and roentgenogram taken 11 years after the acute burn.

does not bridge the joint. In adults, resorption tends to be slow, and resection is recommended because it will restore joint motion quickly.

Surgical excision of heterotopic bone must be adequate—even generous. This is particularly true in patients with posterior bridging of the elbow. In such cases it is advisable to resect as much as 0.5 cm. or more of normal olecranon.

SCOLIOSIS

Among burned children, scoliosis occurs as a result of severe scar contractures of the skin of the trunk or groin (Fig. 193). Knee and hip flexion contractures and leg length discrepancies due to other reasons have caused temporary functional curves. Most of the scoliosis observed following burns is transient and will disappear as the scarred skin regains its elasticity. If contractures are severe, correction of the curve depends upon surgical release. Curves of long standing may not correct spontaneously after skin release. Simple shoe lifts correct scoliosis which is secondary to permanent leg length discrepancy.

ABNORMALITIES OF GROWTH

Epiphyses may close prematurely near joints which become ankylosed because of septic arthritis. The younger the patient, the greater will be the eventual functional significance of the epiphyseal arrest. Shoe lifts must be used for leg length discrepancies of $1/4$ of an inch or greater.

Acceleration of growth of a general sort or involving only one extremity has been reported by patients and parents. A case has been reported in which there was persisting measurable discrepancy of lower extremity length, the involved extremity being $3/4$ of an inch longer than the uninvolved. Epiphyses were roentgenographically normal.

Occasionally adults, following extremity burns, have found it necessary to wear larger shoes than before. This apparent growth is not skeletal.

AMPUTATIONS

In the severely burned patient an amputation is performed because of nonviability of the part. Occasionally, as a life-saving measure, circumfer-

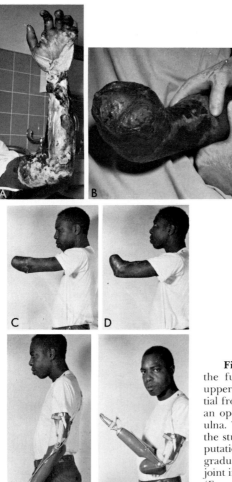

Figure 194. *A*, In this 27-year-old man, the full-thickness burn which extends to the upper one-third of arm medially is circumferential from the elbow to the fingers. *B*, At surgery an open amputation preserved 3 inches of the ulna. The split-thickness skin graft coverage of the stump is shown. *C*, Seven months after amputation the range of motion is 45 degrees and gradually increasing. *D*, The split socket elbow joint increases the useful range of the prosthesis (*E* and *F*). The patient is skilled in the use of his prosthesis and is receiving on-the-job training.

entially burned lower extremities are amputated without strict regard to the level of viability to reduce the extent of burned surface. Usually, it is in the early stage of burn treatment that amputations take place.

Technique

All amputations are open in type. The level of amputation is that most distal point at which there is viable muscle. It need be of little concern that there are areas of skin which are destroyed by full-thickness burn proximal to the level of amputation. This is an interesting reverse of the situation encountered in amputations for major vascular occlusion, in which the skin may be viable for some distance distal to the level of viable muscle. It also differs from a situation encountered occasionally in electrical injuries.

The decision regarding level of amputation becomes quite critical when it relates to preserving an elbow or a knee. As in amputations for other reasons, it is preferable to leave a short below knee stump or a short below elbow stump if there is any possibility that even restricted knee function and elbow function can be retained (Fig. 194A, B). The stump is treated as any other open amputation. Occasionally, if there is excessive soft tissue retraction or advancing muscle necrosis, a revision may be required. Split-thickness skin graft coverage of the stump is all that is necessary to prepare the extremity for a prosthesis. These grafts soften in time and attain sufficient pliancy and thickness to withstand contact with the prosthesis (Figs. 194C, D, E, F and 195).

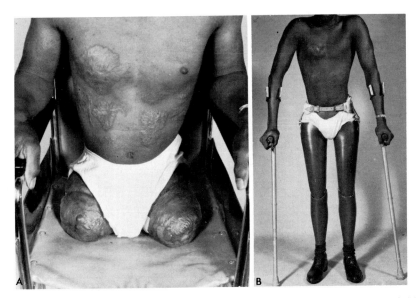

Figure 195. *A*, A 20-year-old man who at age 9 years sustained circumferential third-degree burns of both lower extremities from groin to toe. The original amputations were revised once because of bone growth. Both stumps are completely covered with split-thickness skin grafts. *B*, The patient is functionally independent and currently is attending college.

After skin coverage of the amputation stump, the conditioning of the stump by proper wrapping is routine, and prostheses may be fitted in the routine manner. Burned patients who have prostheses have no problems of a special nature. If the prosthesis is fitted before the lines of scar between the skin grafts have become soft and mobile, there may be a tendency to linear excoriation along the scar lines.

Electrical Injuries

In electrical injuries, early assessment of the extent of damage is impossible if one relies on the appearance of the skin. Even after several days, when the skin around the eschar has become hyperemic, it is extremely difficult to determine the extent to which deeper structures have been damaged. It is a safe practice for those who are called upon to amputate extremities damaged by electrical injury to await positive demarcation of the skin, being aware that damage to the deeper structures may extend proximally beyond the apparent level of superficial viability. Amputations in electrical injury are likewise of the open type, and because of the uncertainty of level, revisions are more commonly necessary than in amputations for thermal burns.

REFERENCES

Boyd, B. M., Jr., Roberts, W. M., and Miller, G. R.: Periarticular ossification following burns. *South. M. J.* **52**:1048, 1959.

Evans, E. B., and Blumel, J.: Bone and joint changes following burns. *In* Artz, C. P. (ed.): *Research in Burns*, Philadelphia, F. A. Davis Company, 1962, p. 26.

Evans, E. B., Larson, D. L., and Yates, S.: Preservation and restoration of joint function in patients with severe burns. *J. A. M. A.* **204**:843, 1968.

Evans, E. B., and Smith, J. R.: Bone and joint changes following burns. A roentgenographic study — preliminary report. *J. Bone & Joint Surg.* **41-A**:785, 1959.

Glover, D. M.: Necrosis of skull and long bones resulting from deep burns, with evidence of regeneration. *Am. J. Surg.* **95**:679, 1958.

Griswold, M. L., Jr.: Extra-articular bone formation as a burn complication. *Plast. & Reconstruct. Surg.* **32**:544, 1963.

Gronley, J. K., Yeakel, M. H., and Grant, A. E.: Rehabilitation of the burned hand. *Arch. Phys. Med.* **43**:508, 1962.

Johnson, J. T. H.: Atypical myositis ossificans. *J. Bone & Joint Surg.* **39-A**:189, 1957.

Koepke, G. H., Feallock, B., and Feller, I.: Splinting the severely burned hand. *Am. J. Occup. Therapy* **17**:147, 1963.

Kólář, J., and Vrabec, R.: Periarticular soft-tissue changes as a late consequence of burns. *J. Bone & Joint Surg.* **41-A**:103, 1959.

Miller, J., Hardy, S. B., and Spira, M.: Treatment of burns of the hand with silicone dressing and early motion. *J. Bone & Joint Surg.* **47-A**:938, 1965.

Moncrief, J. A.: Complications of burns. *Ann. Surg.* **147**:443, 1958.

Owens, N.: Osteoporosis following burns. *Brit. J. Plast. Surg.* **1**:245, 1949.

Rabinov, D.: Acromutilation of the fingers following severe burns. *Radiology* **77**:968, 1961.

Reiss, E., Pearson, E., and Artz, C. P.: The metabolic response to burns. *J. Clin. Invest.* **35**:62, 1956.

Tidrick, R. T.: Bone and joint changes associated with thermal burns (Abstract). *J. Bone & Joint Surg.* **42-A**:907, 1960.

Yeakel, M. H., Gronley, J. K., and Tumbusch, W. T.: A fiberglass positioning device for the burned hand. *J. Trauma* **4**:57, 1964.

Chapter
Seventeen

TREATMENT
OF BURNS
IN DISASTER

Within the past three decades several civilian disasters have occurred in the United States in which large numbers of burned casualties were seen. The experiences in these disasters and the experiences of the armed forces during World War II and the Korean War have greatly improved our understanding of the problems of disaster care for burns.

The fire at the Cocoanut Grove night club in Boston on November 28, 1942, took the lives of 491 persons. Excellent care for the survivors was made possible by planned organization for such an emergency. Injury of the respiratory tract presented the most pressing problem of therapy. Valuable information was obtained about the diagnosis and treatment of respiratory tract irritation from noxious gases.

There were 125 persons burned to death on the lot, and 150 others were burned and admitted to various hospitals after the circus fire at Hartford, Connecticut, on July 6, 1944. This unusually large number of burned patients could be managed effectively because of prior planning by the Hartford Hospital staff. There were no deaths in the first 48 hours because vigorous fluid therapy was instituted promptly.

Approximately 560 persons were killed and 800 persons were hospitalized when two ships exploded at the docks at Texas City, Texas, on April 16, 1947. Most of the patients received mechanical injuries but many were burned. In his discussion of the experience gained in this disaster, Blocker pointed out that a great many doctors are unaware of disaster problems. Local physicians in a disaster region, rather than medical assistance brought to the scene of disaster from the outside, are primarily responsible for the care of the sick and injured. Blocker expressed the conviction that a detailed disaster program for physicians should be active in every community.

On March 31, 1954, 20 burned casualties were admitted to the Edward J. Meyer Memorial Hospital in Buffalo, New York, from the Cleveland Hill School fire. Eleven patients were estimated to have burns in excess of 20 per cent of the body surface. In reporting on this disaster, Schenk pointed out the need for rapid screening of cases. He noted that 50 per cent of the cases required 95 per cent of the personnel's time. The efficient use of personnel and facilities was accomplished only after proper sorting.

Enyart and Miller have given a detailed report on the disaster in which 203 casualties resulted from an explosion on the aircraft carrier USS Bennington on May 26, 1954. The patients were treated at the Newport Naval Hospital, Newport, Rhode Island. All but eight of the 82 hospitalized patients had severe burns. Dextran and serum albumin were used effectively as resuscitative agents. The exposure method of local care was applied in the treatment of all patients, apparently with great success.

All of these experiences emphasize the need for organization and planning for disasters. Since the development of thermonuclear weapons, there is an even greater need for physicians to become acquainted with disaster care. When Hiroshima, with a population of 300,000, was devastated by an atomic bomb, there were 80,000 to 100,000 injured, 15,000 missing and 70,000 dead. The highest percentage of the casualties were burns. Thermonuclear weapons now are capable of producing approximately 10,000 times the explosive force of the bombs used at Hiroshima. A thermonuclear weapon is accompanied by the release of an enormous amount of kinetic energy. At least 80 per cent of this energy is in the form of ordinary heat. It might be expected that tens of thousands of burn casualties would result from a major thermonuclear attack.

A SURVEY OF THE PROBLEM

It is obvious that certain compromises in ideal therapy must be made. The quality of therapy varies in accordance with the number of casualties and the available personnel and supplies (Fig. 196).

Different compromises in therapy may be necessary with each disaster. Under conditions of thermonuclear warfare, it is apparent that a wide disparity would exist between the medical load imposed and the surviving medical assets, at least during the early postdetonation period. In meeting the problem, the extent of medical care given must be determined by two basic considerations: (1) provision of maximum care for the maximum number of patients and (2) avoidance wherever possible of any procedures that might reduce a patient's ability to care for himself.

Although it is difficult to specify definite details of therapy, some generalizations may be made.

1. Policy decisions concerning the compromises that are necessary must be made by the person who is most experienced in casualty care. The surgeon available at the scene of the disaster who has the greatest experience in the management of burns should accept the leadership for deciding and outlining necessary compromises in therapy.

2. Proper medical sorting is of paramount importance. With improper sorting, hospitals close to the scene are often swamped by the less severely injured who could well withstand transportation to more distant points.

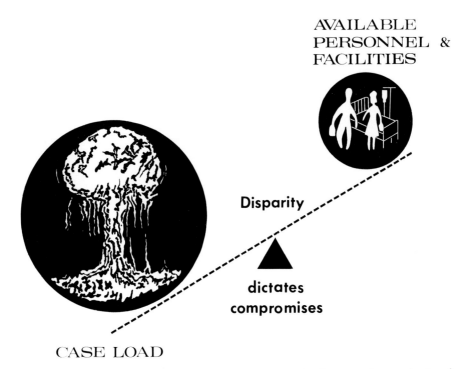

AVAILABLE
PERSONNEL &
FACILITIES

Disparity

dictates
compromises

CASE LOAD

Figure 196. In any disaster situation a disparity exists between the case load and available personnel and facilities. The degree of this disparity dictates the compromises that must be made in patient care. If the case load is not too great and available facilities are good, almost ideal care can be given. When, however, the case load is far greater than the available facilities major intelligent compromises in ideal therapy must be made.

3. Patients with minor injuries who can be easily rendered effective must be returned to duty.

4. There should be a maximum conservation of medical effort. Trained medical individuals should not be assigned to first aid or rescue operations.

5. Essential supplies should be rigidly conserved.

6. Every hospital should be organized for disaster, and regular periodic drills should be held so that the staff is familiar with the plan. Prior planning has been extremely effective in all civilian disasters; of course, it is of greatest importance in all military medical operations.

7. The organization of ancillary personnel, such as the police, communication workers, supply workers and volunteers is extremely important.

TYPES OF BURNS

In most civilian burn disasters, the injury is due to contact with the heat source, such as flame or heated object. Thermal injuries resulting from thermonuclear blasts would be predominantly flash burns involving the exposed portions of the body. The source of the heat is the weapon itself, which on detonation not only produces a huge fireball but also radiates heat in the form of electromagnetic radiations. Similar radiant energy is released in gasoline explosions with resultant flash burns of those not in actual contact with the flame. The radiant energy travels in a straight line but is reflected from smooth surfaces and the rays diffused by dust or moisture particles in the atmosphere. The electromagnetic radiant energy from a weapon may travel many miles before it is attenuated to the point of being harmless. Flame burns may occur after thermonuclear explosions because of ignition of clothing and contact with burning materials.

Evidence has been presented that radiation injury and thermal burns act synergistically in increasing mortality in experimental animals. A thermal burn and exposure to radiation, each of which alone is nonlethal in most of the animals tested, can produce a high percentage of mortality when combined. Death appears to be due to sepsis in the combined injury, and the mortality can be substantially reduced by antibiotic therapy.

The frequency with which combined thermal and radiation injury might be expected to occur in thermonuclear warfare is not known. In general, the small, tactical weapons of 10 kiloton range (i.e. equivalent to 10,000 tons TNT) will have primarily a blast and radiation effect. As the yield of the weapon increases, the amount of radiant energy released greatly increases. Soon the limits of blast and irradiation are so far exceeded by thermal effects that the only immediate survivors of injury will be those sustaining only burns. Treatment would have to be directed primarily toward the thermal burn. There is no specific therapy for radiation injury. Antibiotics and blood transfusions, which are valuable in the treatment of burns, are also of supportive value in radiation injury. The principles of treatment of burns resulting from thermonuclear explosions are the same as those applied in the common forms of burns.

Studies have been made to predict the effectiveness of troops exposed to thermal radiation from nuclear weapons. Langevin has presented methodology which makes it possible to use such data as are available on the exposure of troops, their susceptibility to burns and their effectiveness following burns—in conjunction with types of evasive action they may employ—to determine in quantitative fashion what their effectiveness will be following exposure to thermal radiation from nuclear weapons. Such data are available in detail in the reference of Langevin, Greenstone and Elder listed at the end of this chapter.

MEDICAL SORTING

Sorting, screening and triage are synonymous terms that refer to the categorizing of casualties on the basis of urgency and type of condition presented for the purpose of proper routing to medical units appropriately situated and equipped for therapy. *Sorting is the key to the effective manage-*

ment of large numbers of burned casualties. Without sorting, an orderly and efficient utilization of available medical means is impossible.

Sorting is a process that must be continued through each stage of care. It is a flexible procedure and should be directed by the most experienced surgeon in the area. His decisions are based not only on the condition of a particular patient, but also on the number of injured requiring treatment and on the available facilities and personnel. For example, a hospital with a limited supply of blood should utilize the blood to aid in the recovery of the largest number of injured. On this basis, a critically injured man who would require all of the 10 pints of blood available would be assigned a lower priority for transfusion than five casualties who could probably recover if each received 2 pints of blood. On the other hand, if large supplies of blood were immediately available, priority for treatment would be established by the severity of the wound.

Sorting in a Mass Casualty Situation

In most disaster situations, the most seriously injured patient receives the greatest priority. However, such a priority system is based on an unfailing source of supplies and on an abundance of medical personnel. In an atomic disaster, some modification of the usual priority system would have to be established.

Percentage of body surface burned is the easiest method of determining the over-all severity of the injury. However, each patient should also be evaluated according to the depth of burn, the area of involvement and the ambulatory state. Since most of the burns are expected to be of the flash variety, burns of exposed areas of the body will predominate. While in burns that occur following secondary fires, the depth and extent of injury would be greater.

Available knowledge points toward the fact that, in a mass casualty situation, the patient with second- and third-degree burns involving more than 40 per cent of his body would probably not survive. This percentage might be a little smaller in persons under 18 months of age or over 50 years. If mechanical and radiation injuries are also present, considerably less than a 40 per cent burn may be incompatible with survival. In the initial sorting, such casualties should be placed in the group designated as expectant treatment and made as comfortable as possible. They should be given adequate doses of morphine if available and placed in the lowest priority group for definitive treatment. They should not receive definitive therapy until all patients in higher priority groups are cared for.

The major effort should be directed toward administering therapy to the casualties having 15 to 40 per cent involvement. Some casualties with 20 per cent superficial burns might be discharged to self care. Casualties with burns involving less than 15 per cent of the body surface could be discharged to self care if the location of the burn does not interfere with ambulation. Although many individuals with burns of 15 per cent of the body

surface are hospitalized in usual practice, there is evidence that most of
these patients could take care of themselves, if they were supplied with
water, food and electrolytes. However, self care is not feasible if the casualty has a severe burn of the face or if an extensive burn of the leg makes
ambulation impossible. Such casualties would have to be referred to a holding facility where untrained personnel could care for their daily needs. Individuals with minor burns might be utilized to help care for the more
seriously injured.

In the event of atomic disaster, it is expected that most of the survivors
would have burns of such configuration that they could care for themselves. Many casualties with full-thickness involvement of small extent
might be expected to care for themselves initially and then receive treatment later in a medical installation where grafting could be performed. It
would be hoped that those who could continue to carry on some type of
work might make themselves most useful and not overburden the medical
facilities.

COMPROMISES IN THERAPY FOR DISASTER

There are several phases of emergency medical care in burns that are
highly important. These include (1) relief of pain, (2) supportive therapy,
(3) management of the burn wound and (4) antibiotic therapy to aid in the
prevention of infection.

Relief of Pain

Full-thickness burns are relatively painless, but partial-thickness burns
are quite painful for the first hour or two after injury. If personnel and
facilities are available, intravenous morphine should be given to allay pain
and apprehension. In a more extensive disaster, it would be impossible to
administer a narcotic. Fortunately, an exposed burn becomes relatively
painless after a few hours. If time permits and supplies are available, the
burn wounds might be covered with a dressing, which leads to the prompt
relief of pain and discomfort. In some situations a simple bland water-
soluble ointment might be applied for the temporary relief of pain. In any
extensive disaster, it would be wise to disseminate the information that
partial-thickness burns become painless as soon as a dry crust has formed.

Supportive Therapy

Proper supportive therapy includes the infusion of adequate amounts
of plasma or dextran, electrolytes and water. The use of a formula for
computing the approximate amount is very helpful. The best formulas
for use in the disaster situations are the Parkland regimen or the 8 hour
attach two zeros rule described in Chapter Five.

Supportive therapy in a thermonuclear disaster could be initiated by supplying water and electrolytes for oral use. A solution of salt and soda made by placing 3 gm. of salt and 1.5 gm. of sodium bicarbonate in a liter of water is an effective solution for replacement therapy. To provide such a solution, it might be possible to have salt, soda and some type of water purification tablet placed in small packages to be given to patients for mixing with water. Such a solution is well tolerated by burned patients. Almost all casualties with less than 20 per cent of the body surface burned can be resuscitated by the oral route. Patients with burns of 20 to 30 per cent can be resuscitated by oral means if they are not ambulated; if resuscitation is borderline, hypotension will develop when the patient is upright. In a few days this is no longer a problem.

The protein losses in burns, especially in the first few weeks after injury, are extremely high. In any disaster situation it might be impossible to provide the usual hospital diet for burned patients. Some type of special high protein feeding would be essential. Developments in this field have yielded palatable high protein powders that would be beneficial in a disaster situation. Powder can be mixed with water so that 250 ml. of the solution will provide approximately 40 gm. of protein and 300 calories. A high protein formula similar to that described under supplemental between-meal feedings in Chapter Thirteen might be very useful.

Blood transfusions for the correction of anemia could be given several days after the disaster.

Management of the Burn Wound

Under ideal circumstances cleansing of the burn with a mild soap or detergent is recommended, but under disaster conditions this procedure would be impossible. There is ample evidence that the lack of cleansing is a minor compromise, especially when burns are exposed. In the event of a disaster, all burned areas would have to be treated by the exposure method because the few dressings available would have to be saved for mechanical injuries. If available, some type of topical antibacterial agent would be very helpful. Should the disaster occur in a cold region, it would be necessary to furnish blankets and some type of covering for the injured surface. If time permits and dressings are available, they should be utilized on individuals who would benefit most by their use. If flash burns occur on the hands and face, the burn casualty discharged to self care would be more effective if he is encouraged to utilize his hands at all times to maintain function. Though initially painful, utilization of the hands is one aspect of therapy which should not be compromised.

Antibiotics

Although burns of moderate size may be treated in a hospital without administering any antibiotics, it would seem wise to use antibiotics in a disaster situation. The main reason for such prophylactic therapy is to prevent infections caused by beta hemolytic streptococci. A broad spectrum antibiotic should be given orally for the first few days after injury. At the same time the casualty received the salt and soda solution, he could be provided with a sufficient supply of an oral antibiotic to last him for several days. Regardless of the type of antibiotics used, the development of resistant bacterial strains and secondary infections could be expected. Provisions should be made for the utilization of additional antibiotics at a later date.

BURN CENTERS

In any disaster, it is advisable to group similarly injured casualties in the same installation. Certain hospitals should be designated as burn centers. Among the supplies that should be available at the centers are blood, dressings and high protein liquid feedings.

Major problems in dealing with a large number of burn casualties are sufficient space in an operating room and time for the multiple grafting procedures that are necessary. Another phase of sorting might be necessary within the burn center. Casualties whose wounds could be closed by one grafting procedure should be taken into the operating room first so that they might return to duty.

In grafting procedures, it is generally desirable to place large sheets of skin over flat surfaces. The grafts may be applied without dressings on the areas which may be exposed. This not only saves on supplies but also gives superior graft results. Since it might be difficult to cover all the areas with autografts, homografts or heterografts might be used for supplementary temporary skin cover. In some instances, homografts could be applied at the time of dressing change and thereby serve as a biological dressing until space becomes available in the operating room for grafting.

REFERENCES

Armstrong, G. E., Schaeffer, J. R., and Artz, C. P.: Treatment of burns in atomic disaster. *U.S. Armed Forces M. J.* **7**:320, 1956.

Artz, C. P., and Reiss, E.: Calculator for estimating early fluid requirements in burns. *J.A.M.A.* **155**:1156, 1954.

Blocker, V., and Blocker, T. G., Jr.: The Texas City disaster; a survey of 3000 casualties. *Am. J. Surg.* **78**:756, 1949.

Callahan, J. L., and Segraves, J. E.: Treatment of fire victims: Lady of the Angel School disaster. *Am. J. Surg.* **29**:814, 1960.

Enyart, J. L., and Miller, D. W.: Treatment of burns resulting from disaster. *J.A.M.A.* **158**:95 1955.

Langevin, R. A., Greenstone, R., and Elder, C.O.: Effectiveness of troops exposed to thermal radiation from nuclear weapons. *Operations Research* **6**:710, 1958.

Management of the Cocoanut Grove Burns at the Massachusetts General Hospital. *Ann. Surg.* **117**:801, 1943.

Pillsbury, R. D., and Artz, C. P.: Necessary compromises in therapy of burns sustained in nuclear warfare. *J.A.M.A.* **162**:956, 1956.

Schenk, W. G., Jr., Stephens, J. G., Burke, J., Hale, H. W., Jr., Eagle, J. F., and Stewart, J. D.: Treatment of mass civilian burn casualties; care of Cleveland Hill School fire victims. *A.M.A. Arch. Surg.* **71**:196, 1955.

Wells, D. B.: The circus disaster and the Hartford Hospital. *New England J. Med.* **232**:613, 1945.

Index